MW01106265

Science and Medicine in Dialogue

SCIENCE AND MEDICINE IN DIALOGUE

Thinking through Particulars and Universals

Edited by Roger Bibace, James D. Laird,
Kenneth L. Noller, and Jaan Valsiner

Praeger Series in Health Psychology
Barbara J. Tinsley, Series Editor

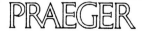

Westport, Connecticut
London

Library of Congress Cataloging-in-Publication Data

Science and medicine in dialogue : thinking through particulars and universals / edited by Roger Bibace . . . [et al.].
    p. cm.—(Praeger series in health psychology, ISSN 1543–2211)
    Includes bibliographical references and index.
    ISBN 0–275–97872–9 (alk. paper)
    1. Medicine and psychology.   2. Medicine—Decision making.   3. Medicine—Philosophy.   4. Psychology—Philosophy.   I. Bibace, Roger.   II. Series.
R726.5.S375   2005
616′.001—dc22   2004025207

British Library Cataloguing in Publication Data is available.

Library of Congress Catalog Card Number: 2004025207
ISBN: 0–275–97872–9
ISSN: 1543–2211

First published in 2005

Praeger Publishers, 88 Post Road West, Westport, CT 06881
An imprint of Greenwood Publishing Group, Inc.
www.praeger.com

Printed in the United States of America

The paper used in this book complies with the Permanent Paper Standard issued by the National Information Standards Organization (Z39.48–1984).

10 9 8 7 6 5 4 3 2 1

CONTENTS

ILLUSTRATIONS

FIGURES

TABLES

SERIES PREFACE

The fields of health psychology experienced tremendous growth in the last two decades. This growth reflects an increasing recognition of the many social and psychological factors affecting health and illness and the realization that physical health can no longer be addressed solely from a biomedical perspective.

The books in this series focus primarily on how social, psychological, and behavioral factors influence physical health. These volumes will serve as important resources for layreaders as well as students and scholars in psychology medicine, sociology, nursing, public health, social work, and related areas.

UNIVERSALS AND PARTICULARS IN THE PRACTICES OF PSYCHOLOGY AND MEDICINE: ENTERING A DIALOGUE

Roger Bibace, James D. Laird, Kenneth L. Noller, and Jaan Valsiner

The casual observer of the fields of psychology and medicine would find few commonalties. The first deals with the mind and its processes, while the second is concerned primarily with the body. Yet, it only requires slightly more intense observation to find myriad areas in which the two overlap. Psychological processes often rely on physical input, and medical problems always have a noncorporeal component. Despite these facts, few published works have attempted to explore these commonalties.

We began our process of exploration by convening two workshops composed of members of both disciplines, including both experimentalists and clinicians from each field. We gave the presenters little guidance beyond telling them that we were interested in the interactions between "The Universal" and "The Particular." While the presentation titles suggested that we were likely to fail to find common ground, the discussions that followed each paper began to identify our mutual areas of interest and our common problems.

We also discovered that we shared at least two goals. The first is that both disciplines seek a basic understanding about how human beings exist in their ordinary biological and psychological worlds. The second is the attempt to describe and treat disruptions of each person's healthy state of being. These goals would seem to divide rather than unite the scientific and applied factions. On the one side is the world of experimental psychology and the basic medical sciences. On the other are clinical psychology and the clinical practice of medicine. What we found, however, is that both the scientists and the clinicians were interested in the same concepts: While scientists are interested in uncovering universal truths, they must use data from individuals. Likewise, while clinicians are primarily motivated to treat the particular individuals who are seeking care, they must rely on universal truths to initiate treatment.

This book is also an experiment on a different level. Not only were we—the four co-editors—attempting to uncover areas of mutual interest between the two disciplines, we were also hoping to uncover the basis for the conflicts that have arisen in our fields. In both psychology and medical practice, schisms have emerged that need to be bridged if we are to develop the most effective science and practice. Most generally, the problem appears to be how to relate universal principles and particular cases. This remains a perennial problem for all science and its applications.

CONSTRUCTING KNOWLEDGE: BEYOND THE OPPOSITIONS GIVEN

It is not difficult to sense the tension between the adherents to the "generalized knowing" and "particularist practices" ideas in our book. Clearly, the chapters reveal that the distance between these positions has not narrowed. One group has "solved" the problem by arguing that universal principles are at best crude approximations and perhaps are no more than illusions. The richness of context-sensitive phenomena—both in psychology and in medicine—is viewed as a means toward a better understanding of reality. At the extreme, this group urges us to focus only on single cases, studied in intensive, "qualitative" ways that permit us to know a great deal about a single person. While this approach results in rich descriptions of the most minute details of the specific case, all generalizing power is lost. Losing that means the end of science and professional self-extinction.

Yet there is a different way to view specific cases, that is, to look for universality within a single, systemically organized case. This is a focus of both basic science and medicine in its practice. In both cases, the object of inquiry—be it a far-away planet in astrophysics (a single case) or the particular Mr. Smith who feels that he has a health problem—is singular and unique. In both cases, the knowledge base that allows the scientist or practitioner to make sense of how the planet or person is functioning is that of a generalized kind. That knowledge comes from the study of other cases, under different conditions, yet in ways that allow for transfer of previously acquired knowledge to the new, not yet understood case.

The other, "quantitative" group seems relatively unconcerned by the problem of universals versus particulars and proceeds to generate general principles that characterize groups of people. These general principles are assumed never to fit any single individual precisely. Yet, from the quantitative perspective, individuality is inevitable, with each individual representing a potentially unique intersection of a potentially infinite array of dimensions.

Both perspectives may be limited when any of the knowledge obtained from groups is to be put to the service of intervention in the case of a particular individual. The transfer of sample-based generalized (averaged) evidence from epidemiology to concrete actions in medicine is a risky undertaking. The "average" condition or treatment may work, but it also is open to errors, due to the lack of knowledge about this particular person whose health is at risk. Correspondingly, too great a focus on the individual may lead a practitioner to ignore evidence-based medicine in favor of the individual's intuitions. Rigid reliance upon either population-based information or individual variation may lead to treatment errors. Both are "right" and "wrong" at the same time. Successful treatment of any patient depends on the clinician's ability to coordinate relevant information from both.

KNOWLEDGE ABOUT HUMAN BEINGS: THE PRIVATE AND THE PUBLIC

The contrast between the general and the particular is linked with another contrast—that between PUBLIC and PRIVATE. The former corresponds to the universal and the latter to the PARTICULAR. All private information is the particular side of whatever may be seen in public in a different way. Thus, politicians' public speeches reveal next to nothing about their personal, particular worlds.

The ways in which the private and public domains are coordinated differs greatly among societies and within the same society over its history. Private/public boundaries changed drastically in the twentieth century, all over the world. First radio, then television, and more recently the internet have made all information "global."

This fact leads to new challenges for both medicine and psychology. We live in a society where the distinctions between what is private and what is public are increasingly blurred. For example, virtually all Web users have received an e-mail that offers a service that can "find out anything about anyone." Of course, such grand promises are advertising gimmicks, yet the amount of information about any person that is available on-line is enormous. Passwords and firewalls only partly control access to our privacy.

A good example of the extent to which societal attempts to protect personal information can be deleterious to medical practice is the "Health Information Portability and Accountability Act" (HIPAA) that recently became law in the United States. The original purpose of the Act was to ensure that an individual would have access to her/his medical records if they ever moved. However, after the politicians and their staff finished adding their personal touches, HIPAA became several thousand pages of restrictions, rules, regulations, and interpretations. It is now very difficult to obtain medical information from another institution or physician, just the opposite of the original intention of the law.

Different contributions to this book touch upon the tension between the individual's rights to privacy and social institutions' self-proclaimed rights to invade that privacy. The situation is further complicated by the need of society to demand individual information for some benevolent interventions for the sake of the lives of people in the society as a whole. The most obvious example concerns infectious diseases. However, these (macrosocial) dilemmas remain largely beyond the scope of the present book.

Another dilemma—the invasion by the researcher of the privacy of the research participant[1]—is one of the central themes in this book. The issue is the basic question, "How should human beings create knowledge about other human beings?" In science, humans are used in experiments for the sake of scientific understanding. In medicine, the goal is to identify concrete and practical solutions for health problems. We need to transcend the "dialogue" between psychology and medicine and analyze the common process in which they are jointly involved.

PARTICULAR SOCIETIES AND THE UNIVERSALITY OF MEDICINE

The organization of medical practice in any country is always tied to its history and societal structure. A good illustration of this is the different ways countries have chosen to provide medical care. In some areas there is a socially guaranteed access to medical services (e.g., Cuba, Sweden), in others there is a centralized government-run "national health system" (e.g., U.K.), and finally there is medicine operating as a private business (U.S.). Each system has its unique strengths and weaknesses.

Each tries to tie Hippocratic ideology with day-to-day practicality. And once again there is the contrast between the universals of medical know-how and the particulars of its application in the social contexts of society. However, all of the different forms of medical services borrow from the same universal medical knowledge base.

We can use the practice of medicine in the United States at the present time to illustrate the social–personal tug of war that is placed on both the science of medicine and the practice of medicine. The U.S. populace, through its politicians, has supported research in virtually all fields of medicine for decades. The multibillion dollar annual budget of the National Institutes of Health is the best proof that the United States has a commitment to extending the boundaries of medical science. On the other hand, millions of individuals do not have access to the fruits of these investigations. Medical care is expensive, and only those who are fortunate enough to have adequate health insurance receive excellent health care.

The peculiarities of the U.S. medical system are situated within the social history of the United States. de Tocqueville (1848/1966) was one of the first to point out how the history of the United States is responsible for a society where extreme individualism is held together with equally extreme collectivism. That unique history is a kind of historical "natural experiment" in the social psychology of macrocommunities. It has resulted in an economically successful society that functions through a unique system of democratic governance—a transformed model of British community governance (see Mead, 1930). There has been a strong dose of missionary spirit in U.S. society that has helped economic development at home, but this has also led to U.S. attempts to export its ideology worldwide. The U.S. social system has not been adopted by other countries in any successful way, however, and the only case of its explicit exportation (to Liberia) has not resulted in a prosperous and peaceful society.

PSYCHOLOGY'S STRUGGLE: THE ROLE OF THE RESEARCHER

Contemporary psychology is a result of the history of the discipline. It can be roughly divided into "mainstream" and "other" groupings—at least in the context of the United States where political pressures prescribe a fight for "the right" way of being, thinking, and making sense. It is an interesting observation that the specific contents of such a "right way" changes relatively quickly, yet at any instant there cannot be more than one "right way" operating within the same competitive, social enterprise. Minority views are tolerated (and at times even highlighted), yet not beyond the point at which they would supercede the "right way."

Surely different enterprises can flourish in parallel (each with their own "right way"). An outsider who looks at psychology in the United States as a whole would be left with an impression of eclectic parallelism. While parallelism may be present on a national level, it is unusual within local enterprises. That is not merely a result of the social organization of the enterprise. Rather, its roots go to the privacy of the members of such institutions. For example, an American psychoanalyst who works in New York, Japan, and India has given an example from the boundary of societies:

> One Indian colleague, Veena, recounted that she is a member of two private psychoanalytic seminars with radically different orientations as well as leaders, one being quite traditional, the other highly innovative. Veena feels perfectly comfortable in both groups, with no conflict whatsoever, and learns a great deal in each. No American psychoanalyst I know of, woman or man, would ever consider being a member of these two particular seminars simultaneously, because they would experience them as far too dissonant and too disruptive of consistent inner professional identity. Since each group's members would probably disapprove of her being in the other group, Veena keeps her participation in the other group secret in a highly private self, typical of Indians and other Asians. (Roland, 1996, p. 27)

This example may test the limits of the cognitive dissonance theory, at least when applied to an active learner in a divided group context. As a strategy of overcoming unnecessary intergroup rivalry within one's private self, however, the example demonstrates the potential for researchers to transcend the usual intergroup frictions within a discipline.

CONTRIBUTIONS BY SOCIAL PSYCHOLOGY

Social psychology has a long tradition of disbelieving verbal reports as data (Nisbett & Wilson, 1977). This idea came to the forefront at almost the same time that cognitive psychology was rehabilitating the use of verbal reports as data (Ericsson & Simon, 1993). In fact, the last century of social psychology and many of the other branches of experimental psychology has been devoted to demonstrating how limited and error-filled is our understanding of ourselves. The real issue, of course, is not in a political stance—"verbal reports by subjects are correct" versus "verbal reports are faulty"—but a careful consideration of why a person makes one or another statement about oneself, how these statements are coproduced by the researcher who sets up the conditions for the investigation, and how the researcher decides to create data from all of the evidence. In the long run, the researcher assembles the scientific picture of the objective phenomena, often using language that is far beyond the comprehension of the participant.

Here we face another tension in the research process: the use of the specialized (universal) language of science versus the particular languages—or idiolects—of the participants. Scientific language necessarily goes beyond the language used in everyday life. Yet, if the researcher has the final word, then that word also can be deceptive. In fact, experimental techniques are meant to bring out conditions where the researcher had made a generalized—yet deceptive—claim. In the case of adequate uses of experimental methods in social psychology (Milgram, 1974; Zimbardo, 1969), the value of experiments in correcting the researcher's delusions is well documented. The driving force behind the development of various aspects of the prevailing methodology is to figure out ways to minimize the impact of the researcher's values and expectations on the outcome. The standard assumption is that one can never entirely remove that bias, but one can minimize it, or sometimes measure it, or, by converging methods, find a way to see the reality that is only dimly reflected in the actual observations.

Deception, or the researcher leading the participant's thinking in a direction so that some other phenomenon can be studied, is a necessary part of science. It is not only the participant who can be misled, often it is also the research assistant who sets up the study whose understanding of what is being investigated is selectively directed. It is precisely the desire to minimize the experimenter's impact on the observations that is behind the use of blind and double-blind studies. It also leads to attempts to standardize the experimenter's behavior as much as possible, so that the participant is not led by the experimenters' nonconscious influences. Such standardization is fraught with problems. Often the interviewer/researcher begins to sound and act like an automaton. Normal personal interactions are lost. The research participant may answer a question, but there is no way to know if it was understood, as it is often believed that each study participant should hear exactly the same words, no more and no less.

DISTANCING FOR THE SAKE OF GAINING A PERSPECTIVE

Among the methods adopted to minimize the impact of the observer, one of the most common is to ask questions in writing rather than in person. It is assumed that the questioners will inevitably influence the answers they receive, without either the questioners or the answerers knowing that the influence has occurred. Of course, pursuant to the guiding assumption that the observer's influence can only be minimized, not removed, the further assumption is that questions themselves influence the answer, even when written. (Of course, in one sense, if they did not produce some sort of relevant answer, they would not be questions.) Norbert Schwartz and others study how question features influence answers by systematically varying the questions (see also chapter 17). While questionnaires may be no more (and perhaps less) biased than interviews, they are imperfect and at least involve a different set of potential biases. If we understand the effects of different formats, we might be able to ask questions in a number of different ways and better converge on the "truth." This book contains several chapters that examine the benefits and shortcomings of both questionnaires and interviews.

FROM RESPONSES TO DATA

In any research, the originally collected specimens of evidence are processed further to become data. Usually, participants' responses must be categorized. The first task is to identify the categories of response. This can be done in advance, and then the response categories can be provided to the participant, as in a multiple choice questionnaire format. Conversely, it can be done after the data are collected by coding responses into categories. Doing it beforehand has the advantage that the participant is the one who decides which of the experimenter's categories best fit his or her response. The disadvantage is, of course, that the experimenter may fail to include one or more important response alternatives in the category system. This problem may be overcome to some extent by providing an "Other" category. The greatest advantage of establishing categories after the data are gathered is that everything the participants say may be included, including responses the experimenter would never have considered.

Potential bias is again introduced when the researcher begins to interpret the responses, whether from interviews or questionnaires. In most experiments that deal with more than a handful of participants, there is no way to use all of the participants' responses in a pure, uninterpreted way. While the use of a complete transcript of every interaction, without categories or any attempt to characterize the responses, will eliminate interpretation bias, it is impractical. Therefore, it comes down either to providing the categories and letting the participant decide what is best or establishing the categories later and having the experimenter make each response fit into a category.

HOW ARE GENERALIZATIONS MADE?

Generalization is the process through which a universal principle is developed from a set of existing evidence (data). Traditionally, this can be accomplished either by qualitative or quantitative methods. Both methods have strengths, and both have weaknesses. Often, the method is chosen because of the tradition of that field or branch of science to which the researcher belongs. The quantitative method moves from responses to classification. For these researchers, the "law of large numbers" reigns. Generalizations here move from samples to populations. The issues of representativeness of samples, randomness of sampling, and sample size are all important.

The qualitative route to generalization does not rely on the notion of a sample (nor of population). Each system under study is treated as a microcosm of its own and is studied as a complete system. Hypotheses are tested on the basis of a single case, but with varying conditions. Here the "law of small numbers" ($N = 1$) prevails. The classic experiments in the history of psychology—such as those of B. F. Skinner, M. Sherif, S. Milgram, and others—did not need at least 29 standardized replication efforts (note: the "magic number" of subjects needed is often said to be 30). Instead, in the many studies conducted by the classic researchers, the experimental procedures were varied as to their particulars in order to test the boundaries of the general principle. If the general principle is adequate (valid), then it will be replicated in every single case that is selected and studied. If there is no replication, then the general principle itself requires modification.

OVERVIEW OF THE BOOK

The structure of this book oscillates between the general and the particular. In Part I we address the issues of how human thinking—in everyday life and in medicine—reaches relevant decisions. Much is at stake in those decisions, and it remains a remarkable testimony for human adaptation that the heuristic means—models for thinking—are robust and available for very speedy decision making. These "fast and frugal" heuristics (chapter 1 by Gigerenzer and Kurzenhäuser) are examples of universal human cognitive mechanisms. Yet it is important to remember that the way an individual makes a decision may vary greatly depending on the context of the need for the decision. For example, the factors involved in deciding how much to bet in a casino are quite different from deciding how to treat a critically ill person. The actual mental processes of decision making are socially guided, as Salovey (chapter 2) shows. The specific ways in which messages are framed make a profound difference in the outcome that is reached. The specific life situation of the individual also changes the decision process. Furthermore, a specific social discourse mode—talking about risks—can lead to either general escalation or de-escalation of the societal concerns about health issues and feed an individual's actual feelings about their own health-related actions (Heyman, chapter 3) and, in Part II, perceptions (Heyman, chapter 4 and Hoffrage et al., chapter 5).

In the context of medical practice, all the cognitive and social conditions for human thinking are subordinated to the goals of the health care system—the recovery or maintenance of health. Clinicians remain central in the decision processes despite the advances in medical science. Only the clinician has the knowledge about the individual that is necessary to treat an illness. Chapters by Noller and Bibace (chapter 6) and Chelmow (chapter 9) provide the readers with an overview of the current state of affairs in the American medical system, where—together with great technological advancements—the possibilities for medical errors are enhanced. The critical issue is how to prevent such errors. In this endeavor, psychology can make a contribution. The No-Fault Learning Program (chapter 7 by Bibace and Noller, and chapter 8 by Bibace, Leeman, and Noller) demonstrates how a focus on an individual clinician's decision making can help to reduce both errors of omission and commission.

Part III of our book is dedicated to case studies in human health-related conduct. The very act of seeking medical assistance is a socially guided practice that—as Bäärnhielm shows in chapter 10—is overdetermined by meanings. Such overdetermination is situated in the ordinary social discourses—and Amorim and Rossetti-Ferreira demonstrate how intricately a child's ordinary illness experience in a day-care setting is socially constructed (chapter 11). A more dramatic story unfolds in the case of a child fighting leukemia (Silva, in chapter 12).

In Part IV, the reader is shown that the interface between universals and particulars can lead to the development of new methodologies. It is demonstrated how all four of the psychologists' favorite measurement scales—nominal, ordinal, interval, and ratio—form an ascending sequence of quantitative sophistication (Laird, in chapter 13). Much real-life decision making takes place without full information and under conditions of rapid change. Toomela (chapter 14) promotes a systemic perspective for looking at decision making without full information.

Contributions to Part V outline the different meanings of the notion of participation. It begins from the initial consent to participate and follows the process over years and even decades. Chapter 16 by Kerllenevich et al. illustrates the intricacies of the process. The research participant has principled autonomy, and no instruction can reduce it. Furthermore, that autonomy extends to the level of each particular question that a clinician or researcher asks. Informed consent can cover a wide range of interpretations (chapter 17). Similarly, all psychological questionnaires—such as personality inventories like the MMPI or NEOPI—are vulnerable to high inter-individual variability, even in seemingly simple items (Valsiner et al., chapter 18).

We have attempted to examine the widely disparate concepts of the universal and the particular in the context of modern society. We have uncovered both friction and accord, but mostly we have found that we have changed our "feelings" about them. We no longer see the universal as one globe on the end of a barbell and the particular on the other, neither do we see the concepts as a continuum. Rather, these concepts are more like the colors of a rainbow. At no point is there only red, or blue, or yellow. Each layer of color extends from one end of the spectrum to the other. Neither is there only universal nor only particular anywhere in science or medicine. Each is inexorably intertwined with the other. To examine one is to examine both. No universal truth is discovered without the data from individuals, and no particular person is healed without knowledge of the universal (Leeman et al., 2003).

We hope you enjoy our "experiment."

NOTE

1. The use of language is interesting here. Both psychology and medicine have changed the way they refer to the persons—or animals—that are being studied. For years these persons were subjects. Now they are research participants.

REFERENCES

de Tocqueville, A. (1848/1966). *Democracy in America*. Garden City, NY: Doubleday.

Ericsson, K. A., & Simon, H. (1993). *Verbal reports as data.* Cambridge, MA: MIT Press.

Leeman, R. F., Szetela, A. E., & Bibace, R. (2003, June). *Speaker to listener: "No! That's not what I said. Furthermore, you do not appreciate what I mean!"* Paper presented at the 10th Biennial Conference of the International Society of Theoretical Psychology (ISTP), Istanbul, Turkey, June 24, 2003.

Milgram, S. (1974). *Obedience to authority.* New York: Harper.

Nisbett, R. E., & Wilson, T. D. (1977). Telling more than we can know: Verbal reports on mental processes. *Psychological Review, 87,* 231–259.

Roland, A. (1996). *Cultural pluralism and psychoanalysis: The Asian and North American experience.* New York: Routledge.

Zimbardo, P. (1969). The human choice: Individuation, reason, and order versus de-individuation, impulse, and chaos. In W. Arnold & D. Levine (Eds.), *Nebraska Symposium on Motivation: Vol. 17* (pp. 237–307). Lincoln, NE: University of Nebraska Press.

Part I

BETWEEN GENERALITIES AND PARTICULARS: AVAILABILITY OF COGNITIVE HEURISTICS

Chapter 1

FAST AND FRUGAL HEURISTICS IN MEDICAL DECISION MAKING

Gerd Gigerenzer and Stephanie Kurzenhäuser

How do doctors solve the challenging task to make treatment decisions under time pressure? Consider the following situation: A man is rushed to the hospital with serious chest pains. The doctors suspect acute ischemic heart disease and need to make a decision, and they need to make it quickly: Should the patient be assigned to the coronary care unit or to a regular nursing bed for monitoring? The decision to admit a patient to a coronary care unit has serious medical and financial consequences. How do doctors make such decisions, and how *should* they?

One way to do it is to rely on experience and intuition. For instance, in a rural Michigan hospital, doctors sent some 90 percent of the patients to the coronary care unit. This behavior can be understood as defensive decision making—physicians fear malpractice suits if they do not send a patient into the care unit, and he subsequently has a heart attack, but less so if they send a patient into the unit unnecessarily, and he dies of an infection. This indiscriminate use of the coronary care unit causes unnecessary costs (too many people in the coronary care unit, which results in high per-day costs), decreases the quality of care, and adds additional health risks (such as serious secondary infections) to patients who should not be in the unit. Only 25 percent of the patients admitted to the coronary care unit did actually have a myocardial infarction (Green & Mehr, 1997; Green & Smith, 1988). Similar rates were found at larger hospitals (ranging from 12% to 42%).

Researchers at the University of Michigan Hospital tried to solve this overcrowding problem by training the physicians to use a decision-support tool based on logistic regression, rather than relying on their intuitive judgment (Green & Mehr, 1997).

Physicians were trained to use the Heart Disease Predictive Instrument (Pozen, D'Agostino, Selker, Sytkowski, & Hood, 1984), which is a

Figure 1.1
The Heart Disease Predictive Instrument (HDPI), a decision-support tool, in the form of a pocket-sized, plastic-laminated card. The reverse side of the card gives the following definitions:

Chest Pain = Chief Complaint
EKG (ST, T wave Δ's)

History	ST&T Ø	ST⇔	T⇑⇓	ST⇔	ST⇔&T⇑⇓	ST⇑⇓&T⇑⇓
No MI& No NTG	19%	35%	42%	54%	62%	78%
MI or NTG	27%	46%	53%	64%	73%	85%
MI and NTG	37%	58%	65%	75%	80%	90%

Chest Pain, NOT Chief Complaint
EKG (ST, T wave Δ's)

History	ST&T Ø	ST⇔	T⇑⇓	ST⇔	ST⇔&T⇑⇓	ST⇑⇓&T⇑⇓
No MI& No NTG	10%	21%	26%	36%	45%	64%
MI or NTG	16%	29%	36%	48%	56%	74%
MI and NTG	22%	40%	47%	59%	67%	82%

No Chest Pain
EKG (ST, T wave Δ's)

History	ST&T Ø	ST⇔	T⇑⇓	ST⇔	ST⇔&T⇑⇓	ST⇑⇓&T⇑⇓
No MI& No NTG	4%	9%	12%	17%	23%	39%
MI or NTG	6%	14%	17%	25%	32%	51%
MI and NTG	10%	20%	25%	35%	43%	62%

Chest pain: Patient reports chest or left arm pressure or pain.

Chief complaint: Patient reports chest/left arm discomfort is most important symptom.

NTG: Patient reports a history of PRN use of nitroglycerin for relief of chest pain. Not necessary to have used NTG for this episode.

MI: Patient reports a history of definite myocardial infarction.

ST⇐⇒: Initial EKG shows ST segment "barring," "straightening," or "flattening" in a least two leads excluding aVR.

ST⇑⇓: Initial EKG shows ST segment elevation or depression of at least 1 mm in at least two leads excluding avR.

T⇑⇓: Initial EKG shows T waves that are "hyperacute" (at least 50% of R-wave amplitude) or inverted at least 1 mm in at least two leads excluding aVR.

Ø: None of the above ST segment or T-wave Δ's are present.

Source: (Green & Mehr, 1997).

decision-support tool that tries to weigh and combine the relevant information. The Heart Disease Predictive Instrument (HDPI) as used in the Michigan Hospital consists of a chart with some 50 probabilities (Figure 1.1). The physician has to check the presence or absence of combinations of seven symptoms and insert the relevant probabilities into a pocket calculator, which determines the probability that a patient has acute heart disease. The probability score is generated from a logistic regression formula that combines and weighs the dichotomous information on the seven symptoms. These symptoms were chosen out of 59 clinical features about which information is available to emergency room physicians (Pozen et al., 1984). However, physicians are generally not happy using this and similar systems (Corey & Merenstein, 1987; Pearson, Goldman, Garcia, Cook, & Lee, 1994). Physicians typically do not understand logistic regression, and even if they do, they are uncomfortable with being dependent on a probability chart. The dilemma the doctors in the Michigan hospital now faced was as follows: Should patients in life-and-death situations be classified by intuitions that are natural but in this case suboptimal or by complex calculations that are alien but possibly more accurate? This dilemma arises in many contexts, from financial advising to personnel recruiting: Should we rely on experts' intuition or on a fancy statistical model?

There is, however, a third alternative: smart heuristics. They correspond to natural intuitions, but they can have the accuracy of fancy statistical models. It was an unexpected observation that initially led the hospital researchers to try a heuristic model. The researchers had employed an ABAB reversal design. That is, they had let the physicians make the decision first by intuition (condition A), then given them the HDPI (condition B), then withdrew the instrument and left the physicians to their intuition once more (condition A), and so on. The researchers had expected that the quality of decision making would be relatively low in condition A and high in condition B, and would oscillate. Quality first increased from A to B, as expected, but then surprisingly stayed at this level, even when the instrument was withdrawn. Figure 1.3 shows that physicians initially had a false-positive rate of over 90 percent (condition A), which improved after they first encountered the HDPI to less than 60 percent (first condition B) and subsequently stayed at this level (all further conditions A and B). It was out of the question that the physicians could have memorized the probabilities on the chart or calculated the logistic regression in their heads. So why did the decision-support system only help the first time? The suspicion was that the probabilities and the logistic computations may have mattered little, and that physicians might have simply learned the important variables. This interpretation opened up the possibility of deliberately constructing a decision heuristic that uses only a minimum of information and computation. Green and Mehr (1997) constructed a simple decision heuristic by using three building blocks of heuristics: ordered search, a fast stopping rule, and one reason decision making (Gigerenzer, Todd, & the ABC Research Group, 1999). Before we turn to the decision heuristic of Green and Mehr, let us first consider its building blocks in more detail.

FAST AND FRUGAL HEURISTICS

There are several classes of heuristics (the term "heuristic" is of Greek origin, meaning "serving to find out or discover"). Green and Mehr (1997) based the construction of their decision heuristic on fast and frugal heuristics (Gigerenzer & Selten, 2001). These heuristics do not try to compute the maximum or minimum of some function, nor, for the most part, do they calculate probabilities. They are fast, because they do not involve much computation, and frugal because they only search for part of the information. They rely on simple building blocks for searching for information, stopping search, and finally making a decision (Gigerenzer & Goldstein, 1996; Gigerenzer, Todd, & the ABC Research Group, 1999).

Building Blocks for Guiding Search

Alternatives and cues are sought in a particular order. For instance, search for cues can be simply random or in order of cue validity.

Building Blocks for Stopping Search

Search for alternatives or cues must be stopped at some point. Fast and frugal heuristics employ stopping rules that do not try to compute an optimal cost–benefit trade-off. Rather, heuristic principles for stopping involve simple criteria that are easily ascertained, such as halting information search as soon as the first cue or reason that favors one decision alternative is found.

Building Blocks for Decision Making

Once search has been stopped, a decision or inference must be made. Many models of judgment and decision making ignore the search and stopping rules and focus exclusively on decision: Are predictor values combined linearly as in multiple regression, in a Bayesian way, or in some other fashion? Instead, fast and frugal heuristics use simple principles for decisions (such as one-reason decision making, see below) that avoid expensive computations and extensive knowledge by working hand in hand with equally simple search and stopping rules.

FAST AND FRUGAL DECISION TREE

Using these building blocks, Green and Mehr (1997) constructed a simple decision heuristic for the coronary care unit allocation problem. The resulting heuristic is shown in Figure 1.2 in the form of a fast and frugal decision tree. It ignores all 50 probabilities and asks only a few yes-or-no questions. If a patient has a certain anomaly in his electrocardiogram (the so-called ST segment change), he is immediately admitted to the coronary care unit. No other information is searched for. If that is not the case, a second variable is considered: whether the patient's primary complaint is chest pain. If this is not the case, he is immediately classified as low risk and assigned to a regular nursing bed. No further information is considered. If the answer is yes, then a third and final question is asked to classify the patient.

This decision tree employs fast and frugal rules of search, stopping, and decision. First, it ranks the predictors according to a simple criterion (predictor with the highest sensitivity first, predictor with the highest specificity second, and so on). Search follows this order, similar to the Take The Best heuristic (Gigerenzer & Goldstein, 1996, 1999). Second, search can stop after each predictor; the rest is ignored. Third, the strategy does not combine—weight and add—the predictors; for instance, a change in the ST Segment sends the patient immediately into the coronary care unit, whether or not his chief complaint is chest pain, and independent of what other factors the patient has. In general terms, predictors that are lower in the tree cannot compensate for one higher up in the tree. Only one predictor determines each decision. This decision rule is an instance of *one-reason decision making*. The entire heart disease tree is a realization of a *fast and frugal tree,* which is defined as a decision tree with a small number of binary predictors that allows for a decision *at each branch* of the tree.

HOW ACCURATE IS THE FAST AND FRUGAL TREE?

The simple tree, just like the Heart Disease Predictive Instrument, can be evaluated by multiple performance criteria. Accuracy is one criterion,

Figure 1.2
Fast and frugal decision tree for coronary care unit allocation. For explanations, see Figure 1.1.

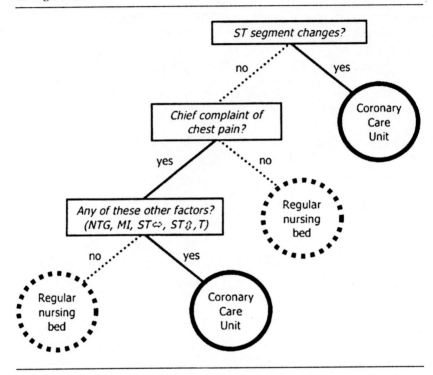

Source: Based on Green & Mehr, 1997.

which includes two aspects: The decision strategy should have (a) a high sensitivity, that is, it should send most of the patients who will actually have a serious heart problem into the coronary care room; and (b) high specificity, that is, it should send few patients into the care unit unnecessarily. Being able to make a decision fast is a second criterion, which is essential in situations where slow decision making can cost a life. A third criterion is frugality, that is, the ability to make a good decision with only limited information. The second and third criteria are not independent, and the fast and frugal tree is, by design, superior in both of these aspects to the HDPI decision-support system, as may be physicians' intuition. A fourth criterion is the transparency of a decision system. An accurate system is worth little when it is not accepted. Unlike logistic regression, the steps of the fast and frugal tree are transparent and easy to teach. But how accurate is one-reason decision making? Would you want to be classified by a few yes-or-no questions in a situation with such high stakes? Or would you rather be evaluated by the HDPI, or perhaps by physicians' intuition?

Figure 1.3 shows the performance of the three forms of decision making. On the Y axis is the proportion of patients correctly assigned to the coronary care unit, as measured by a subsequent heart attack. On the X axis is the proportion of patients incorrectly assigned. The diagonal line represents chance performance. A perfect strategy would be represented by a point in the upper left-hand corner, but nothing like that exists in an uncertain world.

As one can see from the triangle, the physicians' initial performance turns out to be at the chance level, even slightly below. The HDPI did

Figure 1.3
Coronary care unit decisions by physicians, the Heart Disease Predictive Instrument (HDPI), and the fast and frugal tree. Accuracy is measured by the proportion of patients correctly assigned to the coronary care unit and the proportion of patients incorrectly sent to the unit. Correct assignment is measured by the occurrence of myocardial infarction. Physicians' initial performance is represented by the right point, and their performance after they encountered the HDPI for the first time is represented by the left data point, which shows a smaller false-positive rate. An ideal diagnostic instrument would be represented by a point in the upper left-hand corner, but in the real world, no such performance exists.

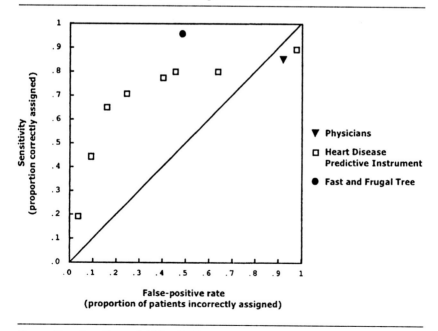

Source: Based on Green & Mehr, 1997.

much better than the physicians' intuition. Its performance is shown by the open squares, which represent various trade-offs between the two possible errors.

How did the fast and frugal tree perform? The counterintuitive result is that the fast and frugal tree was more accurate in classifying actual heart attack patients than both the physicians' intuition and the HDPI. It correctly assigned the largest proportion of patients who subsequently had a myocardial infarction into the coronary care unit. At the same time, it had a comparatively low false-alarm rate. Note that the expert system had more information than the smart heuristic and could make use of sophisticated statistical calculations. Nevertheless, in this complex situation, less is more.

The potentials of fast and frugal decision making are currently being discussed in the medical literature, and some medical researchers see in it a powerful alternative to the prescriptions of classical decision theory for patient care (Elwyn, Edwards, Eccles, & Rovner, 2001). The crucial question is, when does simplicity pay and when does it not?

WHEN LESS IS MORE

How can it be that a heuristic that ignores information and forgoes computation can be not only faster, more frugal, and transparent but also more accurate? A comparison between the logistic regression (HDPI) and the fast and frugal tree can help to understand the secret of less is more.

Consider the error-free case in which a decision strategy can classify all objects correctly, that is, where a point in the upper left-hand corner of Figure 1.3 exists. In an error-free world, what is the relation between a fast and frugal tree and a logistic regression? The answer is: If an error-free fast and frugal tree exists in an environment, then an error-free logistic regression always exists as well (Forster, Martignon, Masanori, Vitouch, & Gigerenzer, 2002; Martignon, Vitouch, Takezawa, & Forster, 2003). But can one prove the converse, that for each logistic regression there exists a fast and frugal tree that is error-free, or equally accurate? This is not the case. Thus, although this analysis shows that in the error-free case, some fast and frugal trees can be as accurate as logistic regression, it cannot explain *why* they are more accurate. For this, we need to look at more realistic situations in which error-free decision making is impossible.

ROBUSTNESS

In situations where decisions are liable to error, the twin concept of robustness and overfitting can predict situations in which less is more. Robustness is the ability to generalize well to new environments, specifically those whose structure is not known in advance. The important distinction here is between data fitting and prediction. In the first case, one fits a model to the empirical data, that is, the training set is the same as the test set. In prediction, the model is based on a training set but is tested on new data. A good fit to the new data may be deceptive because of overfitting. In general, a model A overfits the training data if there exists an alternative model B, such that A has higher or equal accuracy than B in the training set but lower accuracy in the test set. Consider two diagnostic systems, one with more adjustable parameters (e.g., predictors) and one with only a subset of these, that is, with fewer adjustable parameters. Both systems fit a given body of data (e.g., a sample of patients) equally well. When making predictions about a new sample, the general result is that the simpler system will make more accurate predictions than the system with more parameters. This form of less-is-more has been mathematically proven for specific situations (Akaike, 1973; Forster & Sober, 1994; Geman, Bienenstock, & Doursat, 1992). With a sufficient number of parameters, one can always force a model to fit a sample of observations. However, part of this fit involves overfitting, that is, explaining noise and idiosyncrasies that do not generalize to a new sample, such as new patients. In an uncertain world, only part of the information available today will generalize to new situations; therefore, good decision making implies ignoring part of the information. The more unpredictable the situation is, the more information should be ignored. The art of good decision making is to focus on that part of the information that generalizes and to ignore the rest.

Predicting heart attacks is far from error-free. In the original sample of several thousands of patients on which the HDPI was validated (Pozen et al., 1984), the latter may very well have provided a better fit than a fast and frugal tree. But it was subsequently applied in different hospitals to new groups of patients who deviated in unknown ways from the original sample. As a result, the model that was best in the original population was no longer guaranteed to be the best in those new situations; it may suffer from overfitting. A fast and frugal heuristic that focuses only on the key variables is likely to be more robust, and it has a chance of performing better than the system that used more information. As Figure

1.3 amply illustrates, assigning heart disease patients is one of these difficult tasks.

HEURISTICS CAN BE FRUGAL BY EXPLOITING STRUCTURES OF ENVIRONMENTS

A second reason why heuristics that ignore information can nevertheless be accurate is their ecological rationality. A heuristic is ecologically rational to the degree it is adapted to the structure of information in an environment, whether the environment is physical or social. Heuristics that employ one-reason decision making can exploit environments in which the importance (e.g., beta weights in regression) of the cues available are exponentially decreasing, that is, noncompensatory. An example are binary cues with weights 1, 1/2, 1/4, 1/8, and so on. If this is the case, one can prove that a simple heuristic called Take The Best can perform as well as any optimal linear combination of binary cues (Martignon & Hoffrage, 1999). Similarly, the fast and frugal tree can exploit noncompensatory environments. If the environment, in contrast, has a compensatory structure, tallying heuristics can exploit this type of information. A tallying heuristic has the following structure: If you find n ($n \geq 2$, say 3) positive indicators of a heart disease, then stop search and send the patient into the care unit; otherwise, into the nursing bed (Forster et al., 2002). In contrast to the fast and frugal tree, tallying does not employ one-reason decision making: It uses more than one cue, but its simplicity is in the fact that it uses only few cues and does not order or weight them, and it can search for cues in any order.

To summarize, the reasonableness of fast and frugal heuristics derives from their ecological rationality, not from following the classical definitions of rationality in terms of coherence or internal consistency of choices. Indeed, some of the fast and frugal heuristics can produce intransitive inferences in direct violation of standard rationality norms, but they still can be quite accurate (Gigerenzer, Czerlinski, & Martignon, 1999).

THE UNAPPRECIATED VIRTUES OF SIMPLICITY

Consider a physician who uses the fast and frugal tree in Figure 1.2 to allocate patients. She makes more accurate decisions than her colleagues who rely on intuition and defensive decision making do, and ones that are as good as or better than with the logistic regression classification. However, one of the patients whom she sent into a nursing bed had a heart attack and died. The relatives ask why the patient wasn't in the care unit, and their lawyer finds out that the doctor had only checked two predictors (the two predictors in Figure 1.2), ignoring the rest. The relatives sue the doctor for malpractice. Do physicians want to run this risk?

The irony in this situation is that physicians often feel pressed to hide how their decisions were actually made and to pretend they have made them on the basis of something different. The virtue of less-is-more is not yet fully understood. As a consequence, the quality of treatment can suffer by the covert and uneducated use of heuristics. For instance, Figure 1.3 shows that whatever intuitive heuristics physicians used before they encountered the researchers, their performance was dismal.

There is growing empirical evidence that physicians rely on fast and frugal heuristics when they make treatment decisions. For instance, a recent study on decisions of British general practitioners to prescribe lipid-lowering drugs suggests that doctors do indeed use only very few cues for their decisions (Dhami & Harries, 2001). But in private conversations, physicians indicate that they often cannot risk admitting to using heuristics. At the same time, there is growing evidence that heuristics can be powerful tools for clinical judgments under uncertainty (Fischer et al., 2002; Forster et al., 2002). Medical researchers have begun discussing fast and frugal decision making as an alternative to classical decision making (Elwyn et al., 2001). The systematic study of fast and frugal decision making can help to bridge the worlds of intuitive heuristics and classical decision making. Furthermore, it can teach physicians what heuristics to use, as well as when and how to improve the decisions they make.

REFERENCES

Akaike, H. (1973). Information theory and an extension of the maximum likelihood principle. In B. N. Petrov & F. Csaki (Eds.), *2nd International Symposium on Information Theory* (pp. 267–281). Budapest: Akademiai Kiado.

Corey, G. A., & Merenstein, J. H. (1987). Applying the acute ischemic heart disease predictive instrument. *Journal of Family Practice, 25,* 127–133.

Dhami, M. K., & Harries, C. (2001). Fast and frugal versus regression models of human judgement. *Thinking and Reasoning, 7,* 5–27.

Elwyn, G., Edwards, A., Eccles, M., & Rovner, D. (2001). Decision analysis in patient care. *The Lancet, 358,* 571–574.

Fischer, J. E., Steiner, F., Zucol, F., Berger, C., Martignon, L., Bossart, W., et al. (2002). Use of simple heuristics to target macrolide prescription in children with community-acquired pneumonia. *Archives of Pediatrics and Adolescent Medicine, 156,* 1005–1008.

Forster, M., Martignon, L., Masanori, T., Takezawa, M., Vitouch, O., & Gigerenzer, G. (2002). *Simple heuristics versus complex predictive instruments: Which is better and why?* Unpublished manuscript.

Forster, M., & Sober, E. (1994). How to tell when simpler, more unified, or less ad hoc theories will provide more accurate predictions. *British Journal of Philosophical Science, 45,* 1–35.

Geman, S. E., Bienenstock, E., & Doursat, R. (1992). Neural networks and the bias/variance dilemma. *Neural Computation, 4,* 1–58.

Gigerenzer, G., Czerlinski, J., & Martignon, L. (1999). How good are fast and frugal heuristics? In J. Shanteau, B. Mellers, & D. Schum (Eds.), *Decision research from Bayesian approaches to normative systems: Reflections on the contributions of Ward Edwards.* (pp. 81–103). Norwell, MA: Kluwer Academic Publishers.

Gigerenzer, G., & Goldstein, D. G. (1996). Reasoning the fast and frugal way: Models of bounded rationality. *Psychological Review, 103,* 684–704.

Gigerenzer, G., & Goldstein, D. G. (1999). Betting on one good reason: The Take The Best heuristic. In G. Gigerenzer, P. M. Todd, & the ABC Research Group, *Simple heuristics that make us smart* (pp. 75–95). New York: Oxford University Press.

Gigerenzer, G., & Selten, R. (Eds.). (2001). *Bounded rationality: The adaptive toolbox.* Cambridge, MA: MIT Press.

Gigerenzer, G., Todd, P. M., & the ABC Research Group. (1999). *Simple heuristics that make us smart.* New York: Oxford University Press.

Green, L., & Mehr, D. R. (1997). What alters physicians' decisions to admit to the coronary care unit? *The Journal of Family Practice, 45,* 219–226.

Green, L., & Smith, M. (1988). Evaluation of two acute cardiac ischemia decision-support tools in a rural family practice. *The Journal of Family Practice, 26,* 627–632.

Martignon, L., & Hoffrage, U. (1999). Why does one-reason decision making work? A case study in ecological rationality. In G. Gigerenzer, P. M. Todd, & the ABC Research Group, *Simple heuristics that make us smart* (pp. 119–140). New York: Oxford University Press.

Martignon, L., Vitouch, O., Takezawa, M., & Forster, M. (2003). Naive and yet enlightened: From natural frequencies to fast and frugal decision trees. In L. Macchi & D. Hardmann (Eds.), *The psychology of reasoning and decision making: A handbook.* Chichester, U.K.: Wiley.

Pearson, S. D., Goldman, L., Garcia, T. B., Cook, E. F., & Lee, T. H. (1994). Physician response to a prediction rule for the triage of emergency department patients with chest pain. *Journal of General Internal Medicine, 9,* 241–247.

Pozen, M. W., D'Agnostino, R. B., Selker, H. P., Sytkowski, P. A., & Hood, W. B. (1984). A predictive instrument to improve coronary-care-unit admission practices in acute ischemic heart disease. *The New England Journal of Medicine, 310,* 1273–1278.

EDITORIAL COMMENTARY

The word "heuristic" is not commonly used in medical circles in the United States. However, the concept of "triage" and the use of algorithms are well-accepted and used every day. "Fast and frugal heuristics" are a bit—but only a bit—different from these. It was battlefield medicine that first gave us the concept of triage. In that setting, nearly instantaneous decisions regarding a combatant's ability to survive needed to be made based on very little information.

The typical algorithm uses some data reference set, often based on complex mathematical models. While some are useful, others are so complex and take so much time to go through the various branches that they become cumbersome and are often ignored. Such overfitting should be avoided—a point made well by the authors—whenever clinical algorithms are developed.

—Kenneth L. Noller

Simplicity is nice, but it needs to be substantive. What we see in this chapter is an argument in favor of the fast and frugal heuristics—in comparison with probability calculations. Yet it seems to replace one black box with another—we still do not know the precise ways in which these fast and frugal heuristics work. We do know that (a) they do work, and (b) they work quickly and relatively efficiently (compared to others). However, unless the actual mechanisms that operate—frugally and fastly—are clarified, we only have a demonstration of effectiveness and not of the reasons for such effectiveness.

—Jaan Valsiner

Chapter 2

PROMOTING PREVENTION AND DETECTION: PSYCHOLOGICALLY TAILORING AND FRAMING MESSAGES ABOUT HEALTH

Peter Salovey

One area in which the science of human decision making could make contact with medicine is in the development of public health campaigns designed to persuade individuals to engage in health-promoting behaviors or to cease health-damaging behaviors. Yet many public health campaigns are designed by advertising and marketing professionals with little attention to underlying research on preference, choice, and motivation and its obvious application in this arena. It should not be surprising, therefore, that many appeals to engage in behaviors from daily dental flossing to consuming more fruits and vegetables fall on deaf ears.

It is the purpose of this chapter to explore research on two aspects of health message design—psychological tailoring and framing—in order to understand how these mechanisms can be applied to the creation of more effective health messages. By tailoring messages to psychological styles and needs, and framing risk information in understandable ways, health professionals may be able to transcend some of the challenges involved in communicating statistical information, so aptly described in the chapter of this volume by Hoffrage, Kurzenhäuser, and Gigerenzer. Although we have focused our attention on health behaviors relevant to the prevention or early detection of cancer and HIV/AIDS, we hope to be able to deduce some rules of thumb about the construction of health messages that generalize beyond these specific behaviors.

MESSAGE TAILORING

Message tailoring is a procedure adopted from the social marketing arsenal. It refers to the customizing of information and interventions to best fit the relevant needs and characteristics of specified target populations or individuals (Pasick, 1997). In this tradition, health messages have been tailored to the demographic characteristics of recipients, especially sex, ethnicity, occupation, and educational background, as well as to stage in the behavior change process (for example, whether the target of the message has ever tried the advocated behavior in the past). Some tailoring interventions create enormous libraries of text messages and accompanying graphics that are matched to complex and nearly unique combinations of previously identified recipient characteristics (Rimer & Glassman, 1999). In recent literature, the term *targeting* is often used for the attempt to match messages to the characteristics of specified populations, while *tailoring* is used to describe the matching of messages to characteristics of individuals (e.g., Kreuter, Strecher, & Glassman, 1999).

Background

Tailoring health messages to individualized needs is generally thought to be a more effective communication strategy than presenting people with generic messages. A directive such as *a fifty-two-year-old, Italian American woman like yourself should obtain a mammogram every year* is thought to be more persuasive than a slogan such as *get a mammogram every year.* Tailoring has for the most part focused on three kinds of variables: personalization, demographic matching, and sensitivity to stage in the behavior change process. The most basic kind of tailoring involves personalizing by including specific identifying characteristics of the recipient of these materials such as name, birth date, residence, health history, family composition, occupation, and the like (Davis, Cummings, Rimer, Sciandra, & Stone, 1992). For personalized print materials, expert systems technology allows investigators to create libraries of text messages tailored to specific survey or interview responses that can then be merged into unique personalized print materials. We distinguish personalized tailoring, which is accomplished at the individual level, from demographic targeting, in which message content varies depending on a recipient's group membership.

Demographic targeting generally involves visual elements in which the age (Morgan et al., 1996; Rimer et al., 1994), gender (Campbell et al., 1994), and ethnic group (Skinner, Strecher, & Hospers, 1994; Yancy,

Tanjasiri, Klein, & Tunder, 1995) of depicted individuals are matched to that of recipients. It may also include themes that are expected to resonate with members of particular social groups or colloquial expressions associated with them (Barg & Lowe, 1996). Demographically targeted messages often combine several of these elements (Hubbell, Chavez, Mishra, Magana, & Veldez, 1995; Mishra et al., 1998).

A frequent target of personalized tailoring is stage of change, the readiness of an individual to adopt a particular health behavior (e.g., Prochaska & DiClemente, 1983). Messages tailored to the recipient's particular stage of change have been effective in promoting smoking cessation (Morgan et al., 1996; Prochaska, DiClemente, Velicer, & Rossi, 1993; Rimer et al., 1994), healthier diets (Campbell et al., 1994), and screening mammography (Rakowski et al., 1998; Skinner et al., 1994). Tailored messages in this tradition often focus on specific perceived benefits and barriers associated with behavior change, because these benefits and barriers vary depending on stage.

Less systematically investigated is personalized message tailoring around specific psychological (nondemographic) characteristics of individuals other than stage of change. We refer to this approach as *psychologically tailoring* messages. For example, there is some evidence that materials that take into consideration a recipient's perceived self-efficacy with respect to a behavioral domain (Brug, Steenhuis, Van Assema, & De Vries, 1996; Campbell et al., 1994), level of social support (Brug et al., 1996), and attributional style (Strecher et al., 1994) may be more effective than generic messages, but neither these nor many other psychological characteristics have been isolated systematically.

A challenge in tailoring research is the precise identification of the "active ingredient" in especially effective messages. Many of the studies cited in the previous paragraphs involve messages in which tailoring is operationalized in several different ways in the same communication. Experimental messages are tailored to several demographic characteristics, stage of change, and psychological needs simultaneously. Such messages are often effective, but it is not possible to attribute this success to a single active ingredient nor to understand the aspects of tailoring that are necessary and/or sufficient to motivate behavior change.

We believe that psychological characteristics representing core interindividual differences in the way people process health information are most important. Findings from such studies broaden the range of variables available for tailoring and suggest priorities for tailoring when practical considerations limit the amount of personalization possible. In this chapter, we summarize findings from field experiments involving the psychological tailoring of messages designed to promote screening mammography and fruit and vegetable consumption (although we expect principles derived from these experiments to generalize beyond these two health behaviors). The experiments conducted thus far have involved tailoring messages around three health information processing dimensions: (a) need for cognition (the willingness to engage in effortful thinking), (b) attribution of responsibility for health (health locus of control, that is, the belief that internal or external forces are largely responsible for health outcomes), and (c) monitoring/blunting (the motivation to seek or avoid threatening health information).

Psychological Tailoring: Dimensions

In the psychological research described here, our strategy was to measure inter-individual differences in each of these three dimensions (one per experiment). For the sake of simplicity, individuals were classified in one of two groups (e.g., high or low in need for cognition, internal or external in health locus of control, or as monitors versus blunters depending on the experiment). Then, health communication materials were designed and tailored to one or the other type of person. In any experiment, two different kinds of people could receive one of two different kinds of messages, yielding four possible combinations or experimental conditions. Before describing the results from these experiments, we review the conceptual and operational definitions of these health information processing dimensions in more detail.

Need for Cognition

Need for cognition refers to an individual's tendency to engage in and enjoy effortful cognitive activities. Although conditions can be created to encourage either enjoyment or avoidance of deep thinking in the same person, most studies of need for cognition treat this dimension as a stable aspect of the individual across time and situations. Inter-individual differences in need for cognition (especially its importance in understanding persuasion and attitude change) have now been the focus of more than 100 empirical investigations in social psychology (Cacioppo, Petty, Feinstein, & Jarvis, 1996). Individuals high in need for cognition tend to actively seek, think about, and reflect back on arguments presented to them. Individuals low in need for cognition are more likely to rely on others (often celebrities and experts), simple rules of thumb, or social comparison processes to understand information presented to them (Cacioppo & Petty, 1982). Need for cognition is typically measured using a brief 18-item scale including Likert-formatted items as, "I would prefer complex to simple problems," and "Thinking is not my idea of fun" (Cacioppo, Petty, & Kao, 1984; Cacioppo et al., 1996).

In studies of attitude change in many different domains, a picture is emerging with respect to the kinds of arguments that are most effective in persuading individuals high versus low in need for cognition. Individuals high in need for cognition are most persuaded by strong arguments about benefits that are clearly articulated and by strong counter-arguments with respect to barriers. Individuals low in need for cognition are more-or-less insensitive to the quality of arguments but pay much more attention to the source of the arguments (public figure or credible authority), the ease with which they can be processed (pictorially rather than verbally), and the number of arguments presented (Cacioppo et al., 1996).

Locus of Control and Attributions of Responsibility

Individuals differ in what they consider the primary determinant of their health: themselves, other people, or just plain luck. Once again, these inter-individual differences are thought to be more-or-less stable across situations. Over several decades, a sizable literature has developed concerning the measurement of what has been called *health locus of control* and its correlates (Wallston & Wallston, 1981, 1982). The construct has been helpful in the study of patient information-seeking, although it has been less systematically used as a predictor in persuasion research. The Multidimensional Health Locus of Control Scale (MHLC) is probably the most widely used measure of causal beliefs relevant to health (Wallston, Wallston, & DeVellis, 1978). The MHLC contains three, six-item subscales (available in three alternate forms) assessing beliefs concerning the self, powerful others, or luck as determinants of health outcomes (Robinson, Shaver, & Wrightsman, 1991).

In general, individuals who endorse internal health locus of control beliefs are more likely to seek information (e.g., pick up free pamphlets), so long as they also report that they value health (Toner & Manuck, 1979; Wallston, Maides, & Wallston, 1976). There is also some evidence that internals have more success in therapeutic interventions requiring active participation, while powerful-other externals do better in programs in which they play a more passive role (Cromwell, Butterfield, Brayfield, & Curry, 1977). It appears to be easier to persuade women with an internal health locus of control to engage in health behaviors that they can control, such as breast self-examination, but that women with a powerful-other orientation seem to gravitate toward physician-controlled screening activities like Pap testing and clinical breast examination (Bundek, Marks, & Richardson, 1993).

In some of our previous work on persuasive health messages (Rothman, Salovey, Turvey, & Fishkin, 1993), we narrowed the emphasis to internal versus external attributions of responsibility for prevention and early detection activities (Michela & Wood, 1986). In a field experiment among about 200 employees of a local telephone company, we examined how altering attributions of responsibility for maintaining one's health affected women's attitudes and behaviors regarding screening mammography. We developed three educational videotape programs about breast cancer and mammography. The three programs contained identical information. However, they varied systematically in terms of the attribution of responsibility for preventing and detecting breast cancer:

> The *internal* tape emphasized a woman's own responsibility for getting a mammogram and detecting breast cancer ("While it is not yet known how to prevent breast cancer, the value and benefits of *your* finding it early are well-known").
>
> The *external* tape emphasized the health care system's responsibility for detecting breast cancer and using mammography ("While it is not yet known how to prevent breast cancer, the value and benefits of a *doctor* finding it early are well known").
>
> The third tape served as a control condition. This *information-only* video communicated the same material about breast cancer and mammography without any particular emphasis on internal (self) or external (medical care system) responsibility ("While it is not yet known how to prevent breast cancer, the value and benefits of finding it early are well known").

The participants were assigned randomly to one of these three conditions. Twelve months after the intervention, women assigned to the internal condition were significantly more likely than women who saw the external or control videos actually to have obtained a mammogram.

Although Rothman, Salovey, Turvey, and Fishkin (1993) demonstrated that internally oriented messages were more motivating than externally oriented messages with middle-class telephone workers, in this experiment we did not attempt to match individuals to messages that reflected their prior beliefs. We suspect, however, that individuals with an internal locus of control may have been persuaded especially well by the internal message; if we could have isolated a group of women with strong beliefs about their health being controlled by powerful-others, we might have found that, at least for these individuals, external messages are persuasive (Harackiewicz, Sansone, Blair, Epstein, & Manderlink, 1987).

Monitoring/Blunting

Monitoring and blunting are personality dimensions pertinent to the processing of threatening information (Miller, Brody, & Summerton, 1988). A given individual might be motivated to seek and attend to information about his or her personal health, even when it is somewhat unsettling; in other situations, the individual might want to avoid this information altogether. In the psychological literature, monitoring and blunting generally have been considered inter-individual difference dimensions. Some individuals are thought to be more likely to seek out and monitor for threatening or stressful information, while others tend to distract themselves cognitively from it in order to blunt its psychological impact.

These inter-individual differences translate into different patterns of interest with respect to health information. High monitors generally prefer detailed and voluminous information (even if it is negative, painful, or dangerous) as well as advice and reassurance about their problems, but high blunters prefer more minimal information and appreciate opportunities to be distracted from the central message.

Monitors and blunters are identified using the Monitor-Blunter Style Scale (MBSS) containing four hypothetical stress-evoking scenes (Miller, 1987). For example, one scene describes flying on a plane, and the respondent is asked to indicate how likely he or she is to "listen carefully for unusual engine noises" and "read and reread the safety instruction booklet" versus "watch the in-flight movie even if I had seen it before." Miller (1987) reports that the MBSS has appropriate reliability and construct validity, especially for cancer-related settings and behaviors (Jacob, Penn, Kulik, & Spieth, 1992; Lerman et al., 1993).

Work on monitoring and blunting has focused on the informational preferences of these two groups of individuals. Rather consistently, monitors desire more thorough information about cancer prevention and detection behaviors (Miller & Mangan, 1983), but blunters are more satisfied with what they already know (Lerman et al., 1993; Steptoe, Sutcliffe, Allen, & Coombes, 1991). This is the case even though cancer knowledge is often quite limited among blunters. Overall, as compared with blunters, individuals with a monitoring style are more concerned and distressed about health risks, report greater treatment side effects, are more knowledgeable about their medical situation yet less satisfied with the psychosocial aspects of their care, and more adherent to medical recommendations (Miller, 1995). However, they also report more intrusive, ruminative thought about their condition (Miller, Rodoletz, Schroeder, Mangan, & Sedlacek, 1996) and are more likely to yield control to another individual who is perceived to be more competent than they are, especially in the face of danger. For example, a blunter may be more likely to let a spouse make health decisions on their own behalf.

Miller (1995) recommends that health information for blunters not be voluminous nor threat-focused, but that information for monitors should be more substantial and comprehensive, especially if it contains clear cues concerning certainty and safety and enables them to prepare emotionally for or find meaning in the situation. For monitors, the key seems to be to provide them with the information that they long to have, but to package it in a way that does not lead to anxiety, ruminative thought, and consequent denial.

PSYCHOLOGICAL TAILORING: WHAT HAVE WE FOUND SO FAR?

We have so far conducted four experiments on the psychological tailoring of health messages. All of these experiments were carried out in collaboration with the New England Cancer Information Service (CIS), a telephone information line supported by the National Cancer Institute. After their request has been addressed, callers to the CIS are assessed for their suitability to receive proactive messages about mammography screening or fruit and vegetable consumption. With very brief questionnaires administered on the telephone, their need for cognition, health locus of control, or monitoring/blunting status is assessed, depending on the experiment. They receive a telephone message matched to their information processing style or not, and then receive follow-up print materials by mail that are similarly tailored. Engagement in the promoted behavior is then assessed through follow-up telephone and mail surveys.

In the first of these experiments, 602 CIS callers who had a spotty history of obtaining mammograms responded to a few items from the Need for Cognition scale and then were assigned randomly to receive a telephone message and follow-up print materials designed for individuals high or low in need for cognition and promoting annual mammography screening. The messages for women high in need for cognition emphasized the facts and details related to cancer and mammography utilization. These messages also included statistics about breast cancer risk. The messages for women low in need for cognition were more succinct and simplistic. There were fewer details on each topic, and they featured celebrity testimonials about the importance of mammography. After six months, 39.3 percent of individuals high in need for cognition who received an appropriate message had obtained a mammogram, but only 29.1 percent of individuals high in need for cognition who had received the mismatched message did likewise. Among women low in need for cognition, both messages were equally effective. These findings provide partial support for the psychological tailoring of messages (Williams-Piehota, Schneider, Pizarro, Mowad, & Salovey, 2003). Further, women low in need for cognition found the phone messages as more educational and the pamphlets as more reassuring than those women high in need for cognition. They also felt more hopeful after reading either of the pamphlets.

We could be more confident about the importance of inter-individual differences in the need for cognition and message tailoring if the effects shown for mammography could also be demonstrated for at least one other health behavior. We attempted to replicate this experiment, but with fruit and vegetable consumption as the target behavior in both women and men (Williams-Piehota, Pizarro, Navarro, Mowad, & Salovey, in press). This time, 517 CIS callers answered the questions from the Need for Cognition scale and were assigned randomly to messages and print materials designed for high versus low need for cognition individuals. Following the intervention, all participants increased their fruit and vegetable consumption by more than one portion per day. Callers high in need for cognition who received the message and materials psychologically tailored for such individuals reported the highest fruit and vegetable consumption one and four months later. Once again, the message matching hypothesis was confirmed, but only partially, for individuals high in need for cognition but not for those who were low in need for cognition.

In another experiment involving women with irregular histories of obtaining screening mammograms, 499 callers to the CIS were provided with information tailored either to individuals with internal or external health loci of control. The information tailored for women with an internal health locus of control underscored the woman's responsibility for her health. The messages for women with external health locus of control beliefs emphasized that the responsibility for maintaining health is in a woman's partnership with her health care provider. In this case, the interaction between participant locus of control and message type was exactly as predicted, meaning that the internally oriented women did best with the internal message and the externally oriented women did best with the external message. Matched messages were more effective than mismatched messages. After six months, among internally oriented women, 50.8 percent of women who had received the materials designed for internals had obtained a mammogram, but only 34.0 percent of such women who had received materials designed for external women had obtained a mammogram. Among the externally oriented women, 41.7 percent who had received materials designed for externals obtained a mammogram, but only 34.9 percent of such women obtained a mammogram if they had received materials designed for internals. These findings held after 12 months as well. Among internally oriented women, 75.9 percent obtained a mammogram when the message matched their orientation, but 60.4 percent obtained a mammogram when the message was mismatched; among externally oriented women, 69.5 percent obtained a mammogram in the matched condition, but only 58.7 percent in the mismatched condition (Williams-Piehota, Schneider, Pizarro, Mowad, & Salovey, under review).

Finally, our most recent experiment on encouraging mammography among CIS callers involved messages and print materials designed for monitors and blunters (Williams-Piehota, Pizarro, Schneider, Mowad, & Salovey, in press). The information for monitors emphasized the evidence and details related to cancer and mammography utilization, including the risk factors for and symptoms of breast cancer and explanations of mammography and early detection. It contained additional statistics related to mammography use and breast cancer. It also included reassuring statements to address the anxiety that is characteristic of monitors. The information for blunters was short and to the point. Nonthreatening, basic information was presented in an outline format and incorporated the use of bold fonts to emphasize key points. We obtained the predicted interaction between participants' monitor/blunter information processing style and the type of materials they received. Among monitors, 43.6 percent who received the monitor message obtained a mammogram after six months, but 37.9 percent did so if they received the message designed for blunters. Among blunters, 48.8 percent obtained a mammogram if they received the blunter materials, but 29.2 percent did so if they received the materials designed for monitors. We are waiting to see if these findings hold after twelve months.

MECHANISMS UNDERLYING THE ADVANTAGE OF PSYCHOLOGICALLY TAILORED MESSAGES

A theoretical orientation known as the social intelligence view of personality (Cantor & Kihlstrom, 1987) guided our selection of dispositional characteristics around which messages could be psychologically tailored. The social intelligence theory of personality argues that differences in information processing styles and competencies are what distinguish individuals from each other more than static personality traits. This approach to individual differences has had enormous impact in the field of personality psychology and has also served as the basis for models of health behavior change. For example, Miller, Shoda, and Hurley's (1996) application of cognitive-social theory to breast cancer screening behaviors fits squarely in this tradition. This theoretical framework focused our attention on variables that differentiate people with respect to how they process new incoming information. We selected for study those variables of this type that appeared most promising for understanding the impact of health information.

Moreover, we believe that the specific mechanism by which psychologically tailored messages exert their especially persuasive impact is by encouraging message scrutiny and central processing. The theoretical framework that integrates work on psychological tailoring with respect to underlying mechanism is the Elaboration Likelihood Model (ELM) of persuasion and attitude change (Petty & Cacioppo, 1986). The ELM distinguishes two ways a person might come to hold and act upon an attitude. The *central* route to persuasion involves carefully thinking about and examining information pertinent to the merits of the topic. The *peripheral* route to persuasion involves reliance on relatively simple cues, such as whether the source of the message seems credible or attractive. Attitudes established through central processes are more persistent and stable over time, more resistant to challenge from competing messages, and more motivating of subsequent behavior because they encourage elaboration, and thinking about new ideas beyond those presented in the message itself (Petty & Wegener, 1991; Petty, Priester, & Wegener, 1994). Attitudes formed by the peripheral route are less persistent, resistant, or tied to behavior because they result from attention to simple cues rather than consideration of substantive arguments. The ELM can be considered an intra-individual model, as the same individual can hold attitudes formed by both the central and peripheral routes. It can also be placed in an inter-individual context; individuals high in need for cognition may chronically form attitudes using central mechanisms more so the peripheral mechanisms (but the reverse is true for individuals low in need for cognition).

The goal of the psychological tailoring experiments was to explore whether providing messages that are matched to the recipient's health information processing style increase the strength of subsequent attitudes by encouraging central rather than peripheral processing. According to the ELM, as the personal relevance of messages increases, they are more likely to be processed centrally (Petty & Cacioppo, 1990). Tailoring messages to health information processing style was expected to increase their personal relevance and thus their likelihood of being centrally processed by all persons.

Message Framing

Our second line of research on the creation of health-promotion messages focuses on their framing in terms of costs or benefits. Framing thus concerns the way in which messages encourage different kinds of representations of risky or probabilistic information. In this context, message framing refers to the emphasis in the message on the positive or negative consequences of adopting or failing to adopt a particular behavior (Rothman & Salovey, 1997). These frames can change recipients' perceptions of risk and feelings about different outcomes, and could be considered psychological risk escalators, analogous to the kinds of risk escalators discussed in Heyman's chapter in this volume.

Gain-framed messages usually present the benefits that are accrued through adopting a behavior (e.g., "eating more fruits and vegetables can keep you healthy"). *Loss-framed* messages generally convey the costs of not adopting the requested behavior (e.g., "not eating fruits and vegetables can lead to illness"). Although these two rather bland messages convey essentially the same information about fruit and vegetable consumption, one of them might be more persuasive than the other one.

Background

Any discussion of message framing must begin with Prospect Theory, the primary framework for understanding preference and decision making under conditions of uncertainty (Kahneman & Tversky, 1979, 1982; Tversky & Kahneman, 1981). Prospect Theory suggests that decision makers represent information relevant to choice options in terms of potential gains (i.e., benefits) or potential losses (i.e., costs) as compared to a reference point (e.g., one's present level of health). Factually equivalent material can be presented to individuals such that they encode it as either a gain or a loss. Prospect Theory characterizes a set of preferences or decision strategies by noting that individuals are, in general, risk-seeking when losses are salient but risk-averse when gains are salient. Prospect Theory assumes that an S-shaped function relates objective outcomes to their subjective values and that the function is concave for gains and convex for losses and steeper in the loss domain. This function suggests that, when behavioral choices involve risk or uncertainty, individuals will be more likely to assume these risks when the downside of a situation is made salient. Alternatively, when behavioral choices involve little risk or uncertainty, individuals are more likely to prefer these options when the upside of a situation is made salient (Rothman & Salovey, 1997; Wilson, Purdon, & Wallston, 1988).

Although loss-framing has been especially effective when promoting breast self-examination (Meyerowitz & Chaiken, 1987), HIV screening (Kalichman & Coley, 1995), and mammography utilization (Banks et al., 1995; Schneider, Salovey, Apanovitch, et al., 2001), gain-framed messages have encouraged preferences for certain surgical procedures (Levin, Schnittjer, & Thee, 1988, Experiment 2; Marteau, 1989; McNeil, Pauker, Sox, & Tversky, 1982; Wilson, Kaplan, & Schneiderman, 1987), the use of infant car restraints (Christophersen & Gyulay, 1981; Treiber, 1986), regular physical exercise (Robberson & Rogers, 1988), and sunscreen utilization (Detweiler, Bedell, Salovey, Pronin, & Rothman, 1999; Rothman, Salovey, Antone, Keough, & Martin, 1993).

From a Prospect Theory point of view, the perceived risk (of finding an abnormality) could make loss-framed messages more persuasive in promoting detection behaviors. However, prevention behaviors may not be perceived as risky at all; they are performed to deter the onset or occurrence of a health problem. Choosing to perform prevention behaviors is a risk-averse option. Because risk-averse options are preferred when people are considering benefits or gains, gain-framed messages might be more likely to facilitate performing prevention behaviors. Therefore, we tested whether the match between a message frame (gain or loss) and the function of the required health behavior (prevention or detection) effectively motivates behavior change. That is, are gain-framed messages more persuasive when promoting prevention behaviors, but loss-framed messages more persuasive when promoting early detection (screening) behaviors.

Loss-Framed Messages Promote Detection Behaviors

Most women pursue screening believing that they are healthy. Obtaining a mammogram, then, is a psychologically risky behavior. Because mammography involves a probabilistic, uncertain outcome, it should be better motivated by loss-framed messages than gain-framed messages.

Our first field experiment focused on mammography screening was conducted as part of a workplace health-promotion program at a large telephone company (Banks et al., 1995). Any woman who had obtained fewer than 50 percent of the mammograms that she should have for someone of her age was invited to view a 15-minute videotape on breast cancer and mammography. One-hundred thirty-three women were assigned randomly to view a video during their lunch hour in which most of the information was presented either in gain-framed terms (titled "The Benefits of Mammography") or in loss-framed terms (titled "The Risks of Neglecting Mammography").

Women who viewed the gain- or loss-framed video did not differ in their liking for the video or knowledge about breast cancer. However, after twelve months, it was clear that the loss-framed video had been more persuasive: 66.2 percent of the women had obtained a mammogram compared to 51.5 percent of the women who had viewed the gain-framed video, and this difference was significant in a logistic regression analysis controlling for mammography behavior at baseline.

Some years later, we replicated this experiment in a different population of women (Schneider, Salovey, Apanovitch et al., 2001). We recruited 752 women from two inner-city health clinics and several public housing developments in the same neighborhoods. About 43 percent were African American, 27 percent white, and 25 percent Latina. Most of the participants were from low-income families. These women viewed a 15-minute video about breast cancer and mammography that was gain- or loss-framed. We produced different pairs of framed videos; one pair emphasized the problem of breast cancer for all women, black, white, or Latina. The other videos were targeted especially for either black, white, or Latina women and provided statistics and pictured models drawn only from those groups. We labeled these pairs of videos multicultural versus targeted. The videos for Latina women could be viewed with either an English or Spanish soundtrack.

When measured six months later, the advantage for loss- over gain-framed messages seen in the telephone company study (Banks et al., 1995) was replicated. With the multicultural messages, 50 percent of the women who viewed the loss-framed message received a mammogram compared to only 36 percent in the gain-framed version. However, there were no differences due to framing when the messages were targeted to the specific ethnicity of the participants, and neither version of the targeted video was as effective as the loss-framed, multicultural one. After twelve months, the pattern of findings was the same, but the effect size had attenuated. Perhaps loss-framed messages that are explicitly targeted to a particular ethnic group elicit some defensiveness that counteracted their expected effectiveness.

Taken together, loss-framed videos designed to promote screening mammography are more effective than gain-framed videos provided they are designed for a multicultural audience rather than specifically targeted for one ethnic group. These findings are consistent with the Prospect Theory prediction that risk (uncertainty) should be preferred over certainty when losses are made salient. Choosing to obtain a mammogram is a behavior with an uncertain outcome.

Gain-Framed Messages Promote Prevention Behavior

In comparison to early detection behaviors such as screening mammography, the use of sunscreen at the beach involves few uncertainties and little psychological risk. Using sunscreen is a low-cost way of reducing skin cancer. Prospect Theory suggests that individuals should prefer options with certain outcomes after considering potential gains, when the advantages of the option are made salient.

We have conducted several experiments involving the manipulation of framed messages and the acquisition of sunscreen, some among college students and others with more diverse samples on public beaches. In one study, 146 undergraduates read gain- or loss-framed pamphlets about skin cancer and sunscreen use (Rothman, Salovey, Antone et al., 1993, Experiment 2). After reading the pamphlets, participants were given postage-paid postcards that they could mail to our laboratory requesting sunscreen samples and more information about skin cancer prevention. Interest in the pamphlet was high and did not differ across the two framing conditions. As Prospect Theory led us to predict, the gain-framed pamphlet motivated more requests for sunscreen. The advantage of gain-framed messages over loss-framed ones was small for the men in the study, but sizable for the women: 79 percent of the women who read a gain-framed pamphlet subsequently requested sunscreen, as compared to 45 percent who read the loss-framed pamphlet. For men, request rates were 50 percent and 47 percent, respectively.

For people sunbathing on the beach, however, skin cancer might be a relatively more involving topic for both men and women. In one experiment, we recruited 217 sunbathers to read either gain- or loss-framed brochures about sunscreen and the prevention of skin cancer. After reading the brochure, they were given a coupon that could be exchanged for a free bottle of sunscreen. When the sunscreen "vender" appeared on the beach, we could observe those who actually turned in their coupons. Seventy-one percent of the participants who read a gain-framed pamphlet subsequently requested sunscreen, but only 53 percent of those who read a loss-framed pamphlet did likewise. This difference remained reliable for both women and men, even when prior intentions to use sunscreen that day were statistically controlled in a logistic regression analysis (Detweiler et al., 1999).

Unlike our experiments targeting mammography, in which an early detection behavior was best promoted using loss-framed messages, the sunscreen experiments suggest that prevention behaviors might be best promoted with gain-framed messages. This was exactly the pattern of effects predicted based on the notions gleaned from Prospect Theory, but this pattern was only obtained across very different experiments targeting very different behaviors. More convincing data require observing both the loss-frame and gain-frame advantages within the same study when participants are randomly assigned to conditions.

Behaviors That Can Be Described as Either Detection or Prevention

Ideally, we would like to show that when a health behavior is described as serving a prevention function, gain-framed messages are more effective than loss-framed messages. But when the same action is described as an early detection or screening behavior, loss-framed messages should be more effective. We have conducted this type of two-way, factorial experiment to encourage, in one instance, the use of mouth rinse and, in the other, annual Pap testing.

Mouth Rinse

In the experiment promoting mouthwash, we described a product to 120 University of Minnesota undergraduates (Rothman, Martino, Bedell, Detweiler, & Salovey, 1999, Experiment 2). Half of these students heard about a typical mouthwash that removes plaque from teeth and prevents tooth decay and gum disease. The other half heard about a slightly more unusual mouthwash that detects the buildup of plaque by leaving red discoloration on teeth where better brushing is needed. As usual, arguments in favor of either the prevention mouthwash or the disclosing mouthwash were framed in gain or loss terms, and participants were assigned randomly to receive one set or the other. Once again, ratings of the quality of the pamphlet were unaffected by either the behavior type or framing manipulations, although participants reported having more positive affective reactions to the gain-framed pamphlet.

Participants were asked about their intentions to buy the mouthwash in the next week. As predicted, intentions to purchase the product were strongest when the preventive mouthwash was described in terms of benefits of using the mouthwash (gain-frame) and when the disclosing (detection) mouthwash was described in terms of costs of not using the mouthwash (loss-frame). For the prevention mouthwash, 67 percent of the participants planned to purchase it after reading the grain-framed pamphlet, but only 47 percent planned to purchase it after reading the loss-framed pamphlet. In the detection condition, 73 percent of the participants said they would buy the disclosing mouthwash after reading the loss-framed pamphlet, but only 37 percent of them said they would purchase it after reading the gain-framed pamphlet.

Pap Tests

Pap testing is generally thought of as a behavior designed to detect cervical cancer. However, Pap tests can be described in two different ways, emphasizing either their precancer detection function or their preventive function. For example, health communicators can emphasize the prevention of cervical cancer through the detection of precancerous abnormalities. We developed four different videotape programs about the benefits of Pap testing. These included gain- and loss-framed versions of a program emphasizing the early detection of cervical cancer and gain- and loss-framed versions of a program emphasizing the prevention of cervical cancer through the detection of precancerous lesions that could be treated (Rivers, Pizarro, Schneider, Pizarro, & Salovey, in press). Although this latter message is not exclusively focused on prevention, it includes more information about cancer prevention than the more typical Pap test-promoting communications.

We showed one of these four videos to 497 women over age 18 attending a community health clinic. Most of these women were from relatively poor families; 59 percent were African American, 26 percent were Latina, and 12 percent were White. Six months later, rates of Pap testing were highest in the prevention-gain and detection-loss conditions. In a logistic regression analysis that included baseline behavior, the main effects for behavior type (prevention/detection) and message framing (gain/loss), the behavior type by message framing interaction just about reached conventional levels of significance.

BEHAVIORS THAT CAN BE CONSTRUED IN DIFFERENT WAYS

Prevention and early detection behaviors differ in terms of the risk or uncertainty typically associated with them. Prevention behaviors are usually construed as safe, risk-averse choices. The decision to initiate a detection behavior often involves uncertainty and risk, as one generally does not know the outcome in advance. Being tested for HIV would seem to be a typical detection behavior with attendant psychological risks and uncertainty and thus should be better motivated by loss-framed messages. However, because HIV is tied to behavior, some individuals might reasonably believe that they are not at risk for HIV, based on their past behavior. For these individuals, HIV testing is a psychologically safe behavior; the behavior has a relatively certain outcome. Therefore, these individuals might be more persuaded by gain-framed messages.

We recently completed a field experiment in which we tested whether individuals who differed in their views of HIV testing in this way would likewise differ in the framed message that would be most effective in motivating them to obtain an HIV test (Apanovitch, McCarthy, & Salovey, 2003). We examined whether gain- or loss-framed messages were more effective in encouraging women living in public housing or attending a community health center to obtain an HIV test (Apanovitch et al., 2003). We expected women who viewed HIV testing as a risky behavior with uncertain outcomes to be more persuaded by a loss-framed message whereas women who viewed HIV testing as a safe behavior with certain outcomes would be more persuaded by gain-framed messages.

All participants were women from a low-income neighborhood of New Haven, Connecticut, either living in one of four public housing developments or attending a community health center. Of the 480 participants included in our analysis, most were either African American or Latina. We developed four videotaped educational programs, identical in informational content but framed differently. Two types of gain-framed and two types of loss-framed videotapes promoting HIV testing were created (Detweiler et al., 1999; Rothman & Salovey, 1997). There were no differences across the two types of gain-framed or loss-framed videos, so they were combined in all subsequent analyses.

At six months, the findings generally conformed to the pattern previously discussed. There was a significant gain-frame advantage among women who viewed HIV testing as a behavior with a certain outcome, such that 38 percent of those who saw a gain-framed video were tested compared to 26 percent who saw a loss-framed video. Participants who viewed HIV testing as a risky behavior with uncertain outcomes showed a trend in the other direction, toward loss-framed messages being more persuasive. Forty percent of participants who saw a gain-framed video were tested compared with 47 percent who saw a loss-framed video. In a logistic regression analysis controlling for prior behavior, this interaction term was significant. (Analyses at three months revealed a marginally significant interaction term; analyses after nine months showed that the messages were no longer differentially effective.) Given the number of unmeasured influences on decisions to be tested for HIV, we consider these findings fairly robust, although they do indicate that brief, message-based interventions can wear off.

HIV, compared to breast cancer, seems to be a unique disease in that individuals have a greater chance of surmising their HIV status without testing, based on their behavioral history. Inter-individual differences in perceptions of the riskiness of being tested for HIV naturally follow, with those engaging in high-risk behavior having more uncertainty as to their HIV status and test outcome and those not engaging in high-risk behavior perceiving the test as an opportunity to confirm their present health status. Loss-framed messages appear more persuasive to the former group of individuals, while gain-framed messages are more effective for the latter group.

CONCLUSION

The research we have been conducting for the last ten years on the psychological tailoring and framing of health messages has demonstrated the importance of matching messages to health information processing styles and of framing messages in accord with the certainty or uncertainty associated with the targeted behavior. The findings in both domains appear robust across different kinds of health behaviors and in different populations. The magnitude of these differences is not only statistically significant in most cases but also represents an increase in desired health behaviors that would have public health impact.

We are less sanguine, however, about the strides we have made in attempting to understand the underlying mechanisms to account for these effects. Nearly all of our experiments were conducted in the field rather than the laboratory, and that provides some confidence that these principles generalize in ecologically complex contexts with truly vulnerable individuals. At the same time, the field does not provide the kind of environment usually needed for the careful scrutiny of mediating variables. Future research will be required to gain a better understanding of the nature of health and illness representations, their alteration in response to framed and tailored messages, and the associations between these cognition changes and health behavior. Moreover, theoretical advances in future work may lead to integrative conceptual views of the determinants of health behavior that move us beyond Prospect Theory or the Elaboration Likelihood Model as ways of understanding the representation of uncertainty and the persuasiveness of health messages.

ACKNOWLEDGMENTS

We thank the graduate students, undergraduates, and, especially, the research staff associated with the Health, Emotion, and Behavior (HEB) Laboratory in the Department of Psychology at Yale University who were instrumental in conducting much of the research reported here. Experiments on the framing of messages about behaviors relevant to the prevention or early detection of HIV and AIDS were conducted under the auspices of the Center for Interdisciplinary Research on AIDS (CIRA) at Yale University.

The research on the framing and tailoring of health messages reported in this chapter was supported by grants to Peter Salovey from the American Cancer Society (RPG-93-028-05-PBP), the National Cancer Institute (R01-CA68427), the National Institute of Mental Health (P01-MH/DA56826), the National Institute of Drug Abuse (P50-DA13334), and the Donaghue Women's Health Investigator Program at Yale University. Some of these experiments have also been described in Salovey and Wegener (in press).

Correspondence concerning this article should be addressed to Peter Salovey, Department of Psychology, Yale University, P.O. Box 208205, New Haven, Connecticut 06520-8205. Electronic mail may be sent to *peter.salovey@yale.edu.*

REFERENCES

Apanovitch, A. M., McCarthy, D., & Salovey, P. (2003). Using message framing to motivate HIV testing among low-income, ethnic minority women. *Health Psychology, 22,* 60–67.

Banks, S. M., Salovey, P., Greener, S., Rothman, A. J., Moyer, A., Beauvais, J., et al. (1995). The effects of message framing on mammography utilization. *Health Psychology, 14,* 178–184.

Barg, F., & Lowe, J. (1996). A culturally appropriate cancer education program for African-American adolescents in an urban middle school. *Journal of School Health, 66,* 50–54.

Brug, J., Steenhuis, I., van Assema, P., & de Vries, H. (1996). The impact of a computer-tailored nutrition intervention. *Preventive Medicine, 25,* 236–242.

Bundek, N. I., Marks, G., & Richardson, J. L. (1993). Role of health locus of control beliefs in cancer screening of elderly Hispanic women. *Health Psychology, 12,* 193–199.

Cacioppo, J. T., & Petty, R. E. (1982). The need for cognition. *Journal of Personality and Social Psychology, 42,* 116–131.

Cacioppo, J. T., Petty, R. E., Feinstein, J. A., & Jarvis, W. B. G. (1996). Dispositional differences in cognitive motivation: The life and times of individuals varying in need for cognition. *Psychological Bulletin, 119,* 197–253.

Cacioppo, J. T., Petty, R. E., & Kao, C. F. (1984). The efficient assessment of need for cognition. *Journal of Personality Assessment, 48,* 306–307.

Campbell, M. K., DeVellis, B. M., Strecher, V. J., Ammerman, A. S., DeVellis, R. F., & Sandler, R.S. (1994). Improving dietary behavior: The effectiveness of tailored messages in primary care settings. *American Journal of Public Health, 84,* 783–787.

Cantor, N., & Kihlstrom, J. F. (1987). *Personality and social intelligence.* Englewood Cliffs, NJ: Prentice-Hall.

Christophersen, E. R., & Gyulay, J. E. (1981). Parental compliance with car seat usage: A positive approach with long term follow-up. *Journal of Pediatric Psychology, 6,* 301–312.

Cromwell, R. L., Butterfield, D.C., Brayfield, F. M., & Curry, J. J. (1977). *Acute myocardial infarction: Reaction and recovery.* St. Louis, MO: Mosby.

Davis, S. W., Cummings, K. M., Rimer, B. K., Sciandra, R., & Stone, J. C. (1992). The impact of tailored self-help smoking cessation guides on young mothers. *Health Education Quarterly, 19,* 495–504.

Detweiler, J. B., Bedell, B. T., Salovey, P., Pronin, E., & Rothman, A. J. (1999). Message framing and sunscreen use: Gain-framed messages motivate beach-goers. *Health Psychology, 18,* 189–196.

Harackiewicz, J. M., Sansone, C., Blair, L. W., Epstein, J. A., & Manderlink, G. (1987). Attributional processes in behavior change and maintenance:

Smoking cessation and continued abstinence. *Journal of Consulting and Clinical Psychology, 55,* 372–378.

Hubbell, F. A., Chavez, L. R., Mishra, S. I., Magana, J. R., & Valdez, R. B. (1995). From ethnography to intervention: Developing a breast cancer control program for Latinas. *Journal of the National Cancer Institute Monographs, 18,* 109–115.

Jacob, T. C., Penn, N. E., Kulik, T. A., & Spieth, L. E. (1992). Effects of cognitive style and maintenance strategies on breast self-examination (BSE) practices by African American women. *Journal of Behavioral Medicine, 15,* 586–609.

Kahneman, D., & Tversky, A. (1979). Prospect theory: An analysis of decision under risk. *Econometrica, 47,* 263–292.

Kahneman, D., & Tversky, A. (1982). The psychology of preferences. *Scientific American, 247,* 160–173.

Kalichman, S. C., & Coley, B. (1995). Context framing to enhance HIV-antibody-testing messages targeted to African American women. *Health Psychology, 14,* 247–254.

Kreuter, M. W., Strecher, V. J., & Glassman, B. (1999). One size does not fit all: The case for tailoring print materials. *Annals of Behavioral Medicine, 21,* 276–283.

Lerman, C., Daly, M., Walsh, W., Resch, N., Seay, J., Barsevick, A., et al. (1993). Communication between patients with breast cancer and health care providers: Determinants and implications. *Cancer, 72,* 2612–2620.

Levin, I. P., Schnittjer, S. K., & Thee, S. L. (1988). Information framing effects in social and personal decisions. *Journal of Experimental Social Psychology, 24,* 520–529.

Marteau, T. M. (1989). Framing of information: Its influence upon decisions of doctors and patients. *British Journal of Social Psychology, 28,* 89–94.

McNeil, B. J., Pauker, S. G., Sox, H. C., & Tversky, A. (1982). On the elicitation of preferences for alternative therapies. *New England Journal of Medicine, 306,* 1259–1262.

Meyerowitz, B. E., & Chaiken, S. (1987). The effect of message framing on breast self-examination attitudes, intentions, and behavior. *Journal of Personality and Social Psychology, 52,* 500–510.

Michela, J. L. & Wood, J. V. (1986). Causal attributions in health and illness. In P. H. Kendall (Ed.), *Advances in cognitive-behavioral research and therapy* (Vol. 5, pp. 179–235). San Diego, CA: Academic Press.

Miller, S. M. (1987). Monitoring and blunting: Validation of a questionnaire to assess styles of information-seeking under threat. *Journal of Personality and Social Psychology, 52,* 345–353.

Miller, S. M. (1995). Monitoring versus blunting styles of coping with cancer influence the information patients want and need about their disease. *Cancer, 76,* 167–177.

Miller, S. M., Brody, D. S., & Summerton, J. (1988). Styles of coping with threat: Implications for health. *Journal of Personality and Social Psychology, 54,* 142–148.

Miller, S. M., & Mangan, C. E. (1983). Interacting effects of information and coping style in adapting to gynecologic stress: Should the doctor tell all? *Journal of Personality and Social Psychology, 45,* 223–236.

Miller, S. M., Rodoletz, M., Schroeder, C. M., Mangan, C. E., & Sedlacek, T. V. (1996). Applications of the monitoring process model to coping with severe long-term medical threats. *Health Psychology, 15,* 216–225.

Miller, S. M., Shoda, Y., & Hurley, K. (1996). Applying cognitive-social theory to health-protective behavior: Breast self-examination in cancer screening. *Psychological Bulletin, 119,* 70–94.

Mishra, S. I., Chavez, L. R., Magana, J. R., Nava, P., Valdez, R. B., & Hubbell, F. A. (1998). Improving breast cancer control among Latinas: Evaluation of a theory-based educational program. *Health Education and Behavior, 25,* 653–670.

Morgan, G. D., Noll, E. L., Orleans, C. T., Rimer, B. K., Amfoh, K., & Bonney, G. (1996). Reaching midlife and older smokers: Tailored interventions for routine medical care. *Preventive Medicine, 25,* 346–354.

Pasick, R. J. (1997). Socioeconomic and cultural factors in the development and use of theory. In K. Glanz, F. M. Lewis, & B. K. Rimer (Eds.), *Health behavior and health education: Theory, research, and practice* (pp. 425–440). San Francisco: Jossey-Bass.

Petty, R. E., & Cacioppo, J. T. (1986). The elaboration likelihood model of persuasion. In L. Berkowitz (Ed.), *Advances in experimental social psychology, Vol. 19* (pp. 123–205). New York: Academic Press.

Petty, R. E., & Cacioppo, J. T. (1990). Involvement and persuasion: Tradition versus integration. *Psychological Bulletin, 107,* 367–374.

Petty, R. E., Priester, J. R, & Wegener, D. T. (1994). Cognitive processes in attitude change. In R. S. Wyer & T. K. Srull (Eds), *Handbook of social cognition* (2nd ed., Vol. 2., pp. 69–142). Hillsdale, NJ: Erlbaum.

Petty, R. E., & Wegener, D. (1991). Thought systems, argument quality, and persuasion. In R. S. Wyer & T. K. Srull (Eds.), *Advances in social cognition: Vol. 4* (pp. 147–161). Hillsdale, NJ: Erlbaum.

Prochaska, J. O., & DiClemente, C. C. (1983). Stages and processes of self-change and smoking: Toward an integrative model of change. *Journal of Consulting and Clinical Psychology, 51,* 390–395.

Prochaska, J. O., DiClemente, C. C., Velicer, W. F., & Rossi, J. S. (1993). Standardized, individualized, interactive, and personalized self-help programs for smoking cessation. *Health Psychology, 12,* 399–405.

Rakowski, W., Ehrich, B., Goldstein, M. G., Rimer, B. K., Pearlman, D. N., Clark, M. A., et al. (1998). Increasing mammography among women aged 40–74 by use of a stage-matched, tailored intervention. *Preventive Medicine, 27,* 748–756.

Rimer, B. K., & Glassman, B. (1999). Is there a use for tailored print communications (TPC) in cancer risk communication (CRC)? *Journal of the National Cancer Institute, 25,* 140–148.

Rimer, B. K., Orleans, C. T., Fleisher, L., Cristinzio, S., Resch, N., Telepchak, J., et al. (1994). Does tailoring matter? The impact of a tailored guide on ratings and short-term smoking-related outcomes for older smokers. *Health Education Research, 9,* 69–84.

Rivers, S. E., Pizarro, D. A., Schneider, T. R., Pizarro, J., & Salovey. P. (in press). Message framing and pap test utilization among women attending a community health clinic. *Journal of Health Psychology.*

Robberson, M. R., & Rogers, R. W. (1988). Beyond fear appeals: Negative and positive persuasive appeals to health and self-esteem. *Journal of Applied Social Psychology, 13,* 277–287.

Rothman, A. J., Martino, S. C., Bedell, B. T., Detweiler, J. B., & Salovey, P. (1999). The systematic influence of gain- and loss-framed messages on interest in and use of different types of health behavior. *Personality and Social Psychology Bulletin, 25,* 1355–1369.

Rothman, A. J., & Salovey, P. (1997). Shaping perceptions to motivate healthy behavior: The role of message framing. *Psychological Bulletin, 121,* 3–19.

Rothman, A. J., Salovey, P., Antone, C., Keough, K., & Martin, C. (1993). The influence of message framing on health behavior. *Journal of Experimental Social Psychology, 29,* 408–433.

Rothman, A. J., Salovey, P., Turvey, C., & Fishkin, S. A. (1993). Attributions of responsibility and persuasion: Increasing mammography utilization among women over 40 with an internally oriented message. *Health Psychology, 12,* 39–47.

Salovey, P., & Wegener, D. T. (in press). Communicating about health: Message framing, persuasion, and health behavior. In J. Suls & K. Wallston (Eds.), *Social psychological foundations of health and illness.* Oxford, England: Blackwell.

Schneider, T. R., Salovey, P., Apanovitch, A. M., Pizarro, J., McCarthy, D., Zullo, J., et al. (2001). The effects of message framing and ethnic targeting on mammography use among low-income women. *Health Psychology, 20,* 256–266.

Skinner, C. S., Strecher, V. J., Hospers, H. (1994). Physicians' recommendations for mammography: Do tailored messages make a difference? *American Journal of Public Health, 84,* 43–49.

Steptoe, A., Sutcliffe, I., Allen, B., & Coombes, C. (1991). Satisfaction with communication, medical knowledge, and coping style in patients with metastatic cancer. *Social Science and Medicine, 32,* 627–632.

Stretcher, V. J., Kreuter, M., Den Boer, D. J., Kobrin, S., Hospers, H. J., Skinner, C. S. (1994). The effects of computer-tailored smoking cessation messages in family practice settings. *Journal of Family Practice, 39,* 262–270.

Toner, J. B., & Manuck, S. B. (1979). Health locus of control and health-related information seeking at a hypertension screening. *Social Science and Medicine, 13,* 823.

Treiber, F. A. (1986). A comparison of positive and negative consequences approaches upon car restraint usage. *Journal of Pediatric Psychology, 11,* 15–24.

Tversky, A., & Kahneman, D. (1981). The framing of decisions and the psychology of choice. *Science, 211,* 453–458.

Wallston, K. A., Maides, S., & Wallston, B. S. (1976). Health-related information seeking as a function of health related locus of control and health value. *Journal of Research in Personality, 10,* 215–222.

Wallston, K. A., & Wallston, B. S. (1981). Health locus of control scales. In H. M. Lefcourt (Ed.), *Research with the locus of control construct: Vol. 1* (pp. 189–243). New York: Academic Press.

Wallston, K. A., & Wallston, B. S. (1982). Who is responsible for your health? The construct of health locus of control. In G. Sanders & J. Suls (Eds.), *Social psychology of health and illness* (pp. 189–243). Hillsdale, NJ: Erlbaum.

Wallston, K. A., Wallston, B. S., & DeVellis, R. (1978). Development of the Multidimensional Health Locus of Control Scales. *Health Education Monographs, 6,* 161–170.

Williams-Piehota, P., Pizarro, J., Navarro, S., Mowad, L., & Salovey, P. (under review). The impact of messages tailored to need for cognition on increasing fruit and vegetable intake among callers to the cancer information service. *Health Communication.*

Williams-Piehota, P., Schneider, T. R., Pizarro, J., Mowad, L., & Salovey, P. (2003). Matching health messages to information processing styles: Need for cognition and mammography utilization. *Health Communication, 15,* 375–392.

Williams-Piehota, P., Schneider, T. R., Pizarro, J., Mowad, L., & Salovey, P. (2004). Matching health messages to health locus of control beliefs for promoting mammography utilization. *Psychology and Health, 19,* 407–423.

Williams-Piehota, P., Pizarro, J., Schneider, T. R., Mowad, L., & Salovey, P. (in press). Matching health messages to monitor–blunter coping styles to motivate screening mammography. *Health Psychology.*

Wilson, D. K., Kaplan, R. M., & Schneiderman, L. (1987). Framing of decisions and selections of alternatives in health care. *Social Behavior, 2,* 51–59.

Wilson, D. K., Purdon S. E., & Wallston, K. A. (1988). Compliance to health recommendations: A theoretical overview of message framing. *Health Education Research: Theory and Practice, 3,* 161–171.

Yancy, A., Tanjasiri, S., Klein, M., & Tunder, J. (1995). Increased cancer screening behavior in women of color by culturally sensitive video exposure. *Preventive Medicine, 24,* 142–148.

EDITORIAL COMMENTARY

No one would be surprised to hear that messages are more persuasive if they are tailored to the nature of the audience and the audience's perceptions of the desired behaviors. But the elegant, powerful demonstrations in this paper exceed anyone's expectations. Across many kinds of health-promoting behaviors, including mammography, sunscreen use, HIV testing, and healthy diet, Salovey has shown the impact of sophisticated, research-based message design on real-world actions. These studies converge from many directions on the conclusion that public health messages can be significantly more effective than they have been. Indeed, the size of the effects reported here suggest that widespread implementation of the message principles would contribute substantially to the health of the nation.

In this book we have seen a wide variety of methods that often seem to align along a single dimension, anchored at one end by conventional psychological laboratory designs and at the other by real-world confrontation with necessarily limited but obviously important samples. Salovey's research represents some kind of middle ground, or perhaps defines a new dimension, since all of his data come from the real world, but his techniques are consistently (and cleverly) experimental.

—Jim Laird

Chapter 3

HEALTH CARE RISK ESCALATORS

Bob Heyman

Give your evidence, and don't be nervous, or I'll have you executed
on the spot.

Lewis Carroll, *Alice's Adventures in Wonderland*

In or around 1993, the present author was discussing some findings from
a qualitative study of day centers for adults with intellectual disabilities
(Heyman & Huckle, 1993, 1995) with a colleague who was supervising
a similar study of sheltered accommodation for older people (Davison
& Reed, 1995). Heyman and Huckle had noticed that parents sometimes
resisted pressure, as they saw it, from day center managers to move their
son or daughter on into a more challenging environment on the grounds
that, if anything went wrong, their child would not be able to return to
the day center for which there was a waiting list.

> I wouldn't want him to get a job and then find that he didn't like it,
> because he couldn't get his place back at the center straight away. It took
> us a year to get [name] a place here in the first place. (Family caregiver,
> interview)

Jan Reed immediately drew a parallel with the situation of older people considering a move to sheltered housing. Because of the shortage of
sheltered housing, older people would often plan their futures proactively, applying for and taking up a place while they could still manage

fully independent living. This proactive strategy made sense in terms of a trajectory of functional decline by removing the risk that they would find themselves trapped in independent living but unable to cope. However, having given up their homes, older people who moved to sheltered accommodation would find it very difficult to return to the wider community, while further moves toward even more institutionalized care became more likely as a result of the disruption caused by the initial move and the ensuing premature increase in dependency.

A number of comparisons between these two observations about health care systems can be made. Each involved the management of uncertainty, respectively, the risk that an adult with intellectual disabilities would not be able to cope with a more demanding environment and that an older person would not be able to continue to cope independently. Both were affected by an internal dynamic, propelling service users further than they might have anticipated, and fueled, in these cases, by resource shortages. At the organizational level, this metaphorical fuel was unintendedly self-enhancing because the shortage management tactics of individuals would increase the pressure on resources and, therefore, the need to obtain them proactively.

In each case, the risk manager thought proactively, anticipating future consequences well beyond the immediate decision. Inclusion of this temporal perspective allows otherwise difficult to explain risk management decisions to be placed in a rational framework. For example, day center managers whom we interviewed for the study of risk management for adults with learning disabilities (Heyman and Huckle, 1993, 1995) regarded parents who resisted the idea of moving the adult into a more demanding environment as overprotective. But this dismissive attitude overlooked the rationality of responding cautiously in conditions of service shortage to the possibility of future failure.

THE CONCEPT OF HEALTH CARE RISK ESCALATOR

The further metaphor of a risk escalator is suggested by the observation that movement in the opposite direction to that in which service users were propelled by the care system became extremely different once the initial move had taken place. The term "risk escalator," discussed further below, refers to a system, designed or emergent, which is oriented toward managing a defined health risk, and which is made up of a set of subsystems, ordered in terms of different trade-offs between autonomy and safety, through which service users may move. The dynamics of risk escalators arise from organizational and personal adaption processes, outlined below, which encourage forward movement and impede reverse movement up or down a risk escalator traveling in one of these directions. The two risk escalators outlined above moved in different directions, up toward increased safety but potential overprotection for older people and down toward increased autonomy but potential neglect for adult day center attendees. Consideration of the dynamics of the latter risk escalator persuaded the parent quoted above not to step onto it in the first place.

The concept of risk escalator can be applied to any risk management system which contains alternative responses differing in intervention intensity. For example, financially suspect companies may be given a reduced credit rating, be placed under bankruptcy protection, or be declared bankrupt. Offenders may be cautioned, fined, placed on probation, subjected to a community order, given a suspended sentence, given a determinate or indeterminate (life) prison sentence, or, in some countries, executed. These upward risk escalators possess their own dynamics. For instance, a reduced credit rating can bring about bankruptcy by increasing the cost of borrowing. The analysis below will identify certain common features of risk escalators in the field of health and social care, namely, ordinally structured trade-offs between autonomy and safety, reflexive recursion, and self-organization. Two case studies, of an upward and downward moving health care risk escalator, will then be offered.

COMMON FEATURES OF HEALTH CARE RISK ESCALATORS

Most domains of health and social care have to be managed in the absence of a magic bullet that can solve a defined problem without serious side effects. Risk managers have to balance the risk or certainty of undesired consequences arising from an intervention against the risk of harm occurring if a sufficiently powerful preventative strategy is not adopted. (This analysis will take for granted the cultural and historical processes underlying risk selection, the theme of chapter 4, "A Qualitative Approach to Health Risk Management," this volume.)

Many examples of autonomy/safety trade-offs in health and social care systems can be offered. Women can give birth at home, in community units, under standard hospital-based maternity care, or under intensive surveillance. Their control over the birth process is progressively reduced at higher levels of intervention intensity, but the potential for medical care is increased. Infirm older people may receive no formal support, get home visits, move into sheltered housing, or be looked after in institutions with increasing levels of staffing and restriction of access to the outside world. People with mental health problems may be cared for by their general practitioners, as outpatients, as voluntary in-patients, or through compulsory detention in a low, medium, or high security hospital. Child protection cases may be managed, in the U.K., through non-intervention, social work, registration of the child as at risk, or physical removal of the child from the family.

The term "autonomy," which, at the level of the individual, has a dictionary definition as personal freedom, is used in the present analysis of health care risk management, more specifically, to refer to the impact of risk management on physical and/or personal integrity. For example, these may be reduced in combination when a forensic mental health patient is both medicated and incarcerated. Risk managers are required to trade off autonomy versus safety because of their essentially tragic relationship. In general, freedom weakens prevention, and vice versa; however, many service providers attempt to mitigate the other side of the dilemma. For instance, the stultifying impact of total institutions (Goffman, 1961) has defeated all attempts to reform them, and side effects of major pharmaceutical interventions such as psychotropic drugs and hormone replacement therapy inevitably come to light. Interference with complex human and social systems is bound to trigger unforeseen, undesired consequences that can only be ameliorated, not eliminated, through measures designed to enhance the quality of care. On the other hand, non-intervention, or inadequate intervention, leaves the risk selected as of concern unprevented. Thus, for example, the damaging effects of child protection measures on families have to be balanced against the risk that children will be abused as a result of inaction or the inadequacy of preventative intervention.

We might expect, therefore, that risk managers will seek autonomy/safety trade-offs that take into account both risk severity and the seriousness of the anticipated consequences of a given preventative strategy. Thus, a mildly infirm older person might be encouraged to remain in their own home because the beneficial effects of familiar surroundings and the damage that can be caused by disruption of routines are recognized. At the other end of the continuum, an older person might be moved into highly staffed institutional care because their disabilities are considered to place them at risk of serious harm. Such alternative responses to the same perceived need can be viewed holistically as a single system with its own dynamics.

REFLEXIVE RECURSION

The term "reflexive recursion" encompasses feedback processes through which intentional, future-oriented actions change a state, in this case a risk, in ways that affect subsequent actions, thus potentially establishing a complex dynamic system.

Adams (1995) has most forcibly made the point that human actions can change the risks that they are designed to manage. For example, the use of seat belts in cars may cause drivers to feel less vulnerable and therefore able to take greater risks, thus detracting from the overall safety benefit of their compulsory wear. Conversely, a road's reputation as dangerous may cause its users to act more cautiously, thereby reducing its dangerousness. Such changes are possible because the risks in question result from human action, even if they are aggregated statistically. This reactivity within the domain of risks arising from human action undermines the validity of probability estimates induced from historical observations.

Adams discusses one, simple form of a reactive system, a risk thermostat (Adams, 1995, p. 15), in which risk managers seek to maintain a preferred equilibrium. In terms of the autonomy/safety trade-off, drivers who respond to the protective effect of seat belts by taking more driving risks are opting to take this benefit in terms of freer driving, keeping their level of risk at its previous level. Similarly, some individuals may feel able to spend a longer time in the sun because they are covered in sun screen (McGregor & Young, 1996). Some may respond to the availability of new AIDS treatments by taking greater sexual health risks (Catz, Meredith, & Mundy, 2001; Ostrow, Fox, Chmiel, Silvestre, Visscher, Vanable et al., 2002). Although their immediate probability of catching HIV may not be affected, the adversity of the infection is reduced, and they can maintain their overall preferred balance between autonomy and safety while enjoying more risky behavior. Both the causal direction of the relationship between belief in the efficacy of HIV treatments and acceptance of sexual health risk (Huebner & Gerend, 2001) and the strength of the compensatory effect (Pinkerton, 2001) have been questioned. However, insofar as individuals do set their HIV risk thermostats in this way, they contribute to an increase in population infection and, therefore, the longer term probability of becoming infected. *Homo thermostaticus,* a variant of the rational economic actor maximizing individual self-interest, impacts disastrously on public welfare which, according to such models, he is incapable of respecting. Nevertheless, the potential for compensatory risk management does illustrate the need to take into account recursive effects in risk analysis.

Risk thermostats appertain to closed circular systems with feedback between two processes: risk appraisal and risk decision making. In risk escalators, multiple subsystems based on particular balances of autonomy/safety are arranged hierarchically. The risk escalator carries individuals who step onto it up or down these levels and makes reverse movement problematic. Risk escalators are driven by reflexive recursion which, for better or worse, gives movement to what would otherwise be a set of static steps.

REFLEXIVE RECURSION IN UPWARD RISK ESCALATORS

With respect to up escalators, the steps represent procedures of progressively increasing intervention intensity associated with a shift away from autonomy and toward safety. However, lower level interventions may themselves stimulate changes which impel the service user toward greater intervention intensity. For example, serum screening tests for prostate cancer generate a high proportion of false positives or, more accurately, classification of men as being at higher risk although they do not have the condition. A diagnostic biopsy, the next step on the risk escalator, carries both morbidity and mortality risk (Ofman, 1995). Some men who decide to be screened, therefore, will die even though they do not have prostate cancer. But those who screen positive and decide not to undergo a biopsy cannot unlearn that they belong to a higher risk group, making it difficult for them to step off the risk escalator as they would then have to live with their higher risk status unclarified.

The prostate cancer risk escalator is driven by preventative decisions which trigger physical interventions which cause new risks. In addition, because of the importance of psychosocial factors to health, as evidenced by the pervasiveness of placebo effects (Spanos, Stenstrom, & Johnston, 1988), upward moving health care risk escalators may be fueled by increased stress resulting from experience of risk assessment at lower levels. Lane (1995) has argued that the categorization of a pregnancy as high risk can trigger a cascade of intervention, as the woman's distress about her risk status provokes emotional and physiological reactions which, in turn, cause further interventions and more intense alarm until a cesarean section has to be resorted to. Evidence from animal studies (Mansfield, 1988) shows that pregnancy outcomes, such as the incidence of spontaneous abortions, are adversely affected by stressors such as flashing lights and white noise.

An observer's moral stance toward an upward risk escalator will be influenced by their view of the potency of reflexive recursion within the system. Those who believe in the iatrogenic power of an intervention will, at the least, favor more caution in its use than will those who do not take account of such reactive processes. This pattern of reasoning underlies a wide range of controversies including those over the wars on drugs and terrorism and the role of prisons, which may be either seen to work or to breed criminals.

REFLEXIVE RECURSION IN DOWNWARD RISK ESCALATORS

Because upward escalation in intervention intensity is associated with iatrogenesis, reflexive recursion will be associated with increased risk and so will provide grounds for questioning the therapeutic value of a health care risk escalator. Conversely, reflexive recursion has the benign effect in downward risk escalators of leading the service user toward less intense interventions which enhance their autonomy. For example, the use of day centers for adults with moderate intellectual disabilities may prevent them from developing their capabilities in more challenging environments, for example a sheltered workshop, generating a self-proving prophecy. Encouraging them to cope with more challenging environments provides learning opportunities which may enable them to progress still further toward managing normal life.

Critics of downward risk escalators can argue that they generate unrealistic expectations about service user potential and, therefore, de facto neglect. This potential shortcoming arises from the absence of hoped for benign reflexive recursion, a charge that is often raised about community care for people with serious mental illnesses such as schizophrenia. As one family caregiver of an adult with a mild intellectual disability put it:

> Every time I go to the review [at day center], they keep saying it is time she got a job. But she is epileptic, and could not work in a kitchen. I tell them what she is like. I should know. I made her. But the center don't see this. (Mother of adult with a mild intellectual disability, interview)

This instructive disagreement between family and day center caregivers turns on a difference of perspective about the capacity of an individual to cope with a new environment. Both parties must rely on counterfactual reasoning because the only way to test their positions would be to place the service user (who would have her own preferences) in a risky situation. Not surprisingly, day center staff who promoted movement down the risk escalator advocated risk acceptance.

> We are all subject to risk and they [service users with learning disabilities] will not learn without taking risk. (Day center caregiver, interview)

Because risk judgments rely upon an elaborate foundation of usually implicit and not necessarily shared assumptions (see chapter 4, "A Qualitative Approach to Health Risk Management," in this volume), frequent differences of opinion between parties involved in risk management can be expected. Concerns about the direction of costs and benefits often underlie such divergences. For example, several parents of adults with learning disabilities who participated in our study argued that they, not day center staff, would have to manage the consequences if an adult with learning disabilities suffered adverse consequences as a result of risk-taking. Service users and family caregivers who opposed risk acceptance could draw upon idiographic knowledge of a particular individual in order to contest the aggregate formulations of risk analysis that are encoded in epidemiology. The analysis above does not endorse either point of view but illustrates the way in which such differences can be understood in terms of variations in belief about reflexive recursion. Such understanding can, hopefully, contribute to improved communication between paid and family caregivers and direct service users whose aspirations should be paramount.

CASE STUDIES OF HEALTH CARE RISK ESCALATORS

The concept of a risk escalator provides a framework for qualitative analysis of the operational delivery of health care risk escalators in concrete organizational settings. This framework can be applied to health care systems aimed at a defined therapeutic goal in which an ordinal series of levels of intervention intensity, each providing its own autonomy/safety trade-off, is recognized, and in which service users can move between different levels. (Health care systems in which ordinal rankings of intervention intensity cannot be defined consensually [Heyman & Henriksen, 1998, p. 101] raise additional questions worthy of qualitative analysis.)

Below, issues associated with the operation of two health care risk escalators are outlined in relation to their functional definitions. The discussion draws upon case studies of prenatal chromosomal screening (Heyman & Henriksen, 2001) and of forensic mental health services (Heyman, Buswell-Griffiths, & Taylor, 2002; Heyman, Buswell-Griffiths, Taylor, & O'Brien, 2002) to illustrate the operation of upward and downward health care risk escalators, respectively.

AN UPWARD HEALTH CARE RISK ESCALATOR

Prenatal chromosomal screening systems are designed to offer pregnant women and their partners screening and diagnosis of chromosomal disorders followed by termination of pregnancy if an abnormality is discovered. Participation is officially voluntary, and a woman may decide not to start the process or to withdraw from it at any point. However, our case study of a large maternity hospital in northeastern England (Heyman & Henriksen, 2001) showed that some women felt pressured into accepting tests.

> They looked at me history, and then they said, 'Well, you are over 35, so I think we will give you—would you like—the blood test'. They says, 'You don't have to have it'. But, I think, when you are offered something I think you feel, well, guilty, so I took it. (Pregnant woman aged 35, interview, serum screening)

Once organizationally embedded, risk escalators influence risk selection by predefining the contingency they are oriented to as requiring attention.

Prenatal chromosomal screening systems vary substantially in the U.K., and hospital doctors within our research site also diverged in their practice, for example, with respect to the ages at which they would recommend particular options to women. In this hospital, the health care risk escalator had four stages. Women under age 35 were not offered testing but could request it. Women of age 35 and over were offered a choice of serum screening or amniocentesis. Women of age 37–38 would be advised to opt for amniocentesis, as were those whose serum screening test put them in the higher risk category, with an estimated post-test probability of $\geq 1:200$ of carrying a fetus with a chromosomal abnormality. If a chromosomal abnormality was identified through amniocentesis, women would be offered an abortion.

This risk escalator, like that for prostate cancer, discussed above, was powered by a high rate of screen positives, that is, women being categorized into the higher risk group for whom amniocentesis was recommended. This rate itself increases with age, from 12 percent to 38 percent between maternal ages 35 and 40 at our hospital research site (Northern Region Genetics Service, 1995), an artifact of the way in which risk estimates were calculated. Women who screened positive were encouraged to undergo amniocentesis, and thereby to accept the increased probability of spontaneous abortion associated with this invasive procedure, even though most would be carrying normal babies. For example, at maternal age 40, 1–2 percent of fetuses would be born with trisomy 21, the cause of Down syndrome, or other chromosomal problems, but nearly 40 percent would screen positive.

Three issues associated with the operation of both upward and downward health care risk escalators will be briefly outlined: firstly, endemic deviations between the risk escalator design blueprint and operational reality; secondly, inter-professional power struggles; and, thirdly, active navigation of risk escalators by service users.

With respect to operational matters, a survey of pregnant women suggested that 28 percent (30) of those aged 35 and over had not been offered any chromosomal tests.[1] We expected doctors to challenge the validity of this finding, but they readily accepted it, expressing concern at the potential for litigation if a woman of this age gave birth to a baby with Down syndrome but had not been offered testing. They explained that an older woman might be missed if her notes were not available at the consultation, she looked younger than her age, or the doctor was distracted by the telephone ringing. We hypothesize that such gaps between standardized organizational blueprints and concrete practice are endemic in risk escalators and reflect the vagaries of human action, particularly in under-resourced systems over which service users have little direct leverage.

Their complexity guarantees that the operation of health care risk escalators requires multiprofessional collaboration between occupational groups that are likely to have parallel, weakly intersecting management structures. In consequence, the mixing of skills and coordination of professional inputs become issues in such systems. U.K. maternity units manage the service user interface with respect to chromosomal screening in diverse ways, such as through midwives or trained genetic counselors taking responsibility for advising parents. At our hospital, unusually, advice was provided primarily by hospital registrars or consultants. Although uncommon, this structure does illustrate the impact of professional power relations on the operation of health care risk escalators. Some midwives accepted a division of labor in which probabilistic information could only be provided by medical experts.

The consultant will talk about statistics, and will tell you actually how much at risk you are from having a Down's syndrome, and maybe what risk you are from having a miscarriage with the amniocentesis, things like that. I don't actually give them statistics. Usually the doctors pull a chart off the wall and show them all the statistics and everything. (Pregnant midwife, aged 34, interview, no genetic tests)

The quotation and our own observations suggest that doctors' grasp of the complexities of Bayesian inference was rather fragile. But their capture of this body of knowledge had enabled them to regain control of the maternity service, at the price of considerable work pressure. As one midwife put it, "Our role here has eroded. We are not a midwives' clinic anymore. It is a doctor-centered clinic."

Some women accepted the legitimacy of this health care risk escalator, as did the respondent quoted above, who felt guilty about declining offered services. Others, not wishing to be sucked into the system, understood the Bayesian principle (see chapter 4, "A Qualitative Approach to Health Management," in this volume) that they could choose to leave their probability, more accurately their degree of uncertainty, on hold or undergo further tests which would either increase or decrease it. Some women who rejected abortion declined to undergo any form of testing on the grounds that a changed probability of giving birth to a baby with Down syndrome might make it more difficult for them to continue to reject termination.

Would I feel pressure from people out there [if Down syndrome diagnosed] who would say, 'You knew you were having a Down's syndrome child, and you brought it into the world', you know. So, I didn't even want to run the risk of going down that road. (Pregnant woman, aged 36, interview, no genetic tests)

Doctors tended to emphasize the problem of false screen negatives over that of false positives.

False positives don't worry me as much because, even though—I have never actually lost a baby related to an amniocentesis yet. And so, for people who have passed the learning curve, it is possible that the foetal loss rate is smaller than the quoted risk. But the false negatives worry me . . . Now that, I mean the legal aspect, doesn't worry me, but the impact worries me . . . It is such a big thing to take on. And until we can get the false negative rate down, I think I would rather not offer it [serum screening] to everybody, because it isn't perfect. (Hospital doctor, interview)

This argument discounted both iatrogenic physical risk and the distress associated with screen positives, as illustrated in the final quotation drawn from this study.

> I would prefer to give you the results [of serum screening] myself because people who screen positive always think that they have got an abnormal pregnancy. They can't see that it's just a blood test. (Recording of hospital consultation with woman, aged 36, serum screening)

This categorization of the severe anxiety experienced by many women during the testing period as irrational provided legitimation for an upward health care risk escalator, the therapeutic status of which required minimization of reflexive recursion, as noted above.

A DOWNWARD HEALTH CARE RISK ESCALATOR

Hospitals concerned with the rehabilitation of offenders categorized as having mental health problems provide good examples of downward risk escalators. These systems are designed to lead service users toward life in the wider community, normally over a period of years, through a series of small stages linked to risk assessment. For example, service users who progress through the entire system at one of our research sites, a medium/low security hospital for offenders with intellectual disabilities (Heyman, Buswell-Griffiths, & Taylor, 2002; Heyman, Buswell-Griffiths, Taylor, & O'Brien, 2002), might start their hospital career on locked units secured by an external air lock, high staffing levels, and no access to the external world. They would then progress to units with less physical security, progressively lower staffing levels, and greater external contact, such as accompanied and then unaccompanied access to the grounds and supervised and then unsupervised parole for progressively longer periods. Finally, they could reside in unlocked units with low staffing levels prior to discharge. This health care risk escalator connects to the high security hospital system from which patients might be accepted or sent up to, as well as to various forms of community care or complete independence of services at the bottom of the risk escalator. Patients could enter or leave this system at various points, depending upon decisions made about their mental health and risk status.

This forensic mental health service provides a textbook example of a downward risk escalator, with success in more highly structured environments providing the basis for service users to cope with more demanding circumstances in which they were allowed more autonomy. As with the chromosomal screening system previously discussed, the operation of this system will be briefly discussed in relation to three issues: deviations from the risk escalator blueprint; inter-professional power struggles; and active service user management of their movement on the risk escalator.

One common source of disruption of this risk escalator was bed blocking associated with pressure on hospital places. Patients could be trapped in immobilized chains because an individual could only progress if a place became available at the next stage through the success of a patient at *that* location who could, in turn, only move if a place was freed at the next level down. Hence, the progress of a patient ready to move from the highest level might depend upon the discharge of one far down the line into the community, as well as downward movement at all the intermediate levels. Long delays in the movement of patients judged ready to progress could result from this capacity problem.

> The next stage for Rob, if he progressed, would be up to [less restrictive unit] which is a locked ward, but they have more freedom. There is more trips out into the community and such like, and then it would be step up to the houses . . . And this is all classed as rehabilitation. However, there's no places on [next unit down]. (Nurse, interview)

Conversely, patients might have to be quickly promoted in order to create room higher up the risk escalator for a patient whose behavior required more intense risk management. The hospital had attempted to cope with this contingency by maintaining empty beds at the highest security level, but this spare capacity had been overwhelmed by demand and by maintaining a reservoir of spare patients ready for promotion at short notice. At a second research site, an East London medium/low security facility for offenders diagnosed as having mental health problems, staff claimed that extra-contractual patients were admitted to the highest security regime for financial reasons, forcing premature moves of existing residents down the risk escalator.

At both of these hospital research sites, problematic interprofessional collaboration was a major source of conflict and disfunctionality. Doctors, nurses, psychologists, and occupational therapists tended to view their role from distinct perspectives, in terms of medication, daily risk management, psychotherapy, and daily living skills, respectively, and found it difficult to collaborate effectively. The following quotation illustrates one source of problems, in relation to the role of therapy. The

patient quoted below had been caught up in a conflict between the
professions:

> But some of them [staff], they've got to be into me all of the time. Like,
> I'm doing a psychology program with the psychologist . . . And . . . [staff
> are] saying I'm getting my own way, doing that, doing this. (Patient,
> interview)

Nurses, who managed day-to-day risk through a system of incentives
and penalties, could view psychotherapy, for example, for anger management, as a perverse reward for misbehavior, whereas psychologists
selected the most needy cases, for example, those who found it difficult
to control their anger on the ward.

Because the timing of patient discharge depended upon their success
in navigating the risk escalator, some adopted active strategies designed
to control their progress. Some patients, according to staff and their own
accounts, deliberately fouled up because they felt that they could not
handle the demands of a less structured, more autonomous environment.
Downward health care risk escalators can only function as intended if
service users have internalized their designated purpose, in this case, safe
rehabilitation. Patients who wanted to return to a higher, less demanding,
level would find failure rewarding, perversely from the perspective of
system design but sensibly from their own point of view.

Others tried to present themselves in ways which would speed up their
progress and eventual discharge.

> **Patient:** I didn't say nowt, just bottled up for years and years, just let it
> go on top of me and stuff . . .
> **Interviewer:** Why haven't you said your opinions?
> **Patient**: Because I thought it would be wrong, and I might get into trouble
> for saying my opinions, so I kept my trap shut, and just got on with it
> [therapy]. (Patient, interview)

Patients were not judgmental dopes. Some attempted to avoid the trap,
as they saw it, of responding to the license to express feelings in therapeutic situations that could be held against them when their progress
was reviewed. Staff, in turn, understood this tactic and would treat ex-
cessive compliance as an indicator of concealed risk. This type of risk
escalator had the potential to generate information games involving cycles of concealment, discovery, and reconcealment (Goffman, 1959).

ORIGINS OF RISK ESCALATORS

The author was surprised to discover that the elaborate downward risk escalator operating at the hospital for offenders with learning disabilities had not been designed but had emerged from piecemeal developments. Existing low security locked wards had been complemented by the subsequent establishment of a medium security unit funded through a central government grant. Houses close to the hospital site had come onto the market, been purchased, and then employed as rehabilitation units on account of their closeness to living conditions in the wider community. These diverse elements had gradually coalesced into a unified system which service users could move down through standardized reviews.

Similarly, the system or prenatal chromosomal screening and diagnostic testing in use at our maternity hospital site had coalesced from separate developments. Serum screening was originally designed for younger pregnant women whose lower level of risk did not justify an invasive test for chromosomal abnormalities. In the U.K., these systems have now been integrated, with screening a potential first step toward diagnostic testing for those women categorized as at higher risk.

In contrast, the health care risk escalator designed to promote the rehabilitation of offenders with mental health problems in East London was explicitly designed as an overall system, with three main levels, focusing primarily on assessment, treatment, and rehabilitation. Subsequently, a fourth predischarge level was inserted between rehabilitation and discharge. Some staff felt that the addition of this extra level served the function of allowing postponement of the critical, often difficult, discharge decision.

It can be concluded from these examples that risk escalators may develop spontaneously as self-organizing systems that coalesce from smaller service entities which in turn become subsystems or may be invented and reinvented. The practitioners who maintain these systems must then defend them by arguing that the intervention steps contained in upward health care risk escalators do not themselves increase risk and, conversely, that the steps in downward health care risk escalators generate increased ability to handle autonomy. These different stances, which must be defended by their deliverers willy-nilly in emergent risk escalators, correspond to the traditional right versus left political division. Defenders of the therapeutic status of downward risk escalators must legitimate them in terms of faith in human potential, while advocates of upward risk escalators must deny the plasticity of human nature.

DISCUSSION: OPERATION OF HEALTH CARE
RISK ESCALATORS

Late, modern risk societies are becoming ever more committed to screening and the preventative use of risk escalators. For example, in the U.K. at the time of writing, proposed reforms to the laws governing mental health would allow the detention of unconvicted individuals deemed likely to commit serious offenses on account of a personality disorder. Defenders argue that prophylaxis is required for a small minority, and critics argue that the law violates human rights and makes unwarranted assumptions about the validity of psychiatric risk assessment. In the United States, fake internet sites selling child pornography have been set up by the police. Proponents argue that a high proportion of internet offenders go on to commit direct abuse, and critics argue that this procedure entails entrapment. In this new, prophylactic culture, health and social services have become increasingly oriented to the screening of populations for risk factors, as against the treatment of individual cases (Castel, 1991).

The generic organizational form which can be analyzed in terms of the metaphor of a risk escalator arises from the ubiquity of the autonomy/ safety dilemma. In general, multiple human service responses to an identified risk will be developed and differentiated in terms of the balance provided between intervention intensity and reduction in autonomy for service recipients. General service providers will attempt to match risk severity with intervention intensity, while specific providers will develop distinctive autonomy/safety mixes in order to increase their chances of survival in the ecology of care through the establishment of market niches. Risk escalators may evolve without conscious design via the coalescence of subsystems, as in the case of prenatal genetic screening worldwide, and that of the hospital providing rehabilitation for offenders with learning disabilities discussed above. Or they may be consciously designed, as was the hospital providing rehabilitation for offenders with mental health problems also mentioned in the chapter. However, modification of the latter to provide an additional intermediate step for patients before discharge provides an illustration of the self-organizing forces that shape risk escalators.

Whether designed or emergent, health care and other risk escalators generate differences of perception and disagreements about their operation at two levels. Firstly, the existence of risk escalators locks in societal attention selectively to concern with a particular risk. In this sense, risks, although not the causal processes which give rise to adverse consequences, are constituted by risk escalators rather than vice versa. For example, provision of chromosomal prenatal screening services turns chromosomal abnormalities into a risk that parents are obliged to consider. Some will not accept the risk selection made for them, as service users do not always act as passive recipients of risk management or use health care systems in the ways designated for them. Secondly, views about the feedback processes which fuel risk escalators will often differ, with implications for judgments about their therapeutic worth. Upward risk escalators are vulnerable to the charge of iatrogenesis, downward ones to the accusation of neglect. Service providers and users may attempt to anticipate the impact of an initial decision on progress through subsequent stages of a risk escalator or may only consider the first decision required. The length of view adopted will affect decision making substantially. A longer term perspective is also overlooked in laboratory studies of cognitive heuristics (Kahneman and Tversky, 2000) that focus on a single, decontextualized decision. Such studies exclude the complex chains of causality and feedback that real life decision makers may take account of.

The examples discussed in this chapter can do no more than illustrate the dynamics of risk escalators. The analysis presented may convince some readers that qualitative analysis of this organizational form in a variety of health care and historical/cultural contexts can generate insights that illuminate both the pragmatics of human service organizations and the nature of risk societies.

NOTE

1. Only a very small proportion of these cases could be explained in terms of late referral to the maternity unit.

REFERENCES

Adams, J. (1995). *Risk.* London: UCL Press.

Castel, R. (1991). From dangerousness to risk. In G. Burchell, C. Gordon, & P. Miller (Eds.), *The Foucault effect* (pp. 281–298). London: Harvester Wheatsheaf.

Catz, S. L., Meredith, K. L., & Mundy, L. M. (2001). Women's HIV transmission risk perceptions and behaviors in the era of potent antiretroviral therapies. *AIDS Education & Prevention, 13,* 239–251.

Davidson, N. and Reed, J. (1995). One foot on the escalator: elderly people in sheltered accommodation. In Bob Heyman (Ed.), *Researching user per-*

spectives on community health care (pp. 150–164). London: Chapman & Hall.

Goffman, E. (1959). *The presentation of self in everyday life.* New York: Doubleday.

Goffman, E. (1961). *Asylums: Essays in the social situation of mental patients and other inmates.* New York: Anchor.

Heyman, B., Buswell-Griffiths, C., & Taylor, J. (2002). Risk escalators and the rehabilitation of offenders with learning disabilities. *Social Science & Medicine, 54,* 1429–1440.

Heyman, B., Buswell-Griffiths, C., Taylor, J., & O'Brien, G. (2002). Risk management in the rehabilitation of offenders with learning disabilities: A qualitative approach. *Risk Management: An International Journal, 4,* 33–46.

Heyman, B., & Henriksen, M. (1998). Probability and health risks. In B. Heyman (Ed.), *Risk, health and health care: A qualitative approach* (pp. 65–105). London: Edward Arnold.

Heyman, B., & Henriksen, M. (2001). *Risk, age and pregnancy: A case study of prenatal genetic screening and testing.* Basingstoke, England: Palgrave.

Heyman, B., & Huckle, S. (1993). Not worth the risk? Attitudes of adults with learning difficulties, and their informal and formal carers, to the hazards of everyday life. *Social Science & Medicine, 37,* 1557–1564.

Heyman, B., & Huckle, S. (1995). How adults with learning difficulties and their careers see the community. In Bob Heyman (Ed.), *Researching user perspectives on community health care* (pp. 165–182). Chapman & Hall.

Huebner, D. M., & Gerend, M. A. (2001). The relation between beliefs about drug treatments for HIV and sexual risk behavior in gay and bisexual men. *Annals of Behavioral Medicine, 23,* 304–312.

Kahneman, D., & Tversky, A. (2000). *Choices, values and frames.* Cambridge, England: Cambridge University Press.

Lane, K. (1995). The medical model of the body as a site of risk: a case study of childbirth. In G. Gabe (Ed.), *Medicine, Health and Risk: Sociological Approaches* (pp. 53–72). Oxford: Blackwell.

Mansfield, P. K. (1988). Midlife childbearing: Strategies for informed decision-making. *Psychology of Women Quarterly, 12,* 445–460.

McGregor, J. M., & Young, A. R. (1996). Sunscreens, suntans and skin cancer. *British Medical Journal, 312,* 1621–1622.

Northern Region Genetics Service (1995). *Maternal serum screening in the northern region: Information for health care professionals.* Newcastle-upon-Tyne: Author.

Ofman, U.S. (1995). Sexual quality of life in men with prostate cancer. *Cancer, 75,* 1949–1953.

Ostrow, D. E., Fox, K. J., Chmiel, J. S., Silvestre, A., Visscher, B. R., Vanable P. A., et al. (2002). Attitudes towards highly active antiretroviral therapy are associated with sexual risk taking among HIV-infected and uninfected homosexual men. *AIDS, 16,* 775–780.

Pinkerton, S. D. (2001). Sexual risk compensation and HIV/STD transmission: Empirical evidence and theoretical considerations. *Risk Analysis, 21,* 727–736.

Spanos, N. P., Stenstrom, R. J., & Johnston, J. C. (1988). Hypnosis, placebo and suggestion in the treatment of warts. *Psychosomatic Medicine, 50,* 245–260.

EDITORIAL COMMENTARY

This chapter focuses on the effects that each decision in a medical system has on the individual. I found myself dividing the many good examples into two categories: Those where a person (patient) was able to make the decision to enter the escalator or not and would have full use of the resources needed for follow-up (e.g., maternal testing for Down syndrome) and those where the decision needed to take into account the fact that there was a paucity of resources that limited further choices. The person with limited abilities who gives up a place in an assisted-living arrangement to take a job loses the position in the home, as the slot will immediately be given to another. If there were unlimited resources the decision might not be easier but certainly would be fairer.

—Kenneth L. Noller

Part II

DIALOGICALITY WITHIN MEDICAL PRACTICE: GENERALIZED KNOWLEDGE AND INDIVIDUALIZED DECISIONS

Chapter 4

A QUALITATIVE APPROACH TO HEALTH RISK MANAGEMENT

Bob Heyman

The revolutionary idea that defines the boundary between modern times and the past is the mastery of risk: the notion that the future is more than the whim of the gods and that men and women are not passive before nature.

P. L. Bernstein, *Against the Gods: The Remarkable Story of Risk*

This chapter will focus on health risk. I will argue that, although a risk framework undoubtedly plays the starring role in modern science-based cultures which Bernstein outlines, its limits need to be acknowledged. Risk analysis provides a crude, value-laden remedy for a core design limitation of science-based cultures, the limited applicability of scientific principles in conditions of real-life complexity.

The chapter will first delineate a distinction between quantitative and qualitative approaches to risk. I will then offer a qualitative approach to the analysis of risk judgments that will be decomposed into four elements: categories, values, uncertainty, and time. Qualitative data, drawn from a study of chromosomal risk management in pregnancy (Heyman & Henriksen, 2001), will be used to illustrate the analysis. Along the way, some methodological implications of qualitative approaches to health risk will be briefly mentioned.

QUANTITATIVE AND QUALITATIVE APPROACHES TO HEALTH RISK

Skolbekken (1995) uses the term "risk epidemic" to depict the exponential growth of medical, particularly epidemiological, papers concerned with risk, a growth which, he implies, is damaging to intellectual health. He notes a number of instructive patterns in the risk epidemic. The volume of research employing related language, such as "danger" and "hazard," has not increased in line with that on "risk." The increase has been particularly marked in certain fields, such as obstetrics and gynecology. The incidence of articles about iatrogenic risks has not expanded. Heyman and Henriksen (2001, p. 3) identified a similar rapid growth in the number of papers concerned with health screening. This research explosion can be understood within a Foucauldian framework which treats risk knowledge as a form of governmentality (Lupton, 2000). This approach depicts naturalistic depictions of risk as assertions of medical power which both derive from and reinforce the authority of science. Direction of analytic attention away from the tacit, debatable assumptions on which risk analyses are predicated underpins this power structure and, therefore, represents a political act.

Quantitative approaches treat risks as natural phenomena, existing independently of risk managers,[1] which can be observed and measured. A qualitative approach, in contrast, views risk judgments as entailing complexes of contextualized values and beliefs which inescapably incorporate the perspective of the risk manager. This distinction is not offered in an attempt to demonize the prevailing quantitative approach. Although hardly the unalloyed blessing implied by Bernstein (1996) in the opening quotation, the quantitative approach to risk provides a valuable heuristic for decision making in conditions of complexity. The naturalistic approach to risk can be welcomed providing that the price paid for simplification is acknowledged and that value assumptions embedded in risk management are articulated.

The act of projecting risk managers' values and beliefs onto the world, so that they are experienced as natural phenomena, can be observed in the following standard definition of risk as "the probability that a particular adverse event occurs during a stated period of time, or results from a particular challenge" (The Royal Society, 1992, p. 2). The definition draws together four elements, each of which can be reframed to articulate the judgmental role of the risk manager, as shown in Figure 4.1.

The synthesis of four distinct ingredients in the Royal Society definition is done casually, without analytic comment. The resulting com-

Figure 4.1
Two views of risk elements.

Risk viewed as referencing natural phenomena	Risk viewed as referencing knowledge
Event	Category
Adversity	Value
Externally defined time scale	Time frame
Probability	Expectation

Source: Adapted from Heyman, Henriksen, & Maughan, 1998, pp. 6–7.

pound concept does not describe a natural phenomenon but represents a cultural institution which, for better or worse, "defines the boundary between modern times and the past" (Bernstein, 1996, p. 1). This transition has involved an expansion of the scope of the causal–mechanical framework at the expense of personalistic explanations, to the point where hyperactivity in children (now, apparently, an epidemic) can be deemed a medical problem requiring pharmaceutical intervention. However, as will be argued below, real-world prediction requires a simplifying process of induction. Heuristics are built into applied science.

RISK CATEGORIZATION AND SELECTION

Risk management requires a double act of categorization of a contingency as an event and its selection as worthy of preventative scanning. These two acts, usually implicit, unconscious, and unreflective, are intimately connected because a risk class cannot be selected unless a range of nonidentical phenomena has been homogenized and foregrounded in a category. Conversely, a risk category will not be selected unless it resonates with personal and/or cultural concerns that risk managers consider important.

Categories lump together diverse phenomena, highlighting their distinctiveness while discounting their differences. Risk management requires that such cognitive structures are maintained. For example, probability estimates for mental illnesses and child abuse are predicated on the assumption that the extremely variable sets of events within a category can be deemed equivalent so that their incidence can be observed. Recategorization, or differentiation into subcategories, will generate many alternative epidemiologies, each requiring assumptions about similarity and distinctiveness.

Committed risk managers may resist definitional inquiries about the classification in use which would undermine the knowledge base for the prevailing risk management system. For example, doctors in a U.K. maternity hospital offering prenatal screening for Down syndrome and related chromosomal disorders appeared puzzled by their own reluctance to discuss the highly variable clinical manifestations of the syndrome (Heyman & Henriksen, 2001).

> **Interviewer:** Do you talk to them [pregnant women] about Down syndrome, about what Down syndrome is?
> **Doctor:** No, I don't actually . . . interesting. And yet, of course, that is addressed in the film [provided for pregnant women], isn't it? Perhaps I should do. (Doctor, interview)

The next quotation illustrates the way in which the definition of a risk entity can be backgrounded and removed from consideration as potentially problematic.

> **Doctor:** Have you read anything about DS [Down's syndrome] yet?
> **Pregnant woman:** No. Just what was in the booklet.
> **Doctor:** I think there are two ways we can look at what we are going to do about it. There is the blood test. What the BT [blood test] does, it tells you if you are at high risk or at low risk. (Transcript of hospital consultation with woman, aged 38, who chose serum screening)

Doctors could not have discussed this topic adequately without describing the immense clinical variability of the syndrome. But the prevailing epidemiology only allowed probabilistic or diagnostic prediction of the presence of the condition, not of its disabling impact. By not discussing this variability, doctors avoided having to acknowledge an inherent limitation of their prognostic knowledge base. This instructive quotation well illustrates the operation of governmentality in medical/patient interactions which sustain the legitimacy of a risk management system by keeping problematic issues off the agenda. The unquestionability of Down syndrome, and of the testing process employed to assess its risk of occurrence, is reinforced by the use of abbreviation to initials which conveys the routine, familiar status of these entities.

Similarly, a couple, who after agonized consideration, had decided to terminate the life of a fetus with Down syndrome defined its nature in a way that justified their decision.

I mean, you can't get away from the fact that they are . . . I mean their eyes come out, they have floppy tongues . . . It's just endless. (Interview with a woman, aged 46, after pregnancy termination following amniocentesis)

This imagery, which discounts the possibility of a child having mild Down syndrome, helped the couple to justify a distressing decision. Despite adopting this strategy, both parents were traumatized by the experience of pregnancy termination (see the section "Risk and Time," below).

Risk selection involves selective attention to a limited set of prioritized contingency categories and blindness to others. Selective attention cannot be avoided because life contains too many potential dangers for it to be possible for any society or individual to worry about more than a small proportion of them. All cultures selectively attend to dangers (Douglas, 1994), such as possible future adversity, while risks can only be managed, selectively, in cultures which, as a result of a highly specific and recent historical process, understand uncertainty probabilistically (Hacking, 1975).

Risk categorization/selection is shaped by the dialectical interplay of societal, organizational, interpersonal, and individual concerns. Risks may be adopted as contingencies of concern unreflectively, without reference to degree of harm. For example, accidents involving passenger trains have received massive publicity following the recent botched privatization of the railways in the U.K., while the greater number of injuries and fatalities suffered by railway workers receive little media attention (Hutter, 2001). This selective focus may result from a combination of media amplification of rarer but larger accidents and social class bias in favor of middle class commuters over manual railway workers. In the U.K. and many other societies, child murders lead the headlines, while the much larger number of children killed as a result of the failure to introduce a 20-mile-per-hour speed limit in urban areas is tolerated with relaxed indifference. The intensity of the public response suggests that child murders threaten the social order in a way that preventable child deaths caused by motorists do not. The U.S. administration is, in 2003, leading a war against the risks posed by terrorism but barely recognizes the risks associated with global warming and world poverty, contingencies which may cause at least as much loss of life.

Macroscale governmentality operates by attempting to push certain contingencies to the top of the national or international agenda. Its successful operation determines the risk questions that are asked, transforming them into issues which, in principle if not in practice, can be technically resolved. Risk selection can be subverted by challenges based on arguments about equivalence (ignored contingency X causes more harm than selected contingency Y), or, indirectly, through arguments about interest (institution A is promoting contingency Y because it will benefit economically or politically).

The notion of a "particular" event in The Royal Society definition begs the question of how an event class comes to be foregrounded as homogenous and special and so smuggles in the culturally mediated value prism leading to its selection.

RISK AND VALUES

Adversity is the second ingredient in the risk compound put together in The Royal Society definition. To count as a risk, in this sense, a contingency must be judged adverse. The judgmental labors of categorization/selection and adversity attribution are intimately associated, because a risk entity would hardly be categorized and selected unless its consequences were judged more than trivially adverse.

The attribution of adversity logically entails a value judgment, which may be externalized as an intrinsic property of an event. It may be objected that serious health problems, such as plagues and cancers, are universally abhorred, and that, therefore, their adversity can be taken for granted. Against this view, it may be countered that even such apparent ills can be viewed differently. For example, early Christians welcomed suffering as a test from God. Some proponents of the Gaia thesis maintain that AIDS represents a homeostatic response of the biosphere to the threat posed by overpopulation. From an evolutionary perspective, pandemics and other hazards can contribute to the development of species. Moreover, acknowledged adversities can differ on a wide range of other dimensions, over and above their badness, including distribution and imminence (Rescher, 1983), cost benefit direction, voluntariness, and moral acceptability (Heyman & Henriksen, 1998, p. 42). Differences in cost benefit direction, for example, make those who benefit directly from risk acceptance more tolerant of possible adversity than those who face collateral damage without the prospect of gain.

Even if it is granted that many health conditions are so universally detested that they can be pragmatically treated as adverse events, it must still be recognized that this attribution entails a heuristic simplification. However, the status of events as adverse becomes problematic in at least three circumstances: where their negative value is contested, historically or culturally; where the meaning of an event is affected by contextual factors; and where multiple positively and negatively valued consequences follow from the same event.

The value of some personal attributes is contested, making problematic their categorization as medical conditions. Many people, including the present author, regard with abhorrence the historic stigmatization of homosexuality as a medical condition. The disability movement (Oliver, 1990) has challenged the prevailing, often implicit, "personal tragedy theory" of such conditions and is associated with the assertion of the positive value of, for example, deafness. Down syndrome provides a good example of a condition which may or may not be thought of as adverse because, with modern medical care, many of those with the syndrome can expect to enjoy a close to average life expectancy with reasonable prospects of good health. A conflict of values giving rise to distinctive assessments of the adversity of an event class is evident in the following quotation.

> I had a time with the Down's syndrome. That was horrendous . . . because of the age thing, people telling you that if you're a certain, well, over 30, there's a risk, and over 35, there is, like, a bigger risk and everything, you know. So we thought, 'We'll look into it'. And we'd decided that, if the baby was Down's, we would keep the baby, no question, you know, and we were both happy with that. (Interview with woman, aged 38, no rejected genetic tests)

The above account well illustrates the power of a risk framework as a form of governmentality, as the categorization of the birth of a baby with Down syndrome as a risk is heard as prescriptive in societies that treat risk as a forensic device (Douglas, 1990). This categorization carries with it the unstated assumption that such a birth is adverse, eliding probability into risk. Tacitly prescriptive governmentality contrasts with the surface liberalism which presents the application of the new genetics as simply an extension of patient choice (Petersen & Bunton, 2002).

The contextualization of values represents the most important process leading to different evaluations of the same event class. When respondents reflect on real-life, meaningful events, they usually locate them within a rich biographical framework from which their significance is derived, as illustrated in the following example.

> I would have got rid of the baby, because . . . I felt that I've got three kids . . . It shouldn't be their responsibility to look after their younger brother or sister if they were Down's syndrome or whatever . . . But I

think I've got my kids into such a way. They are very compassionate, they are caring kids. You know that they would feel the way I would feel, that, if anything would happen to mum and dad, I would look after. And I wouldn't want that for them, to have that responsibility. (Interview with woman, aged 37, amniocentesis)

This respondent derived the adversity, for her, of giving birth to a baby with Down syndrome from reasoning about the expected future behavior of her children. By implication, this event would have been more acceptable to her if her children had not been brought up to be so compassionate.

Such contextual influences will not be captured by research methods which investigate hypothetical risk decision making involving abstract values, for example, by the prisoner's dilemma paradigm relied upon by many cognitive psychologists such as Kahneman and Tversky (2000) and their followers. These authors define the research focus of Prospect Theory as "choices between simple monetary gambles with objectively specified probabilities and at most two nonzero outcomes" (p. x). Extrapolation to richly contextualized, multiple outcomes involving health outcomes which raise major life and death or quality-of-life issues with ill-defined probabilities is highly problematic.

A third issue in the attribution of adversity arises when, as is usually the case, an adversely viewed consequence occurs within a multitude of linked effects, of which some are rated as beneficial. In principle, this type of situation is covered by a utilitarian approach which defines rational action as the sum total of values for each consequence, multiplied by their probabilities. Whether decision makers do, or should, reason in this way can be questioned. However, The Royal Society definition does not even make it to the utilitarian starting line because it focuses on the probability of a "particular" adverse event. This decontextualizing of multiple values goes beyond a mere definition, giving rise to misunderstandings of apparently irrational behavior. For example, impoverished mothers may smoke because they feel that they could not otherwise manage to meet the needs of their children (Graham, 1987), not because they have failed to understand health messages about this lethal habit. Similarly, Bloor (1995) has argued that the unsafe behaviors of male sex workers can be explained in terms of powerlessness rather than ignorance or indifference to risk.

When a strong consensus exists within a social group about the negativity of an event class, this judgment may be heuristically projected onto, and experienced as, a property of the event. Such projection also serves the governmental purpose of attempted removal of value contests from the articulated agenda for debate, leaving those who do not share the prevailing perspective, for example, about the adversity of disability, at a disadvantage.

RISK AND TIME

The Royal Society definition of risk acknowledges its temporal dimension by proposing that adversity should be appraised over a "stated time period." The definition begs the obvious questions of who should specify this time boundary and how it should be determined. Varying the length of time over which consequences are considered will change the overall adversity of a risk both quantitatively and qualitatively. For example, the global ecological debate turns crucially on the issue of whether decision making takes into account risks associated with climate change over centuries or focuses on the short-term expense of transforming the carbon economy. Young people may discount health education messages about smoking because they do not feel concerned about health effects that usually take decades to manifest themselves.

The quotation given above, in which a woman discusses the impact of having a baby with Down syndrome upon the adult lives of her existing young children after her death, well illustrates the potential impact of a decades-long time frame on an immediate medical decision. Other women focus on the immediate emotional impact of going through an abortion. One participant in our Down syndrome study avoided chromosomal testing because she did not want her pregnancy experience spoilt by anxiety during the waiting period for test results.

> And I thought, well, if I'm at high risk [from serum screening], then you are waiting. You go and have the amniocentesis, and you are waiting three weeks for that. And then they could say there is something wrong, but, at the end of the day, there might not be. So you've got all those months of chewing and preparing yourself, and then you have a normal baby. So why not have a nine month happy pregnancy, and then worry at the end of the day? (Woman, aged 36, interview, no genetic tests)

Such responses should not be dismissed as short-termist and therefore irrational. Future management in Western societies appears to be tacitly modeled on the decades-long time frame of a traditional middle-class, predominantly male, career, while the immediate present and longer time scales are neglected. Thus, strategies for preventing the birth of children with Down syndrome, and minimizing the requirements which they place on health and educational services, are well-developed. In contrast, the slowly increasing risk posed by, for example, the gradual accumulation of resistance to antibiotics is ignored, while their prophylactic use in animal husbandry is tolerated.

In critical situations, including pregnancy, the present may loom large while the future is backgrounded. Moreover, because events are causally interconnected, they can operate in multiple time frames, blurring the distinction between immediate and longer term consequences. The risk of maternal postnatal depression is as neglected in the Western health care system as that of fetal abnormalities is emphasized (Datamonitor, 2002). However, insofar as stress during pregnancy affects mental health, its consequences may endure long after the pregnancy. One couple whom we interviewed four months after they had opted for a termination were still experiencing severe distress.

> I feel I've aged ten years. I feel shattered. I mean, I am shattered. I've hardly slept, and things like that, chewing over the facts of why of, sort of why, how, you know, could it happen again? And if it does, you know, I mean we've got to through it again. (Husband of woman, aged 46, interview after pregnancy termination, amniocentesis)

Ripples of causality can transform the immediate into the very long-term. Risk management can only be understood in relation to the time frames that the social actors adopt. Stating a time period for assessing adversity merely projects, usually implicitly, the values of those who attempt to impose it.

RISK, PROBABILITY, AND EXPECTATION

The terms "probability" and "risk" are sometimes used interchangeably. However, for a probability to become a risk, a categorized and selected risk entity must be judged adverse within a chosen time frame. Probabilistic reasoning, nevertheless, represents the core of a risk perspective, providing an understanding of the future in terms of the operation of the laws of chance, as against the "whim of the gods" mentioned by Bernstein (1996) in the opening quotation.

Beyond the quantum level, chance operates only metaphorically. Its laws provide a means of predicting outcomes which a risk manager cannot model specifically on account of their causal complexity. Probabilistic induction offers a simplified heuristic which provides limited understanding of two types of complexity: intrinsic and knowledge-based. Intrinsic complexity arises where causal factors interact in non-linear fashion and affect each other through feedback, giving rise to an exponential relationship between the number of determinants and states of the system (Albrecht, Freeman, & Higginbotham, 1998; Griffiths & Byrne, 1998). Health effects usually demonstrate intrinsic complexity, which takes their specific modeling beyond the scope of any feasible computational procedures.

Knowledge-based complexity arises when the risk manager lacks information which would remove the chance element from prediction of a future contingency. A stranger, completely lost in a strange town and deciding to turn left rather than right, faces a 50 percent chance of choosing the right direction, while a local resident may make the same choice with certainty. Intrinsic and knowledge-based probabilistic reasoning differ only in that the former refers to causal processes that could never be totally specified because the number of combinations in questions exceeds any conceivable computing power, while the complexity of the latter depends upon the risk manager's expertise.

Even though complexity, intrinsic or knowledge-based, may preclude specific modeling, some empirically justified absolute or conditional expectations can be generated by aggregating outcomes and estimating their rate of occurrence inductively. For example, the causal processes leading to a trisomy 21 conception and Down syndrome are ill-understood. However, inductive observation shows that, currently in the U.K., about 1:700 live-born babies have the condition. A woman may be told that she faces such a probability of this event, or may be given her age-related probability, for example 1:190 at age 38. These conditional statistics are derived from partitioning the numerator and denominator for rate estimation in terms of the states of one or more marker variables observed to be associated with the outcome in question.

Although not any probability of an event class may be validly induced from the same set of observations, many can, depending upon how the data are partitioned. I have found that exposition of this idea to health professionals usually provokes a shocked reaction because they have learned to think of probability as a property of events rather than of knowledge. The following procedural description exposes the heuristic process through which expectation is reframed as probability in risk analysis. First, take a set of entities, for example, people, and observe which of them possess the risk attribute of interest; then divide the set into subgroups in terms of predictor variables; then observe the rate of possession of the adverse property in each subcategory; then attribute the observed rate in each subcategory to each individual who falls into it. Finally, attribute this rate to new individuals within the subcategory.

The fallacy of inductive reasoning in this procedure (the sun eventually will not rise) may offend purists but can, perhaps, be tolerated in health risk management because many of the complex causal processes that give rise to health needs often remain historically invariant to some extent. However, its operation also depends upon acceptance of the ecological fallacy that aggregated properties, in this case a rate of occurrence within a category, may be attributed to the individuals within that category. The following quotation illustrates the operation of the ecological fallacy in clinical practice.

> What the blood test will do is measure hormone levels. And it will give you an individual risk, right. So it will say, it won't tell you that your baby has got Down's syndrome, or hasn't got Down's syndrome . . . But what it does is, instead of giving you the risk of all women who are 35, it gives you your own risk. (Hospital consultation with woman, aged 35, who chose serum screening)

The notion of an individual risk, or, more accurately, individual probability, is an oxymoron because probabilities, at least inductively derived ones, can only appertain to aggregates. At the individual level, a woman either is or is not carrying a fetus with Down syndrome, as could be determined by an invasive diagnostic test such as amniocentesis. Serum and other forms of screening are used merely to further divide the category of women of a given age into subgroups with probabilities higher and lower than the overall, inductively estimated rate for that age group. (For a discussion of the complexities of Bayesian reasoning, and their misunderstanding by health professionals, with respect to screening, see Hoffrage, Kurzenhäuser, & Gigerenzer, this volume.)

Projection of aggregated attributions onto individuals establishes their apparent facticity, and may make them more persuasive as a guide to conduct. However, this heuristic, deeply embedded in the culture of risk societies, has certain unsatisfactory and even bizarre consequences. Firstly, health service users may feel let down by probabilistic knowledge that applies only to aggregates while they are concerned above all with personal outcomes.

> I felt that that was, like, a bit impersonal, you know, to be told about statistics and that, and things like that . . . I just wanted to know what, what could be done and what couldn't be done, you know. (Pregnant woman, aged 40, interview, amniocentesis)

Other women drew upon the limitations of the probability heuristic in order to undermine its governmental power.

> My husband knows someone who was only in his early 40s now, and he's got a Down's syndrome boy, and he's in his 20s. And both him and his wife were in their early 20s when they had him. And I think, well, it can happen at that age. It can happen any time. (Pregnant woman, aged 38, interview, no genetic tests)

Such apparent anomalies are entirely to be expected because the probability heuristic only specifies overall rates, not individual outcomes. (Moreover, the greater birth rate among younger women counterbalances their lower odds of carrying a fetus with Down syndrome. The probability of a maternal age given Down syndrome cannot be equated with the probability of Down syndrome given a maternal age. Most babies with Down syndrome will be born to younger mothers just because most babies are born to younger mothers.) The above respondent used this limitation in order to invalidate the knowledge base which categorized her as a higher risk case and, therefore, in need of testing.

Second, risk managers can exercise a degree of control over the probability of an adverse event by choosing how much information to obtain about it. Older women could console themselves by considering the overall rate of Down syndrome births at the hospital they were attending.

> That sort of, like, cheers me up . . . 4,500 or something . . . , and only 5 of them were Down's syndrome. (Pregnant woman, aged 39, interview after taped hospital consultation, amniocentesis)

She used this statistic to counter the other probability which she had been given, that a woman of her age had a probability of 1:120 of giving birth to a baby with Down syndrome. The lower overall rate arose from the young average age of women attending the maternity clinic. Different probabilities can be induced for the same numerator (number of fetuses with Down syndrome) depending upon how the denominator (number of pregnancies) is divided.

Some women chose not to undergo screening or diagnostic tests because they did not want to risk changing a prior probability.

> I didn't want to have the, em, I could have had the amnio, because I didn't want to be placed in a position of having to decide about a termination, because I knew I wouldn't want one. But I thought, once you know for a fact that you have a Down's syndrome child, would that change you?

Would you then want to have a termination because you would feel pressure . . . from other people. (Pregnant midwife, aged 36, interview, no genetic tests)

Her age-related probability, around 1:310, would either increase to almost 1 or decrease to almost 0 following an accurate diagnostic test. Having ruled out termination, she preferred to leave her probability at a level which legitimated not taking further action rather than run the risk of changing it.

THE PROBABILITY HEURISTIC AND SOCIAL STEREOTYPES

Probabilistic reasoning represents a way of managing complexity based on induction from observed averages and attribution of such collective statistics to individuals belonging to the event class in question. Because complex health phenomena are associated with multiple, interrelated predictors, many alternative grouping criteria may work well enough, providing some increase in predictive power over the unpartitioned population rate. In this gray zone, choice between alternatives offering some predictive power may be swayed by social attitudes, a point that is best illustrated by examples.

During the early days of the AIDS pandemic, the disease was popularly branded as a "gay plague." However, the increased risk incurred by gay men was mediated by sexual behaviors which, at the time, occurred more frequently among gay men. Monogamous gay men, or those who used barrier contraceptives, were not at higher risk. Those who thought of this risk as a gay plague thus chose to latch onto a proxy variable, sexual orientation, rather than the causal factor, sexual behavior, with which it was only loosely associated (Schiller, Crystal, & Lewellen, 1994). This choice of predictors could be legitimated through the operation of grounded rationality (Gigerenzer & Selten, 1999) as working well enough, albeit suboptimally. However, the choice of a socially marked proxy variable as the predictive indicator of high risk reinforces social prejudices against stigmatized groups. This analysis connects qualitative risk analysis to traditional concerns of classical social psychology, such as inter-group conflict, stereotyping, and racial prejudice.

Other examples of the socially stereotyped selection of proxy variables in risk thinking can easily be identified. For example, the high crime rate among young black men living in impoverished, inner city areas arises because poor young men are more likely to commit crimes, and many such men are black on account of demography and economic discrimination. To the prejudiced, being black, rather than young and poor, becomes the marker of crime (Harris, 2001). Similarly, Bowler (1993) studied the belief of midwives working in one U.K. Midlands maternity ward that women of Asian origin were both less prone to pain in labor and more pain intolerant. The proxy variable in this case was greater average family size and, therefore, higher mean parity. On average, Indian women experienced less labor pain because they were less likely to be having their first baby during a given birth. Those Indian women who were undergoing their first labor experienced as much pain as those from other ethnic groups but were branded as intolerant of pain because of the belief system outlined above. Again, choice of a proxy variable which worked predictively to some extent both reflected and fueled racial prejudice.

CONCLUSIONS: RISK ANALYSIS AS A FORM OF GOVERNMENTALITY

This chapter has outlined a qualitative approach to health risk which explores the complex, usually tacit, assumptions on which the facticity of risks is founded. Risks, which can be recognized only in cultures which reason probabilistically, need selective attention, homogenization, value judgments, time framing, and acceptance of the ecological fallacy before they can become established as cultural entities. Even contingencies cannot exist unless a risk manager groups the events for probabilistic induction. This lukewarm, but not rejecting, attitude to the value of risk management as a strategy for colonizing the future contrasts with the unbridled enthusiasm shown by The Royal Society (1992) and others (Bernstein, 1996). Official risk knowledge derived from the application of science in conditions of ultimately incalculable complexity is merely heuristic. Therefore, lay simplifications, for example, gauging probabilities in terms of single available events, should be considered as heuristics about heuristics, doubly removed from the complexities that are being modeled.

The governmentality approach argues that risk selection provides a form of social control in science-based societies. An indefinitely large range of potentially identifiable contingencies of possible concern languish unrecognized, outside the scope of risk management. The selection of a small proportion entails a form of attempted social control which is sustained through micro-interaction, as illustrated above.

Alternative fast and frugal heuristics may guide decision making well enough, but their selection becomes a matter of serious political and cultural significance once they are taken out of the laboratory and put into the real world. Social scientists interested in the latter can, through qualitative analysis, study a modern governmentality that is internalized in the human mind by analyzing the reification of risks and also their deconstruction by those who are targeted for risk management.

NOTE

1. The term "risk manager" will be used to refer generically to refer to persons who deal with a risk, as accredited experts, through direct involvement or as concerned members of the public.

REFERENCES

Albrecht, G., Freeman, S., & Higginbotham, N. (1998). Complexity and human health: The case for a transdisciplinary paradigm. *Culture, Medicine & Psychiatry, 22,* 55–92.

Bloor, M. (1995). A user's guide to contrasting theories of HIV-related risk behaviour. In J. Gabe (Ed.), *Medicine, health and risk: Sociological approaches* (pp. 19–30). Oxford, England: Blackwell.

Bowler, I. (1993). 'They're not the same as us': Midwives' stereotypes of South Asian descent maternity patients. *Sociology of Health and Illness, 15,* 157–177.

Datamonitor (2002). *Postpartum depression: Overcoming unique barriers to treatment.* Retrieved 2002 from http://www.datamonitor.com.

Douglas, M. (1990). *Risk as a forensic resource.* Daedalus, 119, 1–16.

Douglas, M. (1994). *Risk and blame: Essays in cultural theory.* London: Routledge.

Graham, H. (1987). Women's smoking and family health. *Social Science & Medicine, 25,* 47–56.

Gigerenzer, G., & Selten, R. (Eds.). (1999). *Bounded rationality: The adaptive toolbox.* Cambridge, MA: MIT Press.

Griffiths, F., & Byrne, D. (1998). General practice and the new science emerging from the theories of 'chaos' and complexity. *British Journal of General Practice, 48,* 1697–1699.

Hacking, I. (1975). *The emergence of probability: A philosophical study of early ideas about probability, induction and statistical inference.* Cambridge, England: Cambridge University Press.

Harris, D. R. (2001). Why are whites and blacks averse to black neighbors? *Social Science Research, 30,* 100–116.

Heyman, B., & Henriksen, M. (1998). Values and health risks. In B. Heyman (Ed.), *Risk, health and health care: A qualitative approach* (pp. 27–64). London: Edward Arnold.

Heyman, B., & Henriksen, M. (2001). *Risk, age and pregnancy: A case study of prenatal genetic screening and testing.* Basingstoke, England: Palgrave.

Hutter, B. M. (2001). *Regulation and risk: Occupational health and safety on the railways.* Oxford, England: Oxford University Press.

Kahneman, D., & Tversky, A. (2000). *Choices, values and frames.* Cambridge, England: Cambridge University Press.

Lupton, D. (2000). *Risk.* London: Routledge.

Oliver, M. (1990). *The politics of disablement.* London: Macmillan.

Petersen, A., & Bunton, R. (2002). *The new genetics and the public's health.* London: Routledge.

Rescher, N. (1983). *Risk: A philosophical introduction.* Washington, DC: University Press of America.

Royal Society, The. (1992). Risk: Analysis, perception and management. Report of a Royal Society Study Group. London: The Royal Society.

Schiller, N. G., Crystal, S., & Lewellen, D. (1994). Risky business: The cultural construction of AIDS risk groups. *Social Science & Medicine, 38,* 1337–1346.

Skolbekken, J. A. (1995). The risk epidemic in medical journals. *Social Science and Medicine, 40,* 291–305.

Chapter 5

UNDERSTANDING THE RESULTS OF MEDICAL TESTS: WHY THE REPRESENTATION OF STATISTICAL INFORMATION MATTERS

*Ulrich Hoffrage, Stephanie Kurzenhäuser,
and Gerd Gigerenzer*

Women are generally informed that mammography screening reduces the risk of dying from breast cancer by 25 percent. Does that mean that for every 100 women who participate in screening, 25 lives will be saved? Although many people believe this to be the case, it is incorrect. The percentage means that for 1,000 women who participate in screening, 3 will die from breast cancer within 10 years, whereas for 1,000 women who do not participate, 4 will die. The difference between 4 and 3 is the 25 percent "relative risk reduction." Expressed as an "absolute risk reduction," the benefit is 1 in 1,000.

The topic of this chapter is the representation of information on medical risks. As the case of mammography screening illustrates, the same information can be presented in various ways. The choice among alternative representations can influence patients' hopes and fears, risks and choices, and ultimately their behavior. For example, women were most likely to accept screening for cancer when the benefits of screening were presented as a relative risk reduction, less likely to do so when the absolute risk reduction was used, and least likely when the benefits were presented in terms of the numbers of women that need to be screened in order to save one life (Sarfati, Howden-Chapman, Woodward, & Salmond, 1998). This observation leaves us with a dilemma. According to Sarfati et al. (1998), health professionals have to make a choice. In order to enhance participation rates, they can either frame the benefits of screening in the most positive light, or they can present the information to reduce framing effects—for example, by expressing the benefits in a variety of forms. The authors contend that there may be a tension between these approaches. While the former is arguably manipulative, the latter may enhance informed choice but reduce participation rates in screening programs.

In our view, high participation rates should not be an ideal per se. Instead, each woman should be helped to understand the pros and cons of screening, to clarify her own values, and to consider the decision that would be best for her. Informed consent involves more than signing a form. In the present chapter, we assume that the patient and physician share the same goal, namely, to reach such an informed decision, based on the patient's understanding of the benefits and risks of a treatment or the chances that a particular diagnosis is right or wrong. There are two necessary steps toward this ideal. First, physicians themselves need to understand the statistical information and its implications, and second, they need to learn how to communicate this information to the patients. This double requirement contrasts sharply with the fact that physicians are rarely trained in risk communication. The lack of training may explain why previous research observed that a majority of physicians do not use relevant statistical information properly. Casscells, Schoenberger, and Grayboys (1978), for example, asked 60 house officers, students, and physicians at Harvard Medical School to estimate the probability of an unnamed disease, given the following information:

> If a test to detect a disease whose prevalence is 1/1,000 has a false positive rate of 5 per cent, what is the chance that a person found to have a positive result actually has the disease, assuming that you know nothing about the person's symptoms or signs? (p. 999)

The estimates varied wildly, from the most frequent estimate, 95 percent (27 out of 60), to 2 percent (11 out of 60). The value of 2 percent is obtained by inserting the problem information into Bayes's rule—assuming that the sensitivity of the test, which is not specified in the problem, is approximately 100 percent. Casscells et al. (1978) concluded that "in this group of students and physicians, formal decision analysis was almost entirely unknown and even common-sense reasoning about the interpretation of laboratory data was uncommon" (p. 1000).

In an article on probabilistic reasoning about mammography, Eddy (1982) reported an informal study in which he asked several physicians to estimate the probability of breast cancer given a base rate (*prevalence*) of 1 percent, a hit rate (*sensitivity,* here the proportion of positive mammograms among women with breast cancer) of 79 percent, and a false-positive rate (proportion of positive mammograms among women without breast cancer; the complement of the *specificity*) of 9.6 percent. He reported that 95 out of 100 physicians estimated the posterior probability of breast cancer given a positive mammogram (the *positive predictive value*) to be between 70 percent and 80 percent, whereas Bayes's rule results in a value one order of magnitude smaller, namely, 7.7 percent. Eddy proposed that the majority of physicians confused the sensitivity of the test with the positive predictive value. Evidence of this confusion can also be found in medical textbooks and journal articles (Eddy, 1982) as well as in statistical textbooks (Gigerenzer, 1993).

In 1986, Windeler and Köbberling reported responses to a questionnaire they mailed to family physicians, surgeons, internists, and gynecologists in Germany. Only 13 of the 50 respondents realized that an increase in the prevalence of a disease implies an increase in the positive predictive value. The authors concluded with a puzzling observation. Although intuitive judgment of probabilities is part of every diagnostic and treatment decision, the physicians in their study were unaccustomed to estimating quantitative probabilities. Given these demonstrations that many physicians' reasoning does not follow the laws of probability (Abernathy & Hamm, 1995; Dawes, 1988; Dowie & Elstein, 1988), what can be done to improve diagnostic inferences? In the remainder of this chapter we propose an easy way to help physicians and patients understand statistical information and its consequences, and we report empirical evidence from three studies demonstrating the benefits of the proposed method. We conclude with a discussion of the impact of this research on medical education, AIDS counseling, and DNA fingerprinting.

NATURAL FREQUENCIES HELP IN MAKING DIAGNOSTIC INFERENCES

Each of the three studies, summarized above, presented numerical information in the form of probabilities and percentages. The same holds for other studies in which the conclusion was that physicians (Berwick, Fineberg, & Weinstein, 1981; Politser, 1984) and lay persons (Koehler, 1996a) have great difficulty in making diagnostic inferences from statistical information. Whether the information is presented as probabilities, percentages, absolute frequencies, or another form is irrelevant from a mathematical viewpoint. However, they are not equivalent from a psychological viewpoint, which is the key to our argument.

We argue that a specific class of representations, which we call *natural frequencies,* help lay persons and experts make inferences the Bayesian way. We illustrate the difference between probabilities and natural frequencies with the diagnostic problem of inferring the presence of colorectal cancer (C) from a positive result in the hemoccult test (pos), a standard diagnostic test. In terms of probabilities, the relevant information is a base rate for colorectal cancer [p(C)] of 0.3 percent, a sensitivity [p(pos|C)] of 50 percent, and a false-positive rate [p(pos|¬C)] of 3 percent. In natural frequencies, the same information would read, "Thirty out of every 10,000 persons have colorectal cancer. Of these 30 with cancer, 15 will have a positive hemoccult test. Of the remaining 9,970 people *without* colorectal cancer, 300 will have a positive hemoccult test." Natural frequencies are absolute frequencies, as they result from sequentially encoding and aggregating observations from a population (or a representative sample). Natural frequencies have not been normalized with respect to the base rates of disease and nondisease (Gigerenzer & Hoffrage, 1995, 1999). Natural frequencies should be distinguished from probabilities, percentages, relative frequencies, and other representations where the underlying natural frequencies have been normalized with respect to these base rates. For example, the following representation of the colorectal cancer problem is not in terms of natural frequencies (Gigerenzer & Hoffrage, 1995), because the frequencies have been normalized with respect to the base rates: a base rate of 30 in 10,000, a sensitivity of 5,000 in 10,000, and a false-positive rate of 300 in 10,000.

Why should natural frequencies facilitate diagnostic inferences? There are two related arguments. The first is computational. Bayesian computations are simpler when the information is represented in natural frequencies rather than in probabilities, percentages, or relative frequencies (Christensen-Szalanski & Bushyhead, 1981; Kleiter, 1994). For example, when the information concerning colorectal cancer is represented in probabilities, applying a cognitive algorithm to compute the positive predictive value, that is, the Bayesian posterior probability, amounts to performing the computation shown in the left side of Figure 5.1. The result is 0.048. This equation is Bayes's rule for binary hypotheses (here, C and ¬C) and data (here, positive and negative test result). The rule is named after Thomas Bayes (1702–1761), who is credited with solving the problem of how to make an inference from data to hypothesis (Stigler, 1983). As can be seen from the right side of Figure 5.1, the computations are much simpler when the information is presented in natural frequencies. The equation in the right box is Bayes's rule for natural frequencies, where [C&pos] is the number of cases with cancer and a positive test, and [¬C&pos] is the number of cases without cancer but with a positive test.

The second argument supplements the first. Minds appear to be tuned to make inferences from natural frequencies rather than from probabilities and percentages. This argument is consistent with developmental studies indicating the primacy of reasoning with discrete numbers over fractions, and studies of adult humans and animals indicating the ability to monitor frequency information in natural environments in fairly accurate and automatic ways (Gallistel & Gelman, 1992; Jonides & Jones, 1992; Real, 1991; Sedlmeier, Hertwig, & Gigerenzer, 1998). For most of their existence, humans have made inferences from information encoded sequentially through direct experience, and natural frequencies are

Figure 5.1
Why natural frequencies facilitate the computation of the probability p(C|pos) of cancer given a positive test (a form of Bayesian reasoning). The symbols "C" and "¬C" stand for colorectal cancer and no colorectal cancer, respectively, and "pos" and "neg" stand for a positive and negative test result, respectively. One can see that Bayes's rule for probabilities (left side) involves more calculation than that for natural frequencies (right side).

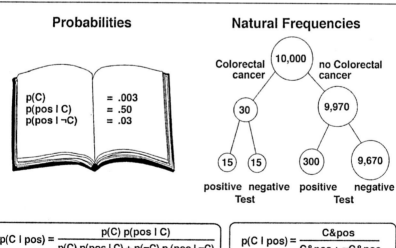

the final tally of such a process. Mathematical probability emerged in the mid-seventeenth century (Daston, 1988), and not until after the French Revolution did percentages appear to have become commonly used, mainly for taxes and interest, and only very recently for risk and uncertainty (Gigerenzer, Swijtink, Porter, Daston, Beatty, & Krüger, 1989). Minds might have evolved to deal with natural frequencies rather than with probabilities.

We tested whether natural frequencies improve Bayesian inference in lay persons, medical students, and physicians.

DO NATURAL FREQUENCIES IMPROVE LAYPERSONS' REASONING?

We first tested students in various fields at the University of Salzburg (Gigerenzer & Hoffrage, 1995). We used 15 problems, including Eddy's mammography problem and Tversky and Kahneman's (1982) cab problem. When the information was presented in natural frequencies rather than in probabilities, the proportion of Bayesian responses increased for each of the 15 problems. The average proportions of Bayesian responses were 16 percent for probabilities and 46 percent for natural frequencies (Gigerenzer & Hoffrage, 1995). Similarly, Cosmides and Tooby (1996) showed that natural frequencies improve Bayesian inferences in the Casscells et al. (1978) problem as well. This hypothetical medical problem is numerically simpler (the hit rate is assumed to be 100%) than the problems in the Gigerenzer and Hoffrage (1995) study, and Cosmides and Tooby reported that 76 percent of the answers were Bayesian (see also Christensen-Szalanski & Beach, 1982). These results lead us to conclude that natural frequencies improve Bayesian reasoning without instruction, at least in laypersons.

But would medical experts also profit from natural frequencies, and do they use them in communicating risks to their clients? The following two studies with medical students and experienced physicians provide an answer to the first question; a study with AIDS counselors addresses the second question.

DO NATURAL FREQUENCIES IMPROVE MEDICAL STUDENTS' DIAGNOSTIC INFERENCES?

We chose four realistic diagnostic tasks and constructed two versions of each. In one, the information was presented in probabilities, and in the other, the information was presented in natural frequencies. The four diagnostic tasks were to infer (a) the presence of colorectal cancer from a positive hemoccult test, (b) the presence of breast cancer from a positive mammogram, (c) the presence of phenylketonuria from a positive Guthrie test, and (d) the presence of ankylosing spondylitis from a positive HL-antigen-B27 (HLA-B27) test. The information on prevalence, sensitivity, and false positives was taken from the literature (Hoffrage & Gigerenzer, 2004; Hoffrage, Lindsey, Hertwig, & Gigerenzer, 2000).

Participants were 87 medical students, most of whom had already passed a course in biostatistics and were, on average, in their fifth year, and 9 first-year interns. Fifty-four studied in Berlin, and 42 in Heidelberg; 52 were female, and 44 were male. The average age was 25 years. Participants were paid a participation fee of 15 DM (approx. $7.50). They worked on the questionnaire at their own pace and in small groups of three to six. The experimenter asked them to make notes, calculations, or drawings, so that we could reconstruct their reasoning. Interviews were performed after the participants completed their questionnaire.

When a participant's estimate was within plus or minus 5 percent of the Bayesian estimate, and the notes and interview indicated that the estimate was arrived at by Bayesian reasoning (Gigerenzer & Hoffrage, 1995) rather than by guessing or other means, we then classified the response as a "Bayesian inference." For each task, the percentages of Bayesian inferences were higher when the information was presented in natural frequencies rather than in probabilities. Across all participants and across all four problems, the percentage of Bayesian inferences was 18 percent when the information was given in probabilities and 57 percent when it was given in natural frequencies (Figure 5.2). Moreover, if we consider only the estimates that were not classified as Bayesian inferences, the absolute deviation from the Bayesian answer was 21 percent lower for the frequency problems than for the probability problems (42%) (Hoffrage & Gigerenzer, 2004). In conclusion, medical students encountered problems similar to those of laypersons when the information was in probabilities, but their reasoning improved more than laypersons when frequency representations were used.

DO NATURAL FREQUENCIES IMPROVE PHYSICIANS' DIAGNOSTIC INFERENCES?

Would these findings generalize to experienced physicians who treat real patients? Forty-eight physicians participated in the following study (Gigerenzer, 1996; Hoffrage & Gigerenzer, 1998). They had practiced

Figure 5.2
Effect of information representation (probabilities versus natural frequencies) on statistical reasoning in laypeople, medical students, and physicians, based on 15 Bayesian inference tasks for laypeople and 4 each for medical students and physicians.

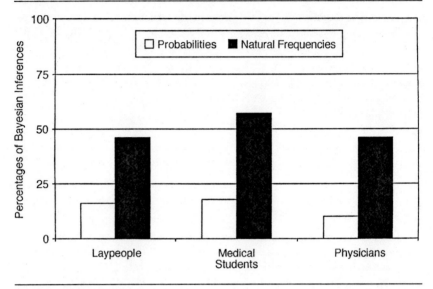

Source: Data from Gigerenzer & Hoffrage, 1995; Hoffrage et al., 2000; Hoffrage & Gigerenzer, 1998.

for an average of 14 years (1 month to 32 years) and had a mean age of 42 years (26 to 59). They worked either in Munich or Düsseldorf. Eighteen were female, and 30 were male. Eighteen worked in university hospitals, 16 in private or public hospitals, and 14 in private practice. The sample included internists, gynecologists, dermatologists, and radiologists, among others. The physicians' status ranged from directors of clinics to physicians commencing their careers.

The interviewer first informed the physician about our interest in studying diagnostic inference and established a relaxed personal rapport. Each physician was then given the same four diagnostic tasks as in the previous study. Each problem was printed on a sheet of paper, and the interviewer asked the physician to make notes, calculations, or drawings so that we could later reconstruct their reasoning. After the physician completed the four tasks, if it could not be discerned how the estimate was made in each task, the physician was asked for clarification. In two diagnostic tasks, the information was presented in probabilities, and in the other two, in natural frequencies. We systematically varied which tasks were in which format and which format was presented first with the constraint that the first two tasks had the same format. To classify a strategy as Bayesian, we used the same criteria as in the previous study.

These physicians reasoned the Bayesian way more often when the information was communicated in natural frequencies than when it was communicated in probabilities. The effect varied among problems, but even in the problem showing the weakest effect (phenylketonuria), the proportion of Bayesian answers was twice as large. For the two cancer problems, natural frequencies increased Bayesian inferences by more than a factor of five as compared to probabilities. Across all problems, the physicians gave the Bayesian answer in only 10 percent of the cases that used probabilities. When natural frequencies were used, this value increased to 46 percent (Figure 5.2).

With probabilities, physicians spent an average of 25 percent more time solving the diagnostic problems than with natural frequencies. Moreover, physicians commented that they were nervous, tense, and uncertain more often when working with probabilities than when working with natural frequencies. They also stated that they were less skeptical of the relevance of statistical information when it was in natural frequencies. Physicians were conscious of their better and faster performance with natural frequencies. We asked the physicians how often they took statistical information into account when they interpreted the results of diagnostic tests. Twenty-six answered "very seldom" or "never," 15 answered "once in a while," 5 said "frequently," and none answered "always."

Their comments suggested two reasons why they used statistical information rather infrequently: the patient's uniqueness and the physician's innumeracy. The first reason can be illustrated by a comment from one of three physicians who refused to participate in the study and did not contribute to the data. This physician explained, "I can't do much with numbers. I am an intuitive being. I treat my patients in a holistic manner and don't use statistics." Similarly, a university professor who seemed agitated and affronted by the test and refused to give numerical estimates remarked, "This is not the way to treat patients. I throw all these journals [with statistical information] away immediately. One can't make a diagnosis on such a basis. Statistical information is one big lie."

The second reason for physicans' reluctance to use statistical information is related to the first. Several physicians perceived themselves as mathematically illiterate, or suffering from a cognitive disease known as "innumeracy" (Paulos, 1988). Six physicians explicitly remarked on their inability to deal with numbers, stating, for example, "But this is mathematics. I can't do that. I'm too stupid for this." With natural frequencies, however, these same physicians spontaneously reasoned statistically as often as their peers who did not complain of innumeracy.

TEACHING BAYESIAN REASONING

Only five of the 48 physicians from the last study stated that they had heard of Bayes's rule. If natural frequencies can foster Bayesian reasoning without instruction, it is straightforward to also use them in statistical education. Statistical information in medical textbooks, newspapers, and other media is most often displayed in a probability or percentage format. Perhaps training should enable participants to translate probabilities into natural frequencies.

Sedlmeier and Gigerenzer (2001) and Sedlmeier (1997) were the first to apply this idea to teaching. They designed a two-hour computerized tutorial where participants could learn to solve Bayesian tasks by translating probabilities into natural frequencies (Figure 5.1, right side). For comparison, participants in another group received the traditional training that teaches how to insert probabilities into Bayes's rule (Figure 5.1, left side). In the group who received the representation training, the proportion of Bayesian inferences in a test taken immediately after the training was substantially higher than in the group who received the traditional rule training.

But how quickly did students forget what they had learned? In several experiments, the students were re-tested between 1 week and 3 months later. The students who had gone through the rule training showed the typical forgetting effect. For example, in one study, performance was down to 20 percent after five weeks. In contrast, when students had learned frequency representations, their performance remained consistently at the level they had achieved immediately after training, which was a median of 90 percent Bayesian responses.

While the use of flexible computer-based tutorial systems has clear advantages, the range of possible applications is still limited. In German universities where traditional instruction in front of a classroom with a blackboard and an overhead projector is customary, the use of interactive tutorial programs is still the exception. Would the representation training approach still be successful when applied in this type of instructional setting? To answer this question, Kurzenhäuser and Hoffrage (2002) developed a one-hour classroom tutorial on Bayesian reasoning, based on the representation training approach, and tested it in a human genetics course for medical students. Participants were 208 medical students in an obligatory all-day course at the Free University of Berlin. To evaluate the relative effectiveness of the new approach in a classroom setting, we also included a traditional rule training condition; 109 participants received the representation training, and 99 participants received the rule training. The two approaches were evaluated two months later by testing the students' ability to solve a Bayesian inference task with information represented as probabilities. While both approaches improved performance compared to pre-test results, almost three times as many students were able to profit from the representation training as opposed to the rule training (47% and 16%, respectively).

AIDS COUNSELING FOR LOW-RISK CLIENTS

An important application of Bayesian reasoning is in AIDS counseling for low-risk clients. In Germany, the prevalence of HIV in heterosexual men who are in no known risk group is approximately 0.01 percent, the specificity of the HIV test is approximately 99.99 percent, and the sensitivity is approximately 99.9 percent. If a counselor communicates these numbers, the client will most likely not be able to work out his chances of having the virus if he tests positive. Most seem to assume that a positive test means infection. For example, in the early days of blood screening in Florida, after 22 blood donors were told they were HIV positive, seven committed suicide (Stine, 1996).

How do AIDS counselors explain what a positive test means to their clients? We studied AIDS counselors in German public health centers (Gigerenzer, Hoffrage, & Ebert, 1998). One of us visited 20 centers as a client to take 20 HIV tests and make use of the mandatory pre-test counseling. The counselor was asked the relevant questions concerning the prevalence of an HIV infection, the sensitivity and specificity of the test, and what the chances were that the client actually has the virus if the test was positive. Not one counselor communicated the risks to the client in natural frequencies. Instead, they all used probabilities and percentages, and in the majority of the counseling sessions, the information was either internally inconsistent or incorrect. For example, one counselor estimated the base rate at approximately 0.1 percent and the sensitivity and specificity at 99.9 percent, and concluded that the client's chance of having the virus if he tested positive is also 99.9 percent. In fact, 15 out of 20 counselors told their low-risk client that it is 99.9 percent or 100 percent certain that he has HIV if he tests positive.

If a counselor, however, communicates the information in natural frequencies, insight is more likely: "Think of 10,000 heterosexual men like yourself being tested. We expect that one has the virus, and this one will test positive. Of the remaining 9,999 uninfected men, one will also test positive. Thus, we expect that for every two men in this risk group who test positive, only one has HIV, or 50 percent."

In real-world contexts such as AIDS counseling, the difference between natural frequencies and probabilities can make the difference between hope and despair.

DNA FINGERPRINTING

The relevance of natural frequencies is not limited to medical diagnosis. As Koehler's work (e.g., 1996b) demonstrates, the difficulty in drawing inferences from probabilities also holds for DNA experts, judges, and prosecutors. Nevertheless, in criminal and paternity cases, the general practice in court is to present information in terms of probabilities or likelihood ratios, with the consequence that jurors, judges, and sometimes the experts themselves are confused and misinterpret the evidence. In a recent study, Hoffrage et al. (2000) demonstrated that both law students and jurists profit from natural frequencies. The percentage of Bayesian inferences rose from 3 percent to 45 percent when the format of the information concerning DNA fingerprinting changed from probabilities to natural frequencies. Possibly even more important, the participants who had seen the information in terms of probabilities had a higher conviction rate than those participants who had been given the same information in terms of natural frequencies (Hertwig & Hoffrage, 2002; Lindsey, Hertwig, & Gigerenzer, 2003).

CONCLUSIONS

Statistical reasoning is indispensable in a modern, technological democracy, similar to the ability to read and write (Gigerenzer, 2002). The last few decades have witnessed much debate on whether minds are equipped with the right or wrong rules for making judgments under conditions of uncertainty. However, the ability to draw inferences from statistical information depends not only on cognitive strategies but also on the format in which the numerical information is communicated. Insight can come from outside. External representation can perform part of the reasoning process. In our studies, natural frequencies improved both laypersons' and experts' statistical reasoning, with and without explicit teaching.

Basic research on reasoning can produce simple and powerful methods of communicating risks that can be of help in various public domains.

ACKNOWLEDGMENTS

We thank Rona Unrau for editing the manuscript and the German Research Foundation (DFG) for their financial support (Ho1847/1–2).

REFERENCES

Abernathy, C. M., & Hamm, R. M. (1995). *Surgical intuition: What it is and how to get it.* Philadelphia: Hanley & Belfus.

Berwick, D. M., Fineberg, H. V., & Weinstein, M. C. (1981). When doctors meet numbers. *American Journal of Medicine, 71,* 991–998.

Casscells, W., Schoenberger, A., & Grayboys, T. (1978). Interpretation by physicians of clinical laboratory results. *New England Journal of Medicine, 299,* 999–1000.

Christensen-Szalanski, J. J. J., & Beach, L. R. (1982). Experience and the base-rate fallacy. *Organizational Behavior and Human Performance, 29,* 270–278.

Christensen-Szalanski, J. J. J., & Bushyhead, J. B. (1981). Physicians' use of probabilistic information in a real clinical setting. *Journal of Experimental Psychology: Human Perception and Performance, 7,* 928–935.

Cosmides, L., & Tooby, J. (1996). Are humans good intuitive statisticians after all? Rethinking some conclusions from the literature on judgment under uncertainty. *Cognition, 58,* 1–73.

Daston, L. J. (1988). *Classical probability in the Enlightenment.* Princeton, NJ: Princeton University Press.

Dawes, R. M. (1988). *Rational choice in an uncertain world.* San Diego, CA: Harcourt, Brace, Jovanovich.

Dowie, J., & Elstein, A. (1988). *Professional judgment: A reader in clinical decision making.* Cambridge, England: Cambridge University Press.

Eddy, D. M. (1982). Probabilistic reasoning in clinical medicine: Problems and opportunities. In D. Kahneman, P. Slovic, & A. Tversky (Eds.), *Judgment under uncertainty: Heuristics and biases* (pp. 249–267). Cambridge, England: Cambridge University Press.

Gallistel, C. R., & Gelman, R. (1992). Preverbal and verbal counting and computation. *Cognition, 44,* 43–74.

Gigerenzer, G. (1993). The superego, the ego, and the id in statistical reasoning. In G. Keren & C. Lewis (Eds.), *A handbook for data analysis in the behavioral sciences: Methodological issues* (pp. 313–339). Hillsdale, NJ: Erlbaum.

Gigerenzer, G. (1996). The psychology of good judgment: Frequency formats and simple algorithms. *Journal of Medical Decision Making, 16,* 273–280.

Gigerenzer, G. (2002). *Calculated risks: How to know when numbers deceive you.* New York: Simon & Schuster.

Gigerenzer, G., & Hoffrage, U. (1995). How to improve Bayesian reasoning without instruction: Frequency formats. *Psychological Review, 102,* 684–704.

Gigerenzer, G., & Hoffrage, U. (1999). Overcoming difficulties in Bayesian reasoning: A reply to Lewis & Keren and Mellers & McGraw. *Psychological Review, 104,* 425–430.

Gigerenzer, G., Hoffrage, U., & Ebert, A. (1998). AIDS counselling for low-risk clients. *AIDS Care, 10,* 197–211.

Gigerenzer, G., Swijtink, Z., Porter, T., Daston, L., Beatty, J., & Krüger, L. (1989). *The empire of chance: How probability changed science and everyday life.* Cambridge, England: Cambridge University Press.

Hertwig, R., & Hoffrage, U. (2002). Technology needs psychology: How natural frequencies foster insight in medical and legal experts. In P. Sedlmeier & T. Betsch (Eds.), *Etc. Frequency processing and cognition* (pp. 285–302). New York: Oxford University Press.

Hoffrage, U., & Gigerenzer, G. (1998). Using natural frequencies to improve diagnostic inferences. *Academic Medicine, 73,* 538–540.

Hoffrage, U., & Gigerenzer, G. (2004). How to improve the diagnostic inferences of medical experts. In E. Kurz-Milcke & G. Gigerenzer (Eds.), *Experts in science and society* (pp. 249–268). New York: Kluwer Academic/Plenum Publishers.

Hoffrage, U., Lindsey, S., Hertwig, R., & Gigerenzer, G. (2000). Communicating statistical information. *Science, 290,* 2261–2262.

Jonides, J., & Jones, C. M. (1992). Direct coding for frequency of occurrence. *Journal of Experimental Psychology: Learning, Memory, and Cognition, 18,* 368–378.

Kleiter, G. D. (1994). Natural sampling: Rationality without base rates. In G. H. Fischer & D. Laming (Eds.), *Contributions to mathematical psychology, psychometrics, and methodology* (pp. 375–388). New York: Springer.

Koehler, J. J. (1996a). The base rate fallacy reconsidered: Descriptive, normative and methodological challenges. *Behavioral and Brain Sciences, 19,* 1–53.

Koehler, J. J. (1996b). On conveying the probative value of DNA evidence: Frequencies, likelihood ratios, and error rates. *University of Colorado Law Review, 67,* 859–886.

Kurzenhäuser, S., & Hoffrage, U. (2002). Teaching Bayesian reasoning: An evaluation of a classroom tutorial for medical students. *Medical Teacher, 24,* 531–536.

Lindsey, S., Hertwig, R., & Gigerenzer, G. (2003). Communicating statistical DNA evidence. *Jurimetrics, 43,* 147–163.

Paulos, J. A. (1988). *Innumeracy: Mathematical illiteracy and its consequences.* New York: Vintage Books.

Politser, P. E. (1984). Explanations of statistical concepts: Can they penetrate the haze of Bayes? *Methods of Information in Medicine, 23,* 99–108.

Real, L. A. (1991). Animal choice behavior and the evolution of cognitive architecture. *Science, 253,* 980–986.

Sarfati, D., Howden-Chapman, P., Woodward, A., & Salmond, C. (1998). Does the frame affect the picture? A study into how attitudes to screening for cancer are affected by the way benefits are expressed. *Journal of Medical Screening, 5,* 137–140.

Sedlmeier, P. (1997). BasicBayes: A tutor system for simple Bayesian inference. *Behavior Research Methods, Instruments, & Computers, 29,* 328–336.

Sedlmeier, P., & Gigerenzer, G. (2001). Teaching Bayesian reasoning in less than two hours. *Journal of Experimental Psychology: General, 130,* 380–400.

Sedlmeier, P., Hertwig, R., & Gigerenzer, G. (1998). Are judgments of the positional frequencies of letters systematically biased due to availability? *Journal of Experimental Psychology: Learning, Memory, and Cognition, 24,* 754–770.

Stigler, S. M. (1983). Who discovered Bayes's theorem? *American Statistician, 37,* 296–325.

Stine, G. J. (1996). *Acquired immune deficiency syndrome. Biological, medical, social and legal issues.* Englewood Cliffs, NJ: Prentice Hall.

Tversky, A., & Kahneman, D. (1982). Evidential impact of base rates. In D. Kahneman, P. Slovic, & A. Tversky (Eds.), *Judgment under uncertainty: Heuristics and biases* (pp. 153–160). Cambridge, England: Cambridge University Press.

Windeler, J., & Köbberling, J. (1986). Empirische Untersuchung zur Einschätzung diagnostischer Verfahren am Beispiel des Haemoccult-Tests [An empirical study of the judgments about diagnostic procedures using the example of the hemoccult test]. *Klinische Wochenschrift, 64,* 1106–1112.

EDITORIAL COMMENTARY

As this chapter clearly shows, many physicians do not understand the meaning of probabilities. The natural frequencies presentation should make sense to these clinicians. However, many patients would still find this concept confusing. Over the past thirty years I have had to tell patients what their findings mean on thousands of occasions. Because of the type of practice I have, I need to explain that they are at an increased risk for cancer, and then must find some way to quantify that risk. For some—a minority of patients—probabilities work well. For others, the natural frequencies are a meaningful method of expression. However, there remains a large fraction for which an analogy may best allow the patient to choose a course of action. For example, when a patient is overly concerned about a minor Pap smear abnormality, I will often tell her, "You are at greater risk driving home from the office than from this abnormality." On the other end of the risk spectrum, it is sometimes necessary to draw a very gloomy picture. On rare occasions I've told a patient that "You won't live to see your children graduate from high school if you don't. . . . " It is always a challenge when it is necessary to explain to a patient the risk of a certain disease or diagnosis, and the astute clinician varies the method of explanation based on a thorough knowledge of the patient.

—Kenneth L. Noller

Chapter 6

THE CENTRALITY OF THE CLINICIAN: A VIEW OF MEDICINE FROM THE GENERAL TO THE PARTICULAR

Kenneth L. Noller and Roger Bibace

It is hard to imagine any profession that must deal more often with both the general and the particular on a regular, daily basis than clinical medicine. Clinicians must constantly deal with the uniqueness of each particular patient. No person is exactly like any other, and each must be cared for as an individual. Physicians practice medicine by applying scientific principles, while biologists search for a universal truth by testing hypotheses. Acknowledgment of this dichotomous role is found in the phrase, "the art and science of medicine." The clinician must address the particular needs of the individual patient while utilizing the latest information from the scientific literature.

The purpose of this chapter is to demonstrate that the clinician (the one responsible for a particular patient, whether a physician, nurse practitioner, physician assistant, clinical psychologist, or other conveyor of medical care) is the only person who is in a position to make decisions about the care of a specific patient, but that this role requires a knowledge of universal principles—those of medical science. While those statements might seem to be straightforward, there is a growing belief held by some individuals that the role of the clinician is an anachronism; that there is no place for the practice of medicine; that the only way to care for illness is through the use of laboratory tests, sophisticated radiological imaging, and what is known as "evidence-based medicine."

THE MULTIPLE CAREERS OF MEDICAL STUDENTS

In the United States, a person who aspires to become a physician must first complete an undergraduate degree. Because medical schools require many credits in various sciences, most pre-meds major in one of the biological sciences. In addition to introductory course work, many will have taken upper-level courses such as "Human Physiology," "Human Anatomy," or any number of other subjects that deal with the human body. Despite these human-oriented courses, it is a shock for most first-year students when they quickly realize that almost nothing they learned in their undergraduate studies has prepared them for medical school. For the first two years, the course work is intense; the language is an arcane mixture of Latin, Greek, and English; and the volume of material that must be committed to memory is overwhelming. Most individuals apply to medical school because they have a genuine desire to help others. They are surprised to find that there is almost no mention of an actual living, breathing human during the first two years. Their professors are scientists who are often leaders in their fields and never miss a chance to make a disparaging remark about the differences between graduate students (true scientists) and professional students (applied scientists). Medical students are indoctrinated in the science of medicine. They eat and sleep the formulas for bizarre biochemical reactions; they puzzle the meaning of infinitesimally small changes in the respiratory gases of rabbits; they learn the names of organs and parts of organs and parts of the parts of organs. In short, they are forced to learn a great amount about all of those fields of scientific endeavor that deal with mammalian organisms.

Beginning, typically, in the latter part of the second year, medical students are first introduced to a course called "Physical Diagnosis." Their professors are no longer basic scientists, but individuals who are experts in the distinctions between "normal" and "not normal" in only one species—the human. Medical students often have trouble with this jump from basic to applied science. They have spent at least six years learning from books and laboratory experiments about the workings of various animals. For example, they have been taught that the muscle that runs from the heel to the back of the shin bone is called the *gastrocnemius*. They've learned about the physiology of muscle fibers and can draw out the chemical equations that result in muscle contraction. Now they must learn how to examine that muscle. For the first time in their fledgling careers, they cannot read a book to find the answer. The muscle must be examined. It must be touched (palpated). It must be observed. To make correct diagnoses, their senses of vision and touch must be trained. When the course moves on to other areas, they must learn how to use olfaction and hearing.

It is at this precise time in medical school that a fundamental decision is made by most students, though few are aware of it. Either they will devote themselves to the art of diagnosis and the care of individuals, or they will withdraw from contact with patients and enter one of the areas of medicine that does not require personal contact with patients. The first group becomes internists, surgeons, obstetricians, family physicians, cardiologists, or enters any one of over twenty other recognized specialties. Many of the second group become pathologists or radiologists. The first group touches patients and cares for them when they are ill. The second group examines tissues and cells and images and dictates reports. The first group has made a clear break with basic science. The second group feels in touch with science. The first group understands that it applies science. The second group believes that it creates science. Everything that the first group has learned about science for six years makes it believe that it is inferior to the second group.

MEDICAL SCIENCE AND EVIDENCE-BASED MEDICINE

It is only in the last two hundred years that there has been a "science of medicine." Even in the late seventeenth century, physicians were still trying to treat illnesses by realigning the balance of the four humors (Noller, 1993). The description of the circulatory system, the discovery of oxygen, the use of the microscope, the invention of anesthesia, and the germ theory of disease were the pilings upon which modern medicine was built. Like most construction projects, the science of medicine quickly rose from its base. Once antibiotics were developed, the field was open to much more aggressive management of diseases that physicians had feared for millennia. Pneumonia, cancer, and tuberculosis were no longer death sentences. When sophisticated laboratory tests became commonplace, the field of endocrinology began to explain many of the most baffling of medical conditions. More recently, the unraveling of the genetic code is leading to the understanding and treatment of even more bizarre human conditions.

Progress in the science of medicine in the last half of the twentieth century was truly remarkable. However, as more and more discoveries were made, it became more and more difficult for the practicing clinician to remain up-to-date. Where once there were a handful of medical journals, there are now thousands, and the number increases each month. In the United States, most physicians practice a specialty, that is, they limit their practice to one specific category of illness. Even with such concentration in one field, it is difficult to keep pace with new information.

Early in the twentieth century, most articles in medical journals were case series. In these papers, physicians reported their experiences with many of the same type of cases. For example, someone would report experience with 500 inguinal hernia repairs. The failure rate, infection rate, length of hospital stay, etc. would be listed. The article would likely be followed sometime later by one authored by a different clinician who would report better results, using a slightly different technique. While case series are useful and are easy to read, they have severe limitations. (For a more complete evaluation of the various types of studies and reports in medicine see chapter 7 by Chelmow, in this volume.)

In the 1960s, studies became more sophisticated and cases series became less common in the literature. Case-control studies, cohort studies, and, on rare occasions, randomized clinical trials (RCTs) became the norm (Grimes & Schultz, 2002a, 2002b; Lilienfield & Lilienfield, 1980; Schulz & Grimes, 2002). In all of these study designs, various methods are employed in attempts to reduce bias. In almost every case, such techniques result in a paper that is superior to a case series. They are also much harder to understand, and take much longer to read. The ever-increasingly sophisticated statistical analyses they use have almost become a game called "See if you can understand what these results mean." This has resulted in great "snobbishness" among some academicians who believe that the only type of report that is worth reading is an RCT. Because so few RCTs are published, those who accept this approach find that they can reduce their monthly scientific reading by many-fold. They often also fail to accept the fact that it is quite possible to perform and report a flawed RCT.

The problem of publication overload was recognized by several universities more or less simultaneously. In an effort to help the overburdened clinician, they proposed a classification system that evaluated the published literature in such a way that a clinician could better choose what to read and what to incorporate into day-to-day practice. Each paper is graded on its quality. Those papers based on the best study design, properly conducted, and appropriately analyzed are graded the highest. This process of grading is now called "evidence-based medicine (EBM)" (Rosenberg & Sackett, 1996). In an ideal world, only the best studies are read and incorporated into clinical practice.

There are several problems with EBM. First, only a very few articles are ever reviewed by an authority and graded. Therefore, the clinician is still left with a mound of literature to read, and many do not themselves have the necessary training to grade the quality of the papers. Secondly, and in our minds more importantly, there is a real limit to the usefulness on a particular (patient) level to the information in even the very best quality paper. In order to understand this statement, a bit of statistical jargon must be reviewed.

MEDICAL STATISTICS AND EPIDEMIOLOGY

Epidemiology is the study of disease in human populations, and those factors that influence that disease. Depending on the way the term "population" is defined, it can be argued that most medical papers other than case series are reports of the results of some type of epidemiologic study. The study group might be the inhabitants of a county, or members of a specific race, or those with a certain disease. The investigator attempts to describe the disease, to determine why it occurs in the population, or the best average way to treat it. Data are collected from the study group, and invariably this involves the use of numbers. The study results are an analysis of these numbers. It is at this point that a medical statistician is consulted.

Medical statistics has become unbelievably complicated. Nonetheless, virtually all of the techniques are based on some variation of the "average" (mean). That is, after all of the manipulations have been complete, the final result of all of the analyses is a description of what will happen to an "average" patient. There is important information to be learned through this process. For example, it is known from many studies that if a person has "Strep throat" a course of penicillin will, most likely, will result in a cure.

Of course, the problem is that there is no such thing as an "average" patient. In any series there are outliers. Not every patient with Strep throat responds well to penicillin. Some will develop septicemia (blood poisoning) and will die. Some will be killed by the antibiotic due to a severe allergic reaction. The universal truth that penicillin cures Strep throat does not apply to each particular patient. How then is the clinician to use the medical literature?

CLINICAL DECISION MAKING

In 1967, Feinstein carefully analyzed clinical decision making. His book, *Clinical Judgment,* remains one of the most important medical publications of the last century (Feinstein, 1967). Feinstein's thesis is that there are three important elements involved in all clinical decisions: the host (the patient), the disease, and the illness (the interaction between the disease and the host). In most of the medical literature, the host is described by reporting a whole list of averaged demographic information. The disease is characterized by listing its most common signs and symptoms. Virtually never does a paper discuss the interaction between these two elements and the fact that the interaction between the disease and the host is unique.

Perhaps the best way to understand Feinstein's concept is to consider that there is no single cause for any illness. The skeptic might immediately suggest that such a concept is folly since, "Everyone knows that poliovirus causes polio!" That statement is untrue! While poliovirus must be present for the disease to occur, it must interact with the host to cause paralysis. In fact, before the development of the polio vaccine, over 90 percent of all individuals in the United States were infected with poliovirus at one time or another, but only a tiny fraction ever developed paralytic polio. Some factor of the host, and perhaps some factor of the virus itself, was responsible for the infection causing only mild viral symptoms in some but tragic paralysis or death in others. The introduction of smallpox and measles to the natives of North and South America by Europeans nearly wiped out their races. However, the operative word in the previous sentence is "nearly." Neither of these diseases killed everyone; some hosts had natural resistance.

There is a further extension of the concept of illness that involves a difference between "cure" and "healed." As an example, a close physician friend of one of us (KLN) was diagnosed and treated for prostatic cancer several years ago. The disease was caught at an early stage, and while he knows that he has virtually a zero chance of having a recurrence of the disease—in other words he has been cured—he is far from healed. He continues to feel assaulted. He recently said, "I feel as though my body has let me down." A medical scientist would have no problem telling this physician that he has been cured and to "forget about it." On the other hand, the accomplished clinician might well have anticipated this reaction (relatively common among physicians) and helped the patient deal with it. In our view, far too much time in medical school is spent on curing and far too little on caring.

Clinicians are continuously bombarded by reports from "Laboratory Science," the field of medicine that deals primarily with the testing of blood. This has become such a routine part of everyday medical practice that even individuals who are in perfect health have blood drawn as a preventative measure to screen for early signs of various illnesses. For example, it is known that in some individuals the thyroid gland functions less and less well with age, and thus it is recommended that patients over the age of 35 have a screening test for thyroid function every 5 years (American Thyroid Association, 2000). But understanding the meaning of the test result for the particular patient is far from straightforward.

It is quite interesting to review how laboratory science establishes a range of values for any specific blood test that are considered to be within "the normal range." Everyone who has spent even a small amount of time in the study of any science will be familiar with the concept of the "normal distribution." This is a mathematical graph that is formed by inserting numbers into a standard formula. The most interesting aspect of this curve is that it is easy to determine the value on the graph where 2.5 percent of the values are higher, and another number where 2.5 percent of the numbers are lower. For some reason, now lost in the history of medicine, it became standard to assume that if a blood test were to be performed on any group of individuals, the results would be "normally distributed." Presently, any value within the central 95 percent of the distribution of values is considered to be "normal" and anything outside of that range is not. The normal distribution—a purely mathematical construct—has become a determinate of who and what is normal.

How then is the "normal range" of a laboratory test determined? While it would make sense that it would be the middle 95 percent of values for all people, it is quite different. The "normal" range is usually determined by drawing blood from a relatively small number (often as few as 100) of volunteers. It should be no surprise to learn that these volunteers are often those who work in and around the medical laboratory. Five percent of the values from these volunteers are considered to be outside of "normal" despite the fact that they are probably all quite healthy. There is likely NO representation of individuals who have the disease or condition for which the test was developed. It would seem to make more sense to conclude that the values of all of the samples from the healthy volunteers are normal. Yet, there is often no attempt to differentiate between "normal," meaning not ill, and "normally distributed."

The astute clinician understands these points and never fails to distinguish between the "normal distribution" and the "normal patient." Laboratory values should be used only as a guideline, not as an absolute diagnosis of a disease process or not. For example, a normal pregnant woman often has a hemoglobin value (a measure of the amount of red blood cell material in a sample) that falls below the lower end of the range of normal values. Every obstetrician knows that normal values (more correctly, normally distributed values) do not apply to normal pregnant women.

There are other areas where the report of the laboratory can cause problems for clinicians. One of these is the reporting of cervical cytology: Pap smears. The Pap smear was originally developed to determine the presence or absence of cancer of the cervix. In populations in which most of the women have had at least one Pap smear, cancer of the cervix is now a very rare disease. Refinements in the technique have enabled it to suggest the presence of cervical cancer precursors, and this is the most common use of the test at the present time. Unfortunately, the consensus conference that determined how cytology reports should be worded suggested that the cytopathology laboratory might make comments or educational notes regarding the management of an abnormal report (National Cancer Institute Workshop, 1989). This makes little sense, even when the laboratory parrots the consensus conference recommendations correctly (a condition that is not always met). The recommendations are not applicable to an individual patient. They only apply to the average patient, an individual who does not exist.

The world of laboratory values and pathology reports belongs to those physicians who, as we have seen, took the nonclinical, medical science oriented path. They describe and compartmentalize individuals based entirely on numbers. They never touch a patient. The information from their areas is vital to the evaluation of individual patients, yet that information alone cannot care for a person with an illness.

CONCLUSION: THE CENTRALITY OF THE CLINICIAN

It should be clear that there are many pieces of information for the clinician to utilize in the care of each individual patient. These include the scientific literature, laboratory reports, radiology reports, and pathology reports, among others. Yet none of this information is directly applicable to any particular patient.

In order to illustrate the centrality of the clinician in the care of patients, an example may be more informative than an abstract discussion. Assume that a healthy 31-year-old woman makes an appointment with a gynecologist for a periodic preventative healthcare examination. When the physician and patient begin their meeting, it is important for the patient to state what she expects from the meeting. The physician must obtain a history from the patient in order to determine what type of care might be appropriate for this person. There is an immediate need for trust between the doctor and her patient: The clinician must trust that she will tell the truth, and she must trust both that the physician will maintain confidentiality and will make the correct medical decisions. Usually, but not invariably, there is a need for an examination. This again requires trust and often some negotiation. The interpersonal exchanges between the patient and the physician are key to the success or failure of the encounter.

During the office visit, several samples might be collected for analysis. These would probably include a Pap smear and perhaps a blood sample for lipid levels including cholesterol. The reports of the analyses of these samples are unimportant unless they are correctly interpreted by the clinician for this particular patient. First, assume that the Pap smear was normal. Even a negative report requires evaluation and discussion. For example, if it was the third normal result in succession over the last three years, it might be suggested to the patient that she need not return for another sample for three years. If, on the other hand, it is abnormal, the clinician must interpret the result for this specific patient. If further evaluation is necessary, it must be negotiated with the patient. The recommendation that might have been added to the report by the laboratory is meaningless without thorough knowledge of the patient.

Even normal values can sometimes present problems of interpretation. Almost all laypersons know that a normal blood pressure is 120/80. There is an international agreement among experts in the area of hypertension (high blood pressure) that any reading above 140/90 is abnormal. The problem is that there is a rather large number of healthy individuals who consistently have blood pressure readings of 90/60. If such a person were to be seen in an emergency department and had a blood pressure of 130/85 it would be considered normal. However, for that particular patient, the reading might indicate important hypertension. Only the clinician who had been taking and recording the blood pressure at regular intervals would be able to spot the sudden increase as a potential health hazard.

There are thousands of possible examples that could be cited. Indeed, every report in the literature, every laboratory test, and every radiological image is only one small piece of information that the clinician has at hand when evaluating an individual patient. The clinician is the focal point for the interaction between the universal (medical science) and the particular (the individual patient) in medicine. It is only through a mutually trusting doctor–patient relationship that the best practice of medicine occurs.

The clinician practicing in the early twenty-first century is able to care for the dozens of patients that appear every day, better than at any time in the past. More is known about more diseases, and more and better treatments are available. There are multiple sources of new information. There are better laboratories, less invasive surgical instruments, and more effective drugs. Never have physicians had it so good.

But some things never change. Each patient must first be evaluated before any of the new technology or information is of any use. The physician must arrive at a diagnosis, and that requires the use of the senses. In some cases, that means that the patient is listened to and observed visually (sight and hearing). In other cases, the patient must be touched. Perhaps an instrument will be used to facilitate hearing (e.g., stethoscope) or seeing (e.g., otoscope). In all cases, the clinician must develop a rapport with the patient, as an examination requires patient consent. In many cases, this is actually a negotiation as the patient may have an entirely different idea of the need for a type of evaluation than the physician. Even more negotiation is necessary when testing and treatment become issues. Physicians begin their education by studying basic science. They learn their profession by serving as the interface between science and their patients.

REFERENCES

American Thyroid Association. (2000). Guidelines for detection of thyroid dysfunction. *Archives of Internal Medicine, 160*(11), 1573–1575.

Feinstein, A. R. (1967). *Clinical judgment.* Huntington, NY: Krieger.

Grimes, D. A., & Schulz, K. F. (2002). An overview of clinical research: The lay of the land. *Lancet, 359*(9300), 57–61.

Grimes, D. A., & Schulz, K. F. (2002). Descriptive studies: What they can and cannot do. *Lancet, 359*(9301), 145–149.

Lilienfield, A. M., & Lilienfield, D. E. (1980). *Foundations of epidemiology.* New York: Oxford University Press.

National Cancer Institute Workshop. (1989). The 1988 Bethesda System for reporting cervical/vaginal cytological diagnoses. *JAMA, 262,* 931–934.

Noller, K. L. (1993). The history of gynecologic surgery: 25 centuries of women's health care. In D. Gershenson, A. DeCherney, & S. Curry (Eds.), *Operative gynecology.* Philadelphia: WB Saunders.

Rosenberg, W. M., & Sackett, D. L. (1996). On the need for evidence-based medicine. *Therapie, 51*(3), 212–217.

Schulz, K. F., & Grimes, D. A. (2002). Case-control studies: Research in reverse. *Lancet, 359*(9304), 431–434.

Chapter 7

A NO-FAULT LEARNING PROGRAM (NFLP) AS LIFE LONG LEARNING

Roger Bibace and Kenneth L. Noller

In this chapter we will propose an innovative educational method that we believe has the potential to reduce medical errors by changing physician behavior. We call this process a No-Fault Learning Program (NFLP).

Although the primary exemplar in this chapter is cervical neoplasia as assessed through colposcopy, we believe that an NFLP can be designed for almost every aspect of clinical medicine that relies on sensory input.

BACKGROUND

Our hypothesis is that an understanding of both the processes (the how) and the outcomes (the what) is required in order to foster the dialogue or integrative links between particulars and universals in science and medicine. The processes relied upon both in science and medicine are very broad. They encompass a breadth that is ordinarily referred to as "levels of organization" in epistemology or a "bio-psycho-socio-cultural" approach in the human sciences (Engel, 1977; Von Bertalanffy, 1968). One of the leaders in U.S. medicine, Alvan Feinstein, has published several books on the importance of careful attention to the processes involved in clinical diagnosis. Feinstein (1967) refers to the "complexity of human data and reasoning" because

> . . . each clinician observes three different types of data. The first type of data describes a disease in morphologic, chemical, microbiologic, physi-

ologic, or other impersonal terms. The second type of data describes the host in whom the disease occurs. This description of the host's environmental background includes both the personal properties of the host before the disease began (such as age, race, sex, and education) and also the properties of the host's external surroundings (such as geographic location, occupation, and financial and social status). The third type of data describes the illness that occurs in the interaction between the disease and its environmental host. The illness consists of clinical phenomena; the host's subjective sensations, which are called "symptoms," and certain findings called "signs," which are discerned objectively during the physical examination of the diseased host. When the diseased host seeks medical attention, he becomes a patient, and the clinician's work begins. (pp. 24–25)

Many scientists and clinicians indicate a preference for either process or outcome. Some journals and federal agencies focus only on either process or outcome. Funding agencies may consider only basic science or applied science. There appears to be some hope that this compartmentalized condition is changing. Attempts have been made recently to create linkages between science and medical practice by establishing centers where there is closer proximity and collaboration between scientists and clinicians who are focusing on a common disease. Such attempts are sometimes referred to as "translational research." Consensus conferences are another effort to bring basic and applied areas of together. Recent examples of such meetings developed guidelines for the care of children with asthma, the evaluation of women with abnormal Pap smears, and the diagnosis and treatment of hypertension.

Both processes and outcomes must be studied because processes complement and are an inherent ingredient of any outcome. Scientists in many areas have demonstrated that many different processes can all lead to the same functional outcome. Such a many-to-one relationship between processes and outcomes is in contrast to the one-to-one relationship between a process and outcome that is often the focus of research. Furthermore, we subscribe to the opinion that understanding how an error comes about in medical practice provides an opportunity to correct that error. An accurate outcome may only yield a score, whereas inquiry into how an error came about is an opportunity to study the mind at work. Paradoxically, accuracy is improved through the study of error because teachers have learned to focus on mistakes.

There are errors in any and all aspects of describing and designating the sensory-driven evidence that leads to a diagnosis through the use of medical devices. Learning a medical procedure, as both process and outcome, can be furthered through the dialogicality of all members of the groups (beginners, experienced, and expert physicians). The paradoxical premise here is that experts also learn from beginners. Our NFLP does not rely solely on the traditional assumption that there is a one-way asymmetrical relationship between the expert teacher and the beginner who is learning a medical procedure. Symmetrical, rather than asymmetrical, relationships among members of these groups are posited as beneficial for all participants in an NFLP.

While processes and outcomes are codependent, for the purpose of explanation we have separated our thoughts into two chapters. The present chapter deals with outcomes as measured by an NFLP, and the companion chapter focuses on the processes that rely upon visual sensory-driven evidence (see chapter 8).

The particulars examined by an NFLP address the ubiquitous issues of consistency and variability of both the phenomenon being examined and of the examiner. Hence, the phenomena selected for examination by physicians in an NFLP can range from very clear cut, textbook examples to the ambiguities of the "same-category" of phenomena in everyday clinical practice. Similarly, the issue of consistency and variability of the examiner can be explored in two distinctive ways across trials of an NFLP: First, an NFLP allows each study participant to become aware of their own intra-individual consistencies and variability for every aspect of the NFLP. Second, the consistency and variability of groups of physicians can be determined.

AMERICAN MEDICAL ASSOCIATION (AMA) CALL FOR LIFE LONG LEARNING (LLL)

In the United States, it is necessary for a physician to complete one or more years of postgraduate training to obtain a license to practice. Most physicians pursue training in a specialty by completing residency training, after which there are diverse requirements for attaining certification by one of several medical specialty boards. Such specialty certification now is time-limited and requires recertification after a variable number of years through completion of some form of "continuing medical education" (CME). However, CME after specialty certification has been shown to be an ineffective means to assess or increase competence. U.S. medicine has felt it necessary to issue calls for Life Long Learning (LLL) to supplement the current recertification practices to ensure competence among practicing physicians.

Why did the AMA and a number of medical specialties issue this call for Life Long Learning? A common answer is that LLL is a response to societal awareness of medical errors. A Presidential order to "reduce medical mistakes," which are "blamed for tens of thousands of deaths," was front page news (Pear, 2000). In 1999, the National Academy of Sciences and the Institute of Medicine issued a report entitled "To err is human: Building a safer health system." The document states, "healthcare providers could reduce the number of errors by 50 percent in the next five years by collecting and analyzing data on unsafe practices, as the aviation industry does" (Pear, 2000).

National reports focus on aggregates indicative of the generality of this issue. For a given individual, however, a medical error becomes a personal issue. A headline such as "the wrong foot, and other tales of surgical error" (Altman, 2001) does not require sophisticated medical expertise to appreciate that an error has occurred. It is the obvious character of the error that elicits intense negative reactions. Many are "outraged" to learn that "150 times since 1996 [to 2001] surgeons and hospitals in this country have operated on the wrong arm, leg, eye, kidney or other body part, or even on the wrong patient" (Altman, 2001). Such mistakes, according to the Joint Commission on Accreditation of Health-Care Organizations, "should never happen, but often they do . . . " (Altman, 2001). As is often the case, these and other errors had been previously recognized and thoroughly discussed by medical experts and national organizations (Bogner, 1994).

These societal, political, and professional factors have led to two possible solutions: changing the medical system in diverse ways and increasing the competence of practicing physicians. The first addresses the complex, impersonal, organizational aspects of health care in hospitals in clinics. The second involves individuals who practice medicine. One aspect of the latter focus has led to a call for LLL. Our plan for LLL involves a no-fault learning program (NFLP).

HISTORICAL ANTECEDENTS OF AN NFLP

Human errors occur in every discipline, in both science and its applications. Unfortunately, errors in the field of medicine can lead to death. In an attempt to identify the causes of such errors and to reduce their occurrence, President Clinton established a Commission in 1999. The Commission's first publication recited Reason's definition of error, " . . . the failure of a planned sequence of mental and physical activities to achieve its intended outcome when these failures cannot be attributed to

chance . . . error is not meaningful without consideration of intention."
(reason, cited in Kohn, Corrigan, & Donaldson, 1999, p. 46). It has long
been recognized that errors in clinical judgment are due to

> the failure of many clinicians to distinguish three different intellectual
> disciplines—description, designation and diagnosis . . . in description the
> clinician gives an account of the sensation, substance or phenomenon
> [which] is observed. In designation [the clinician] . . . gives a name or
> classification to the observed entity. In diagnosis, [the clinician] indicates
> the anatomic or other abnormality that is responsible for the observed
> entity. (Feinstein, 1967, p. 322)

We have observed that there has been little emphasis in medical education on the importance of the elements mentioned above: Sequence is
rarely mentioned; intention is largely ignored; description is taken for
granted and never tested; and classification is limited to gross categories
only. Traditional medical education only asks that the clinician arrive at
the correct diagnosis with no investigation of the processes required to
develop that diagnosis. Usually the learner is credentialed if a certain
"percentage correct" is achieved on a standardized test. The problem with
that approach is that it allows mistakes (even approves a certain percentage of mistakes) to be made as long as the person being tested
achieves the minimum level that has been established. However, it is no
longer appropriate (if it ever were) to accept a margin of error. New
techniques need to be established that require the clinician to evaluate
personal performance consistently with the goal of optimizing performance. We believe that one key to such self-evaluation is a no-fault
approach. This technique has been used in the evaluation of airline pilots
for many years but has not been tested adequately in clinical medicine.

Bogner (1994) argues analogically that licenses are to pilots as medical
malpractice is to physicians. But pilots, unlike physicians, report their
errors to the Aviation Safety Reporting System. Many measures are in
place to ensure the anonymity of the reporter. In actual practice, one
federal agency "de-identifies" the information before forwarding it to
another federal agency. The anonymity of the pilot who is reporting an
error is ensured further by the destruction of the reporting form. Efforts
are made to generalize the information so as to obscure the identity of
the reported incident. Lastly, the reporting pilot is not penalized if certain
criteria are met.

For our purposes, it is important to note that a system as a whole as
well as groups of professionals can improve their performance through

the reports of errors by individuals in that group. We agree with Bogner that at every level of organization, "the key to the viability of this approach is information" (p. 378).

CHARACTERISTICS OF LIFE LONG LEARNING THROUGH A NO-FAULT LEARNING PROGRAM

The objective of an NFLP is to increase accuracy and decrease errors of omission and commission in the performance of a medical procedure. An NFLP addresses Feinstein's requirements for "description, designation, diagnosis" related to any sensory-driven evidence for a physical examination or medical procedure for diverse sensory modalities. Feinstein argues that a main impediment to accurate diagnosis is

> the failure of many clinicians to distinguish the three different disciplines—description, designation, diagnosis—used for the total procedure. In description, the clinician gives an account of the sensation, substance, or phenomenon that [they] have actually observed. In designation, [they] give a name or classification to the observed entity. In diagnosis, [they] indicate the anatomic or other abnormality that is responsible for the observed entity. (Feinstein, 1967, p. 322)

LLL through an NFLP permits both multiple opportunities for learning and repeated measures of learning during the professional lifespan of a participating physician. Learning in clinical medicine often relies on the aphorism "see one, do one, teach one." While there are many advantages to hands-on learning, the NFLP complements clinical practice by making it possible to implement well-known aspects of learning a medical procedure without actual patient involvement. Another aphorism, "practice makes perfect," implies repetition. Such repetition (see "automaticity" in next chapter) is readily available through an NFLP. Further, the many constraints of the clinical encounter, such as time pressure, are eliminated in an NFLP. A physician can choose when to learn or use an NFLP and to take as much time as that physician feels is needed for each of the activities in the NFLP. One or more modules may be repeated as often as that physician considers desirable.

The duration of time for each aspect of an NFLP is personally chosen by each physician. This feature makes it easier for each participant to determine the time "I need" to achieve "my best personal practice." Best practice has become an umbrella term for describing how groups of medical practitioners should practice with respect to a particular disease.

"My best personal practice" complements these normative group practices by increasing a physician's awareness of their own individuality—their range of accurate and erroneous responses and their variability.

An NFLP addresses both the private psychological processes of the physician that are related to an outcome as well as the reported public outcomes in the performance of a medical procedure. Privacy is essential to the "no fault" aspect of an NFLP. In medical school and residency training, the teaching/learning interaction is often evaluated publicly. The approval/disapproval by attending senior physicians varies a great deal. But repeatedly, one hears that it is disapproval that is most frequently experienced by both medical students and residents.

The NFLP facilitates the reporting of the subjective thoughts and feelings of a physician. The report of those psychological processes (e.g., I forgot; I did not see that . . .) is completely omitted when accuracy or error as an outcome is the only indicator of the performance.

AN NFLP IN COLPOSCOPY LLL

The sense of vision is the most used in clinical medicine. It is also the easiest to use as a basis for testing a new approach to medical education that is designed to decrease errors through an NFLP.

We have chosen as our study tool a diagnostic procedure (colposcopy) that relies on the sense of vision and that is widely used by primary care clinicians to evaluate women who have abnormal Pap smears. However, if our educational approach is proven to be effective, the results of this study should be widely applicable to many medical specialties. Examples of such areas include radiology, dermatology, surgery, ophthalmology, and otolaryngology.

In the actual performance of a colposcopic examination, the examiner first places a speculum in the vagina and brings the uterine cervix into view. The colposcope—a low-power binocular microscope—is moved into position. The examiner applies a dilute solution of acetic acid—about the same concentration as half-strength vinegar—to the cervix to bring out those changes that are associated with disease. If acetowhite changes are observed following the application of acetic acid, a clinically significant abnormality may be present. It is then up to the examiner to determine if the observed patterns indicate the possible presence of a precancerous condition (compare Figs. 7.1 and 7.2). If there is such a suspicion, a small biopsy of tissue is taken from the cervix and sent to the laboratory for evaluation. Other findings of interest include "punctation" and "mosaic" changes. The diameter of the vessels that cause the tissue pattern, the

Figure 7.1
Colpophotograph (×10) of a normal uterine cervix. Normal squamous epithelium
(Sq) can be seen at the periphery. Normal columnar glandular epithelium (Gl) can
be seen in and around the cervical os. The space between the Sq and Gl epithelia,
shown here between the white lines which lie 1–3 mm apart, is an area of active
cellular division and replication. This area is the "transformation zone." The great
majority of all cancerous lesions of the cervix occur in this narrow zone.

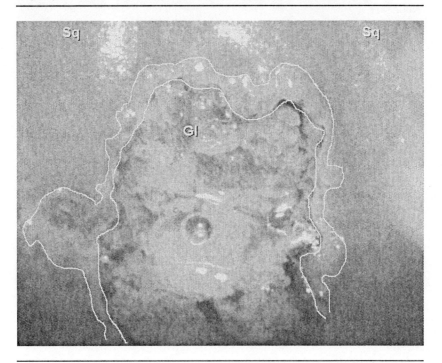

spacing of the abnormalities, and the contour of the lesion all have significance in making a decision about the presence of disease.

"Atypical vessels" represent a special category. When present they
often indicate that invasive cancer is present. It is a fatal flaw not to
identify such vessels.

Because it is relatively easy to obtain high-quality images (colpophotographs) during an examination, these images can be used in an NFLP.

Cycle I

In the first cycle, the participant in the colposcopy NFLP is required
to make a series of judgments on a series of 30 colpophotographs under
two conditions. The first condition limits the length of time the partici-

Figure 7.2
Colpophotograph (×16) of an area of cervical precancer. A mosaic area can be seen in the top/anterior portion of the cervix. The dark lines that form the tiles are blood vessels. A smaller area of punctation is seen in the bottom/posterior section of the figure. The black dots are blood vessels.

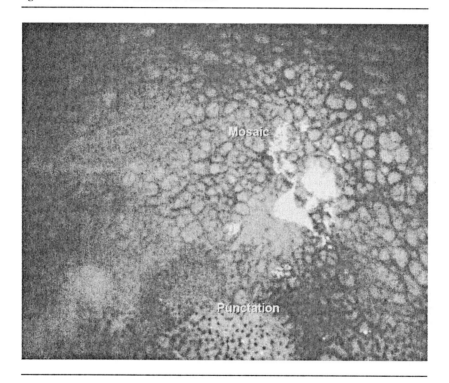

pant has to view the slide and make a decision. This is meant to approximate the conditions in actual clinical practice where decisions are usually made in less than a minute. Upon completion of the first task, the participant is then asked to re-examine the same series of slides without time constraints but with strict adherence to a protocol. In colposcopy, certain decisions must be made before it is appropriate to move on to the next step. For example, the participant is first asked if the entire "transformation zone" can be seen. If "yes," the participant can move on to the next step in the evaluation. Subsequently, the protocol successively focuses the participant's attention on each of four quadrants on each slide.

In the first condition, judgment is based on "an overall, immediate impression." The second condition requires that the judgments be made in a formal sequence, from the whole to the smallest parts.

A participant has completed the first cycle after both series of judgments have been made.

Activities Prior to Cycle II

Prior to Cycle II, the participant will have received feedback regarding errors of omission and commission for both conditions. After reviewing the results from Cycle I, the participant will be asked to complete a form that requires them to state their expected actual performance on Cycle II, for both conditions. These forms can be conceptualized as levels of aspiration, or feed-forward, prior to the task. The participant is being asked, "How realistic is my judgment about my performance?" After Cycle II, the participant will be able to assess how well their expectations matched their actual performance.

Cycle II

Cycle II is a repetition of Cycle I with a different set of 30 slides. At the end of Cycle II, the participant will review the feedback for Cycles I and II, for both series of slides, for both conditions. In addition, the participant will be provided with group data that allows each physician to compare personal performance as a whole, and on each individual slide, with the group.

Each participant will be asked to explain differences between the judgments they made under the clinical practice and the protocol-driven conditions. These explanations will allow the creators of the NFLP to make changes in the program for subsequent cycles. This feedback also allows for a movement toward symmetry between teacher and learner by acknowledging that a learner can teach the teacher. Teachers need to learn which aspects of the task are difficult and which are easy. This complementary relationship develops a partnership between the two. The participant will also be provided with normative data from two other groups of medical practitioners: "beginners" and "experienced" physicians.

These repeated comparisons should be effective in bringing about changes in the performance of the individual participant. These changes are expected to be both in the judgments made by the participant and in the internal representations (psychological processes) that are related to the outcome. The empirical and conceptual work of Irving Sigel on "psychological distancing activities" is the basis for this approach to change (Sigel, 1993 ; see also chapter 8, this volume).

Furthermore, the protocol requires judgments that are organized in a formal sequence from the whole to the smallest parts. This sequence is clinically meaningful and not based on an arbitrary, formal analysis of large compared to smaller body parts.

PARTICULARS OF A COLPOSCOPIC NFLP

This NFLP on colposcopy requires each participant to describe, to categorize, and to diagnose each visual display. While the evaluation of slides is not the same as the actual procedure the only difficult portion of the process is the evaluation of the features that are present. Descriptive features are grouped into several categories that include

1. Transformation zone (T-zone) (part of the whole cervix);
2. Acetowhite epithelium (ACW) (part of the transformation zone);
3. Mosaicism (Mo) (part of the ACW);
4. Punctuation (P) (part of the ACW);
5. Atypical vessels (AV).

The categories in turn lead the physician to classifications that constitute the diagnosis. These classifications, arrived at by consensus conferences among cytologists, colposcopists, and histologists are the basis for a diagnosis (see chapter 6, this volume).

NFLP SUMMARY

Our proposal for an NFLP requires that the participant has absolute confidentiality from governing and credentialing groups. There should be no negative public consequences for errors made by a participant. A participant should not be constrained by time. The participant should be allowed to repeat any aspect of the program that is experienced as difficult by that person. Repeating different versions of an NFLP during the course of a professional career qualifies an NFLP as LLL.

An NFLP allows a participant to compare their performance to two other groups of clinicians (beginners and experienced physicians) using the same set of materials. Comparative evaluations constitute psychological distancing activities (Sigel, 1993) that are known to produce changes in behavior and in the psychological processes related to those behavioral outcomes. An NFLP provides feedback to participants; however, it also requires the participant to provide feedback to the creators of an NFLP regarding ambiguities in the program that should be addressed. Updating a new version of an NFLP requires a group of clinicians and researchers to accommodate such feedback from participants who have used the program. New versions of an NFLP also require the incorporation of new scientific results and technological changes in the use of a medical procedure.

REFERENCES

Altman, L. K. (2001, December 11). The wrong foot, and other tales of surgical error. *New York Times.* Retrieved December 12, 2001, from http://www.nytimes.com.

Bogner, M. S. (1994). Human error in medicine: A frontier for change. In M. S. Bogner (Ed.), *Human error in medicine* (pp. 373–384). Hillsdale, NJ: Erlbaum.

Engel, G. L. (1977). The need for a new medical model: A challenge for bio-medicine. *Science, 196,* 129–136.

Feinstein, A. R. (1967). *Clinical judgment.* Huntington, NY: Krieger.

Kohn, L. T., Corrigan, J. M., & Donaldson, M. S. (1999). *To err is human: Building a safer health system.* Washington, DC: Institute of Medicine, Committee on Quality of Health Care in America.

Pear, R. (2000, February 21). Clinton to order steps to reduce medical mistakes. *New York Times,* p. A1.

Sigel, I. E. (1993). The centrality of a distancing model for the development of representational competence. In R. R. Cocking & K. A. Renninger (Eds.), *The development and meaning of psychological distance* (pp. 141–160). Hillsdale, NJ: Erlbaum.

Von Bertalanffy, L. (1968). *Organismic psychology and systems theory.* Worcester, MA: Clark University Press/Barre Publishers.

Chapter 8

ANALYSIS OF PSYCHOLOGICAL PROCESSES RELATED TO OUTCOMES IN SENSORY-DRIVEN MEDICAL PROCEDURES

Roger Bibace, Robert Leeman, and Kenneth L. Noller

> Much as human behavior in a medical setting is still behavior and not medicine, human error in a medical setting is still error and not medicine.
>
> J. W. Senders, "Medical Devices, Medical Errors, and Medical Accidents" in *Human Error in Medicine*

> If you do not know a thing, you are quite sure not to suspect it; and if you do not suspect a thing, you are almost certain not to find it.
>
> Duncan Matthews

Human errors are a part of everyday life, including medical practice. While people in all walks of life make errors, the potential for deleterious results makes medical errors more severe than most. According to a report issued by the National Academy of Sciences and the Institute of Medicine, preventable medical error lead to the death of as many as 98,000 patients per year with total costs between $17 and $29 billion (Kohn, Corrigan, & Donaldson, 2000). As a response, the American Medical Association has issued a call for life-long learning by physicians, above and beyond requirements already in place, such as board recertification (Bibace & Noller, chap. 7).

In his book titled *Clinical Judgment* (1967), physician and epidemiologist Alvan Feinstein argued that many medical errors result from medical professionals failing "to distinguish the three different intellectual disciplines—description, designation and diagnosis—used for the total (medical) procedure" (p. 322). After conducting field research on clinicians specializing in the diagnosis of rare genetic disorders, Shaw (2003) echoes Feinstein's sentiments by concluding that, for the majority of the clinicians, "diagnostic skill rests to a large extent on the clinician's ability to discern genetic characterization from phenotypic appearance. In this process clinicians speak of the 'gestalt' or 'diagnostic intuition' " (p. 40). However, there is much more involved in medical evaluation than intuition. By failing to acknowledge the multiple psychological processes that constitute the *private* inferences made by these physicians that lead to their *public* diagnostic conclusions, major conceptual and empirical gaps may occur. While the intuition of an experienced clinician is indispensable, it is but one of a number of psychological processes that should be involved in the medical evaluation of a patient. By separating the processes of description, designation, and diagnosis, Feinstein (and we) believe that the diagnostic accuracy of any physician can be improved.

In chapter 7 we described a no-fault learning process (NFLP) that we have developed for physicians who use the technique "colposcopy," which primarily uses the sense of sight. In this chapter, we will explore the various psychological processes that are involved in Feinstein's "description, designation, and diagnosis" (hereafter referred to as the "3 D's"). These psychological processes are illustrated in the realm of sensory-driven medical procedures. We will use the colposcopy procedure as our recurring example of such a procedure as we have preliminary data on how physicians make decisions when they use this technique. Given that vision is the most commonly used sensory modality in medical practice, colposcopy seems to be an appropriate example for examining the psychological processes implicated in Feinstein's 3 D's.

The NFLP was developed as a means of life long learning (LLL) for physicians performing sensory-driven medical procedures (Bibace & Noller, chap. 7). Implementation of an NFLP facilitates the empirical investigation of one source of error resulting from a psychological process, namely misplaced attention. The no-fault aspect of the program is a crucial element as it provides physicians with the opportunity to learn at their own pace with no penalty for errors. Physicians participating in an NFLP are asked to make descriptions, designations, and diagnoses under two very different conditions. In the colposcopy trial, they were first asked to make spontaneous judgments of photographs, similar to the manner in which they likely conduct these examinations in their everyday medical practice. Next, participants were engaged in a sequential, protocol-driven condition. Overlays were placed on the colpophotographs to direct the participant's attention to a tissue feature.

During the spontaneous condition, physicians make use of multiple psychological processes simultaneously (e.g., visual perception, reasoning, memory). This precludes precise evaluation as to where errors in designation and diagnosis may have occurred. In contrast, during the protocol condition, focusing of the physician's attention allows for feedback that specifies where errors may have arisen; for example, there may have been an incomplete description of the contour of a lesion.

Both universals and particulars are addressed in an NFLP. Universals include the importance of distinguishing Feinstein's 3 D's, and recognition that there are multiple psychological processes at work in sensory-driven medical procedures. At the same time, participation in an NFLP in the context of LLL will also help physicians over time to identify the particular psychological processes involved in their own medical practices.

Historically, psychologists have differentiated between simultaneous and sequential mental processes, also referred to as "System 1" and "System 2," respectively (Stanovich & West, 2000). System 1 processes have been viewed as operating rapidly and intuitively in an automatic fashion, typically without conscious awareness on the part of the individual and requiring little in the way of attentional resources with the potential of multiple automatic processes being undertaken in parallel. System 1 processes are considered analogous to, but separate from, sensory perception. However, for our purposes, sensory perception will be grouped together with System 1 processes, such as intuition.

In contrast, System 2 processes are thought of as operating more slowly, in a serial, step-by-step fashion. System 2 processes require conscious awareness and greater attentional resources than System 1 processes. Memory and reasoning are examples of System 2 processes. Debates in psychology (Pashler, 1999) have continued for years as to whether different processes should be classified as System 1 or 2 and whether processes falling under the former or latter category are more significant in the workings of the human mind (Bargh & Chartrand, 1999; Pashler, 1999).

Distinction between System 1 and System 2 is an oversimplification because both types of psychological processes are intimately linked and tend to coexist in many aspects of everyday life and professional (including medical) practice. Furthermore, the number of counterexamples that challenge the historical presuppositions about System 1 and 2 processes are enough to call into question whether this distinction has any value. In the area of economic theory, Kahneman and Tversky (1979) found that people rarely analyze situations to the fullest and instead tend to rely on heuristics or "rules of thumb" in making choices. They suggest that decision making is not a sequential, serial process but rather resembles a simultaneous, parallel process. Further, it is unlikely that most people would be able to describe their own decision-making processes (Nisbett & Wilson, 1977).

We do not to take a position with respect to which psychological processes belong to System 1 or 2. Instead, our position is merely that there are multiple processes involved in sensory-driven medical procedures, and that addressing them can only improve accuracy. For this reason, the NFLP was structured to include both the physician's intuitive, simultaneous judgments, and judgments made as the physician follows a sequential, systematic protocol.

This chapter proceeds with an overview of the psychological processes involved in each of Feinstein's 3 D's as they relate to sensory-driven medical procedures, including visual perception, attention, memory, and reasoning. The two main theoretical approaches that form the basis of the NFLP will then be discussed. These are the Partnership Model outlined by Bibace and colleagues (Bibace, Dillon, & Dowds, 1999) and the necessity of exploring both outcomes and their corresponding psychological processes (Werner, 1948).

DESCRIPTION

The physician's main aim in description is to provide "an account of the sensation, substance or phenomenon he has actually observed" (Feinstein, 1967, p. 322). In colposcopy, visual perception is of particular importance in description, so much so that a number of colposcopists have informally reported their opinion that colposcopy is entirely visual, thus ignoring other relevant psychological processes such as memory. Nonetheless, given its centrality in description, visual perception will be the main focus of this section.

The act of seeing a particular object in the environment can begin either as a conscious, willful act or as an unconscious one. In the former case, one intends to look at a particular object. In the latter case, vision may be directed at aspects of the environment without any conscious intent. This may occur either because an operation is well-practiced (e.g., gazing upward at traffic lights after stopping at an intersection), or because one item in our field of vision is particularly salient. Regardless of how vision is directed initially, its operation from that point on is automatic and unconscious.

There are a number of strengths to the automatic, unconscious nature of psychological processes. First, they tend to operate more rapidly than conscious, effortful processes (Brunswik, 1956; Hoffman, 1998). In addition, Bargh and Chartrand (1999) argue that "automatic mental processes free one's limited conscious attentional capacity." Bargh and Chartrand continue by reflecting on "how impossible it would be to function effectively if conscious, controlled, and aware mental processes had to deal with every aspect of life" (p. 464).

Indeed, as Hoffman points out, visual perception is a prime example of an automatic, unconscious process. "Vision is normally so swift and sure, so dependable and informative, and apparently so effortless that we naturally assume that it is, indeed, effortless" (Hoffman, 1998, p. xi). Despite this air of effortlessness, research points to the conclusion that vision is an active, intelligent process of image construction (Crick & Koch, 1998). The image construction process is described as "uncertainty geared," according to Brunswik (1956), and relies upon "relatively superficial and stereotyped cues" (p. 89). Our visual system makes use of features of objects in the outside world detected on a bottom-up basis, combined with a number of top-down expectations of the visual world regarding object form, content, movement, etc. Rather than passively reporting the contents of the outside world, these cues are used by the visual system to construct the images we see (Logothetis, 1999).

The smooth, automatic manner in which vision functions is not without its drawbacks. The visual system typically produces images that are faithful to the way objects exist in the outside world, yet anyone who has succumbed to an optical illusion is well aware of the "intrinsic 'stupidity' of the perceptual process" (Brunswik, 1956, p. 92). For example, in the classic Müller-Lyer illusion (Figure 8.1), viewers are asked to determine which of two lines is longer. Each line has an arrow at both ends. The arrows are pointed inward on one line and outward on the other. While the lines are of equal length, the one with the arrows pointed inward appears longer. The only way to avoid being fooled by this illusion is with prior knowledge that the lines are equal. This illusion illustrates the power of bottom-up processing, in that the line with the inward arrows always looks longer, despite the top-down knowledge that the lines are actually equal in length.

In colposcopy, the distance between capillaries is an important predictor of lesion severity (Kolstad & Stafl, 1972). This approximation of the length of the distance between capillaries is a bottom-up assessment. Given that estimates are made of adjacent areas, the variant of the Müller-Lyer illusion given in Figure 8.2 in which the lines are side-by-side would seem to provide a particularly relevant analogy for the difficulty involved in judgments of intercapillary distance. As with the Müller-Lyer illusion, top-down processing is also required in that physicians must be aware of the clinical significance of making comparisons involving intercapillary distance (Kolstad & Stafl, 1972).

While the visual system is capable of simultaneously processing disparate information in parallel, there are limitations to this ability, although the severity of these limitations are debated (Pashler, 1999). Due to capacity limitations, once the demands of the visual system exceed a certain threshold, parallel or simultaneous processing becomes less efficient. Capacity limitations are thought to be specific to each sensory modality, which explains why one can watch television, attending to both the images on the screen and the accompanying sound at the same time (Pashler, 1999).

Figure 8.1
The classic Müller-Lyer Illusion.

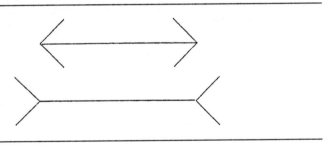

Figure 8.2
A variant of the Müller-Lyer Illusion.

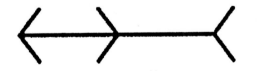

Attention solves some of the problems of perceptual capacity limitations (Broadbent, 1958; Itti, 2000). Attention works in a bottom-up fashion when directed toward particularly stimulating or appealing features of stimuli, whereas top-down attentional processes are at work when prior knowledge is used to direct one's attention to the location of the most crucial aspects of a visual array. Indeed, "while visual selectivity is enormously flexible . . . selection by any criterion seems to be ultimately mediated by location selection" (Pashler, 1999, p. 402). Location is highly relevant to colposcopy, in that not only must abnormalities be detected, but the location of the abnormality must also be assessed (Kolstad & Stafl, 1972).

Recent research conducted by Muller and Hubner (2002) suggests further limitations. For example, "seeing" and "looking" are not one and the same. The "spotlight" metaphor of attention, which argues that the brain processes all objects falling within its "beam," dominated for a number of years (Posner & Peterson, 1990). However, Muller and Hubner's work suggests that visual attention may instead resemble a "doughnut," in that holes of inattention analogous to holes in the center of doughnuts may lie within visual fields to which an individual is attending. This research is highly relevant to colposcopy and other visually driven medical procedures, because looking at a particular area does not necessarily mean that one is processing important aspects of the array. To put this colloquially, looking is not equivalent to seeing.

Data from a pilot study conducted by Bibace and Noller (2003) suggest that directing physicians' attention to important locations in a colpophotograph in a manner similar to the NFLP protocol will reduce errors of omission, but they are not eliminated entirely. In one condition of the study, physicians were asked to give their spontaneous assessments of a series of colpophotographs. In a second, "focused attention" condition, a series of visual overlays and follow-up questions were used to direct physicians' attention to a series of key features in the colpophotograph. While errors of omission were greatly reduced in the "focused attention" condition, some features were still frequently omitted (Table 8.1).

While vision appears to be an effortless process that simply reproduces the contents of the outside world, research has repeatedly shown vision to be an active, intelligent process of image construction. While vision is normally effective and informative, it is not without its pitfalls. For this reason, the aim of the NFLP is to accentuate the physician's immediate, simultaneous psychological processes by properly directing at-

Table 8.1
Errors of Omission under Two Conditions from the Bibace & Noller Pilot Study

	Photograph 1		Photograph 2		Photograph 3		Total	
	Spontaneous	Overlay	Spontaneous	Overlay	Spontaneous	Overlay	Spontaneous	Overlay
Blood	0	0					0	0
Gland	20	3					20	3
Columnar Epithelium	17	15	17	11			34	26
ACW	3	1	14	0	6	0	23	1
Irregular Border	20	19			19	0	39	19
Mosaicism	13	0	16	0	0	0	29	0
Faint Mosaicism	20	18					20	18
Coarse Mosaicism		0		0		0		0
Irregular Mosaic Tiles					19	18	19	18
Variable Width Vessels					20	18	20	18
Punctation within Mosaic Tiles					20	16	20	16
Punctation	8	0			5	4	13	4
Large Punctation			13	11			13	11
Punctation Above Surface			19	8			19	8
Atypical Vessels			13	6			13	6

tention through the use of the sequential protocol in order to improve the physician's skills in description and to reduce errors of omission.

DESIGNATION

The descriptive information discussed in the prior section is an essential ingredient in designation, which according to Feinstein (1967) involves the assignment of "a name or classification to the observed entity" (p. 322). Thus, the physician's task in the designation phase is to integrate the various features they have observed and the locations in which they have observed them, in order to assign an appropriate classification or classifications to a particular patient's condition.

To make a proper designation in colposcopy, a physician must assess a variety of perceptual features of the lesion, including intercapillary distance, surface contour, color tone, and clarity of the demarcation between non-normal and normal tissue. Each of these features must be seen and integrated in order to classify the lesion as containing (or not) abnormalities that are associated with a precancerous condition.

What makes the physician's task more difficult in colposcopy is the importance of the location of the features (Kolstad & Stafl, 1972). One worrisome classification is called "mosaicism," but is only meaningful if it is within a key boundary in the cervix referred to as the transformation zone (T-zone). It is within the T-zone where all abnormalities related to cervical cancer are seen. Unfortunately, locating the T-zone is perceptually difficult, and mistakes in its identification are a common source of errors in colposcopy (Noller, 1993). Location has been shown to be a central factor in determining which attributes (e.g., form, color) of a stimulus an individual will selectively attend to (Pashler, 1999), and this seems to be especially relevant in colposcopy.

System 2 psychological processes, such as reasoning and memory, are the focus of this section due to the shift from System 1 to System 2 processing that occurs when designation is performed according to the NFLP protocol. The use of System 2 processing offers a number of advantages over System 1 and "serves to monitor the quality of both mental operations and overt behavior" (Kahneman, 2003, p. 699). According to Brunswik, "the intellectual approach, using measurement and calculation, thus appears to fulfill the ultimate ends of perception in a way perception itself is incapable of doing" (1956, p. 91). This is because perception is a sort of probabilistic guessing game, making use of bottom-up and top-down cues to construct an image of the world quickly that is likely to be a faithful representation but is subject to a number of potential pitfalls. By relying on various forms of reasoning, physicians are able not only to think through a problem sequentially and rationally but also to call upon memories of past cases that may compare or contrast with the present observation. The NFLP colposcopy protocol aids physicians by directing their attention to each of the key features of the photograph.

Of course, no single psychological process is considered sufficient. Indeed, System 2 processes are accompanied by their own set of possible risks. As Kahneman (2003) points out, the monitoring function undertaken by System 2 is "normally quite lax and allows many intuitive judgments to be expressed, including some that are erroneous" (p. 699). In addition, the conscious operation of attention can lead the mind into misleading tangents. Brunswik (1956) points out that one can be led "off in the wrong direction by being right about something else" (p. 91). Problems associated with forgetting are obvious and are likely faced by each and every person on a daily basis (Neisser, 1982).

The potential problems caused by tangents in reasoning and forgetting highlight the importance of Feinstein's (1967) call for individual physicians and medical staffs to standardize the sequence of steps that make up sensory-driven medical procedures. In her field research conducted among a group of physicians specializing in diagnosing rare genetic disorders, Shaw (2003) observed a number of interactions in which physicians failed to differentiate description, designation, and diagnosis. For example:

> **Consultant 1:** "This girl was referred because the pediatrician thought she was dysmorphic, but when she started walking the parents did not want to pursue it."
> **Registrar:** "She looks chromosomal."
> **Consultant 2:** "She has the look of Floating Harbor."
> **Registrar:** "It is not a 22q nose."
> **Consultant 1:** It is a big nose, with the tip turned down. And note the long philtrum" (p. 41).

Although Consultant 1 provides a description of the case ("It is a big nose, with the tip turned down"), the Registrar and Consultant 2 move right into designation ("chromosomal," "a 22q nose"). In doing so, the Registrar and Consultant 2 fail to differentiate description from designation or to integrate information gathered from these two disciplines.

One can understand physicians' inclinations to speak in designations, as this facilitates communication about abstract or unusual classifications with their peers. In contrast, communication of a description requires greater time and detail. However, to fail to separate description from designation is to turn a blind eye to the complex series of perceptual and cognitive processes that lead to the selection of a particular designation. A colleague is almost certain to make use of a different manner of reasoning and can call upon a different set of prior cases and patients, which could lead to alternate designations.

DIAGNOSIS

Diagnosis is defined by Feinstein as "the anatomic or other abnormality that is responsible for the observed entity" (1967, p. 322). While physicians will likely make use of many of the same psychological processes in diagnosis as they do in description and designation, diagnosis is an inherently different problem. When making designations, physicians can largely remain at the level of the disease "in morphological, chemical, microbiologic, physiologic, or other impersonal terms" (Feinstein, 1967, p. 24), but when making a diagnosis, a broader range of data must be integrated.

Indeed, the term "diagnosis" is ambiguous because it can and does refer to two very different entities. Diagnosis can refer to the results of an examination such as a colposcopic exam, but it can also refer to the individual patient being examined. A correct diagnosis requires the integration of both results from medical procedures and knowledge of the individual patient's life (Noller & Bibace, 2002, chap. 6).

Proper diagnosis requires an integration of all data gathered throughout the examination by means of simultaneous and sequential psychological processes. The optimal endpoint of integration is the conservation of all parts into a coherent whole that takes into account all relevant information. This is a very difficult task. With so many parts to consider, there are many errors that may occur in the process of reasoning. Of particular risk in the medical realm is an error described by the developmental psychologist Piaget and his colleagues, referred to as *pars pro toto* thinking (Piaget & Inhelder, 1969). "Part for the whole" thinking occurs in medicine when a physician makes one designation and bases a diagnosis on this one factor, thus failing to consider fully not only other designations but also factors related to the particular patient being examined.

An example of the potential risk of *pars pro toto* thinking in colposcopy can be found in "a recent survey of family physician colposcopists," in which "approximately one-third formulate a colposcopic impression by a simple guess and otherwise most use a single colposcopic sign" (Ferris, 1999, p. 151).

A number of apt analogies for the type of integration we propose can be found in a recent book by Strogatz (2003) entitled *Sync: The Emerging Science of Spontaneous Order.* In a review, Kopell describes the book as addressing "collections of things—neurons, bosons, fireflies, chemical reactants—that display period oscillations and whose elements have predictable phase relations, often synchrony in the strict sense (i.e., zero phase lags among components)" (2003, p. 1878). Another appropriate analogy for integration from the world of music is provided by Bernstein (1973), who explains that Mozart's G-minor symphony achieves "that classical balance. . . . It's the combination of those two contradictory forces, chromaticism and diatonicism, operating at the same time that makes this passage so expressive" (p. 43). Integration in medical practice requires a similar, synchronous joining of disparate elements into a coherent whole.

In conclusion, multiple psychological processes are involved in each of the three intellectual disciplines involved in a medical procedure (i.e., description, designation, diagnosis) outlined by Feinstein (1967). The importance of accounting for automatic, simultaneous, as well as controlled, sequential processes cannot be overstated. Bargh and Chartrand (1999) point out that "dual process models in which the phenomenon in question is said to be influenced simultaneously by conscious (control) and non-conscious (automatic) processes are now the norm in the study of attention and encoding, memory, emotional appraisal, emotional disorders, attitudes and persuasion and social perception and judgment" (p. 463).

PSYCHOLOGICAL THEORIES UNDERLYING THE NOVEL APPROACH OF THE NFLP TO PHYSICIAN LIFE LONG LEARNING

The No-Fault Learning Program (NFLP) has been improved by the addition of two theoretical approaches: the Partnership Model (Bibace et al., 1999) and the necessity of exploring both outcomes and their corresponding psychological processes (Werner, 1948). A brief background on each approach and a discussion of connections to the NFLP should make the reasons behind certain aspects of the program more apparent to the reader.

The Partnership Model

The Partnership Model, which has been explored previously in the areas of education and research in addition to medical practice, is based on two key attitudes: complementarity and reciprocity. Complementarity in a partnership is the recognition that each partner has a special expertise from which others may benefit (Bibace, 1999). In the feedback they receive as part of an NFLP, both novice and experienced physicians have the opportunity to benefit from the many years of experience of the experts who designed the program. What may seem less obvious is that novices also make an important contribution to more experienced physicians. Those who have been practicing for many years are likely to forget the types of difficulties they faced as beginners. This input can help the experts to relate to those with less experience in subsequent interactions. In addition to the recognition of complementary roles, a spirit of reciprocity is also crucial to a successful partnership. Each partner must be willing to share their expertise with other partners in a back-and-forth, give-and-take series of exchanges. Only with a commitment to reciprocity will partners have the chance to benefit from one another's knowledge (Bibace, 1999).

The NFLP as a partnership is opposed to the traditional instructivist approach, and instead adheres to aspects of constructivism. Jonassen (1994) put forth eight characteristics of the constructivist approach to teaching and learning, a number of which closely pertain to aspects of the NFLP. One of the main aims of a constructivist learning environment is that knowledge should be constructed rather than just reproduced (Jonassen, 1994). In the NFLP, physicians make judgments both spontaneously and sequentially through the use of the protocol. These physicians, in effect, construct their own knowledge of how they can best improve their own skills by examining their errors of omission and commission over time. Inclusion of the spontaneous condition, which mimics everyday medical practice, also fulfills another constructivist mandate, namely, that educational tasks reflect real-world practices.

In constructivist education, learners should be encouraged to reflect on what they have done (Jonassen, 1994). Physicians taking part in an NFLP are encouraged to reflect on the written feedback they receive from the expert physicians.

The commitment to reciprocity and complementarity in an NFLP as a partnership ensures collaborative knowledge construction by means of social negotiation among partners as encouraged in constructivist approaches. The anonymous, no-fault nature of an NFLP precludes competition among learners, which is considered to be detrimental to learning by those adhering to constructivism (Jonassen, 1994). Another important element of constructivism, the provision of multiple representations of reality, will be discussed below.

Importance of Process as Opposed to Outcome

Rather than focusing solely on outcome measures, in an NFLP, emphasis is placed on the processes through which physicians come to make assessments. Rather than receiving only a percentage of correct and incorrect assessments, physicians participating in an NFLP should receive detailed feedback outlining whether errors of omission and commission were made.

A great deal of empirical evidence in psychology points to the conclusion that conscious effort can be used to correct inaccuracies resulting from the use of automatic processes, although these corrections are at times themselves flawed (Kahneman, 2003). For example, Devine (1989) found that most people will exhibit some evidence of stereotypes on unconscious, automatic tasks. It is only on conscious, controlled tasks when low-prejudiced individuals appear to suppress their unconscious leanings, while prejudiced individuals tend to be more likely to allow their unconscious prejudices to show through.

The objective of an NFLP is to make an analogous accomplishment. By making participants aware of the key features that must be addressed in a given diagnostic problem, assessment accuracy will increase and errors will decrease. The use of an NFLP protocol essentially eliminates errors of omission that result from forgetting. While errors of commission resulting from tangents in reasoning are not eliminated, it is likely that they will decrease due to the structure provided by the sequence of steps in the sequential protocol condition. At the same time, the strengths of each psychological process are accentuated. Vision is harnessed and channeled to the most important features in a systematic way. Given that physicians are directed to one feature at a time, the risk of exceeding the limitations of parallel-processing capacity is decreased. On the System 2 side of things, physicians are able to use memory by remembering prior cases without fear of the pitfalls of forgetting and are free to reason about designations (e.g., "is this an example of mosaicism or not?"), with the possibility of tangents being decreased. Therefore, an NFLP targets both psychological processes capable of acting simultaneously and those operating sequentially.

Werner (1948) recognized the importance of considering the process one uses to achieve an outcome rather than just the achievement itself. In this respect, errors can be illuminating because they shed light on the ways in which the mind works to arrive at an error and also on the mental steps taken to correct it. In contrast, a correct answer in and of itself provides little information regarding the way the individual arrived at the response.

An emphasis on process as well as outcome is optimal for a number of reasons. The recognition of process represents an acknowledgment that things are not always black and white, good or bad, especially when dealing with complex tasks like sensory-driven medical procedures. A correct designation or diagnosis may be made despite errors in attention or reasoning. In such a case, taking note of only outcomes would obscure these errors, and possibly lead to a repetition of the same mistake at a later time with unfortunate results. The converse is also possible. Namely, that despite properly directed attention and correct reasoning, an error can still occur. Without taking note of the psychological processes involved, physicians making such an error would not be given the opportunity to recognize the aspects of the assessment they performed correctly, as contrasted to those performed incorrectly. Werner's focus on process runs counter to the medical establishment in that typically, "a favorable result is more important than how it is attained" (Carmichael

& Carmichael, 1981, p. 123). But Carmichael and Carmichael argue that "an understanding of the process of medical care has valuable implications for health care delivery as well as the education of physicians."

In an NFLP, the errors of omission and commission are distinguished, along with the differing psychological processes responsible for them. In the Bibace and Noller trial of an NFLP using colposcopy, errors of omission were common. This type of error is likely to be caused by shortcomings in memory.

Errors of commission could be caused by the type of tangent in cognitive reasoning in which one attends to the wrong aspects of the task (e.g., evaluating a colpophotograph) or it could be caused by faulty reasoning. Either could result in the addition of an unnecessary step into one's plan for making a medical assessment.

Not only do the mental processes that lead to the types of errors differ, individuals' outlooks on errors of omission and commission seem to differ as well. Baron (1994) argues that people tend to view acts as having a greater impact than omissions, since the latter are often confounded with the *status quo.* Therefore it is possible that people may be more vigilant about preventing errors of commission because they are widely viewed as more deleterious than errors of omission. Errors of omission due to a memory deficit can be eliminated by NFLP participants as long as they adhere strictly to the protocol as it should account for all necessary steps in properly assessing a diagnostic task.

An emphasis on process in addition to outcome also can be achieved in an NFLP through a focus on multiple types of communication. Verbal and pictorial modes of representation should be used in an NFLP because both are integral parts of everyday medical practice. However, there are multiple examples (mammography, dermatology, and colposcopy, to name but a few) of visually oriented medical procedures where most communication among physicians is done verbally, either orally or in written documents.

While participants in an NFLP make their responses verbally and receive feedback in written form, another communication tool can be added. The physician can be asked to draw certain key features of the observation. In a colposcopy NFLP, photographs can be used, as previously described, but the participant can also be asked to draw the lesion. The use of multiple modes of communication in this way should reduce error ambiguity. As the success of Sigel's Psychological Distancing Acts (Sigel, 1993) attests, the use of multiple modes of communication is advantageous in conveying information in both formal and informal educational settings. The use of multiple modes of communication also meets one of the requirements of a constructivist learning environment as discussed above (Jonassen, 1994).

As a result of the influence of the Partnership Model, interaction among participants in an NFLP is based on the attitudes of reciprocity and complementarity and thus operates as a two-way rather than a one-way street (Bibace, 1999; Bibace et al., 1999). The necessity of exploring both outcomes and related psychological processes has guided our decision to focus on these processes for physicians participating in an NFLP.

CONCLUSIONS

The No-Fault Learning Program was designed with both the complementarity and reciprocity of the Partnership Model and Werner's emphasis on process in mind. Both universals and particulars of physician practice are addressed in an NFLP. The most central universal is that multiple psychological processes are involved in sensory-driven medical procedures. Separation of a medical procedure according to Feinstein's 3 D's of description, designation, and diagnosis facilitates making these multiple psychological processes explicit. Another key universal is the ubiquity of errors. While they cannot be avoided entirely, participation in an NFLP that attempts to accentuate physicians' intuitive abilities by directing them systematically through the use of a protocol offers an effective means of minimizing errors. The no-fault aspect of the program is considered essential to physician learning.

In addition to these universals, the NFLP also accounts for particulars in physician practice. Not only is every physician different, with varied training, experiences, and working habits, but further, a given physician will not always proceed in exactly the same way. These particulars are acknowledged in an NFLP by providing physicians with an opportunity to assess their own performance over time with the help of written feedback from experts.

While we have attempted to identify psychological processes that are likely at work during sensory-driven medical procedures, we have refrained from making definitive statements, given the presence of both individual and intra-individual differences.

REFERENCES

Bargh, J. A., & Chartrand, T. L. (1999). The unbearable automaticity of being. *American Psychologist, 54*, 462–479.

Baron, J. (1994). Nonconsequentialist decisions. *Behavioral and Brain Sciences, 17,* 1–10.

Bernstein, L. (1973). *The unanswered question: Six talks at Harvard.* Cambridge, MA: Harvard University Press.

Bibace, R. (1999). A partnership ideal. In R. Bibace, J. J. Dillon, & B. N. Dowds (Eds.), *Partnerships in clinical, education and research contexts* (pp. 275–306). Greenwich, CT: Ablex Publishing Co.

Bibace, R., Dillon, J. J., & Dowds, B. N. (Eds.) (1999). *Partnerships in clinical, education and research contexts* (pp. 27–36). Greenwich, CT: Ablex Publishing Co.

Bibace, R. & Noller, K. L. (2003). *A comparison of colposcopic judgments made under two conditions: Spontaneous versus focused attention.* Unpublished raw data.

Broadbent, D. E. (1958). *Perception and communication.* London: Pergamon Press.

Brunswik, E. (1956). *Perception and the representative design of psychological experiments.* Berkeley, CA: University of California Press.

Carmichael, L. P., & Carmichael, J. S. (1981). The relational model of family practice. *Marriage & Family Review, 4,* 123–133.

Crick, F., & Koch, C. (1998). Consciousness and neuroscience. *Cerebral Cortex, 8,* 97–107.

Devine, P. G. (1989). Stereotypes and prejudice: Their automatic and controlled components. *Journal of Personality and Social Psychology, 56,* 5–18.

Feinstein, A. R. (1967). *Clinical judgment.* Huntington, NY: Krieger.

Feinstein, A. R. (1994). *Clinical judgment* revisited: The distraction of quantitative models. *Annals of Internal Medicine, 120,* 799–805.

Ferris, D. G. (1999). *Comprehensive colposcopy.* Kansas City, MO: American Society for Colposcopy and Cervical Pathology.

Hoffman, D. D. (1998). *Visual intelligence: How we create what we see.* New York: W.W. Norton.

Itti, L. (2000). *Models of bottom-up and top-down visual attention.* Unpublished doctoral dissertation, California Institute of Technology.

Jonassen, D. H. (1994). Thinking technology: Toward a constructivist design model. *Educational Technology, 34,* 34–37.

Kahneman, D. (2003). A perspective on judgment and choice: Mapping bounded rationality. *American Psychologist, 58,* 697–720

Kahneman, D., & Tversky, A. (1979). Prospect theory: An analysis of decision under risk. *Econometrica, 47,* 276–287.

Kohn, L. T., Corrigan, J. M., & Donaldson, M. S. (Eds.) (2000). *To err is human: Building a safer health care system.* Washington, DC: National Academy Press.

Kolstad, P., & Stafl, A. (1972). *Atlas of colposcopy.* Baltimore: University Park Press.

Kopell, N. (2003). A tree of fireflies, a flock of boson clouds. *Science, 300,* 1878–1879.

Logothetis, N. K. (1999). Vision: A window on consciousness. *Scientific American, 281,* 68–75.

Matthews, Duncan. (1878). *Medical Times and Gazette,* 1878, p. 729.

Muller, M. M., & Hubner, R. (2002). Can the spotlight of attention be shaped like a doughnut? *Psychological Science, 13,* 119–124.

Neisser, U. (1982). *Memory observed.* San Francisco: Freeman.

Nisbett, R. E., & Wilson, T. D. (1977). Telling more than we can know: Verbal reports on mental processes. *Psychological Review, 84,* 231–259.

Noller, K. L. (1993). *Common colposcopic errors.* Presented at the Northwestern University Advanced Colposcopy Course, Chicago, IL.

Noller, K. L., & Bibace, R. (2002). The centrality of the clinician in the evaluation of patients with abnormal cervical cytologic studies. *American Journal of Obstetrics and Gynecology, 187,* 1533–1535.

Pashler, H. E. (1999). *The psychology of attention.* Cambridge: MIT Press.

Piaget, J., & Inhelder, B. (1969). *The psychology of the child.* New York: Basic Books.

Posner, I. P., & Peterson, S. E. (1990). The attention system of the human brain. *Annual Review of Neuroscience, 13,* 25–42.

Senders, J. W. (1994). Medical devices, medical errors, and medical accidents. In M. S. Bogner (Ed.), *Human error in medicine* (pp. 159–177). Hillsdale, NJ: Lawrence Erlbaum & Associates.

Shaw, A. (2003). Interpreting images: Diagnostic skill in the genetics clinic. *Journal of the Royal Anthropological Institute, 9,* 39–55.

Sigel, I. E. (1993). The centrality of a distancing model for the development of representational competence. In R. R. Cocking & A. Renninger (Eds.), *The development and meaning of psychological distance* (pp. 141–158). Hillsdale, NJ: Lawrence Erlbaum & Associates.

Stanovich, K. E., & West, R. F. (2000). Individual differences in reasoning: Implications for the rationality debate. *Behavioral and Brain Sciences, 23,* 645–665.

Strogatz, S.H. (2003). *Sync: The emerging science of spontaneous order.* New York: Hyperion.

Werner, H. (1948). *Comparative psychology of mental development.* New York: International Universities Press.

Chapter 9

EVIDENCE-BASED MEDICINE: QUANTITATIVELY MOVING FROM THE UNIVERSAL TO THE PARTICULAR

David Chelmow

All interactions between physician and patient involve degrees of uncertainty. The physician must first ascertain both what is important to the patient and what things are unimportant to the patient but of importance to the patient's health. Questions must be asked, and diagnostic methods must be used to uncover the underlying problem. Once the physician has decided, without absolute certainty, on the potential diagnoses, a list of potential treatment options must be drawn up, and these must be presented to the patient with a recommendation. Medicine differs from other fields as the consequences of incorrect decision making can lead to increased morbidity, suffering, or even death.

The knowledge that is used to direct the patient interview, choose the diagnostic strategy, and delineate treatment options is derived from experience, scientific study, and tradition. Physicians use a variety of paradigms to make these decisions (Figure 9.1). Frequently used paradigms include logic based on understanding the pathophysiology of the presumed disorder, prior personal experience, common sense, and now "evidence-based medicine." In this chapter, we will describe evidence-based medicine (EBM), with particular emphasis on its use as a tool to move from the universals of medical knowledge to the particulars of an individual patient, as well as its limitations.

HISTORY

"Evidence-based medicine" is a term that Guyatt and Rennie (2002) attribute to David Sackett. During the late 1970s, epidemiologists at

Figure 9.1
The place of EBM in the clinical universe. Medical decision making involves a number of paradigms. The large oval includes all current medical knowledge. The surrounding rectangle includes all potential medical knowledge, including things not yet discovered, and things no longer practiced. Within clinical medicine is a much smaller group of knowledge, evidence based knowledge (small oval). Here the oval has been drawn relatively large, mostly for the ease of visualization. Many practitioners would argue that actual medical decision making supported by rigorous scientific evidence is a much smaller proportion than depicted here. As noted in the graph, some of medicine is currently practiced incorrectly (area to right of line); this includes areas of evidence based medicine (5), which will be supplanted by better evidence. The parts of the clinical medicine that are not practiced as part of EBM (2 and 4) comprise decisions made based on tradition, the practitioner's training, or presumed understanding of the disease pathophysiology.

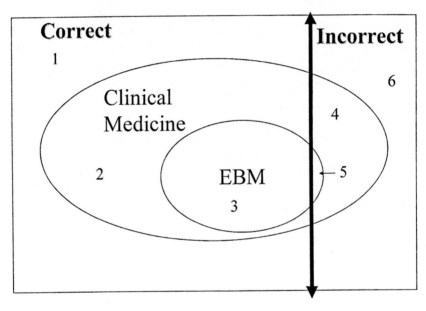

The Clinical Universe

McMaster University in Canada wrote a series of articles advising clinicians on how to interpret the vast medical literature and at the same time began to teach residents how to make this a routine part of their practice. They initially called this "critical appraisal." In 1990, they created a document for their residents in which they used the term "evidence-based medicine" (EBM). The goal was to teach their residents to be aware of the actual scientific evidence on which they were basing decisions, to evaluate the quality of this evidence, and to determine how reliable a decision they could make on the basis of this information. The ultimate goal was to ensure that patients always received the best-proven, most efficacious care and at the same time avoided ineffective or unproven treatments. Guyatt published an article in the *ACP Journal Club* (1991), which appears to be the first time the term "EBM" appeared in a publication. The concept has spread to the point where it has become a required part of medical school curricula and most lectures.

EBM DEFINED

More explicitly, EBM requires that, whenever possible, decisions be made and management strategies be implemented based on scientific evidence. Further, it stipulates that this scientific evidence be the result of carefully done, methodologically sound, and carefully presented studies. Ideally, these studies are published in the peer-reviewed literature. Randomized placebo-controlled clinical trials should be the basis for decisions whenever possible.

EBM is a process of formulating a clinical question in a way that the medical literature can be searched. It then involves finding studies that have been reported that potentially provide an answer to the question. These studies are critically evaluated based on their design and the quality with which they were performed. EBM practitioners have developed techniques, such as meta-analysis, to combine results when there are multiple studies on the same topic.

They then review this evidence to answer their clinical question. Ideally, they restrict their practice to diagnostic techniques and management strategies that are supported by well-constructed studies.

IMPETUS FOR EBM

The impetus for EBM comes from the desire to rationalize and improve patient care, but it is particularly driven by two concerns: attempts to make medical decision making rational and consistent and to minimize cost.

A large body of literature suggests that major medical procedures are used very differently by different practitioners in ways that cannot be explained. The first of these studies (Wennberg & Gittelsohn, 1973) used Medicare reimbursement and population data to study health care in Vermont. The study noted wide variations in hospital usage and procedures such as tonsillectomy, appendectomy, prostatectomy, and hysterectomy in different regions throughout the state. These could not be explained by population density, number of physicians, insurance, or patient age. Procedures varied as much as ten-fold between the areas of lowest and highest utilization. Similar results were noted for the management of myocardial infarction (Pilote et al., 1995), carotid endarterectomy (Wennberg, Lucas, Birkmeyer, Bredenberg, & Fisher, 1998), and use of psychiatric outpatient services (Kessler et al., 1997). These variations seem to bear no relation to the relative health of the local community, training of the provider, or availability of resources. In fact, this variation suggests that many providers use very expensive procedures in very different ways for completely unclear reasons. Unfortunately, these studies are unable to determine what the correct utilization of the procedures should be. It is unclear if they are underutilized in areas of low utilization or overused in areas with high utilization.

Another important motivation cited by EBM advocates is controlling cost. The Office of the Actuary at the Centers for Medicare and Medicaid Services (http://www.hcfa.gov/stats/nhe-oact/nhe.htm) projects that U.S. national health care expenditures will grow at a mean annual rate of 7.3 percent and reach $2.8 trillion by 2011. In 2000, these expenditures represented 13.2 percent of the gross domestic product, a fraction projected to reach 17.0 percent by 2011. These costs pose a serious burden on society, and the continued increase needs to be controlled. The data suggest that procedures with potential large cumulative costs and unproven benefit are being performed. EBM is attractive to the government, payers, and consumers of health care as there is a much greater rationale for focusing payment on proven, effective, screening and diagnostic procedures and treatments.

THE EVIDENCE

Evidence is derived from studies that may be published or not. There are literally thousands of English-language medical journals and thousands more in other languages. PubMed, a service of the National Library of Medicine, is a searchable computer database that contains references to over 12 million articles in 4,500 medical journals dating back to the 1960s (http://www.ncbi.nlm.nih.gov/entrez/query.fcgi). Journals vary widely in quality and circulation. The *Journal of the American Medical Association* (JAMA) and the *New England Journal of Medicine* (NEJM) receive high-quality manuscripts which are reviewed by physicians knowledgeable in the field (peer reviewed) as well as the journal editors. They tend to restrict publication to quality articles of general interest. Most other journals receive little attention outside of their field and have limited readership. Published studies are of a variety of methodologies, each with advantages, disadvantages, and limitations in quality.

Many studies are presented at conferences but never published, and a significant fraction are neither presented nor published. Despite the large amount of time required to complete a project, manuscript preparation can be prohibitive, and studies show that a result of "no effect" for a treatment is deemed less interesting and less often published. Unpublished studies contain potentially valuable information. Egger and Smith (1998) reviewed publication bias and noted that studies showing that a treatment has an effect were three times more likely to be published than studies showing no effect and that the time from manuscript submission to publication was shorter for these studies. They also noted other differences; for example, studies that were publicly funded were more likely to be published than those that were privately funded.

The provider must search for relevant information from this vast array of medical journals, make assumptions about unpublished data, evaluate the quality of the evidence, and suggest a treatment plan for a particular patient.

HIERARCHIES OF EVIDENCE

Published medical studies are usually categorized into a number of different types (Figure 9.2), each with its own strengths and weaknesses (Hulley, Cummings, & Browner, 2001). It has become clear that use of the study types at the top of this hierarchy, especially randomized clinical trials (RCTs), is particularly important. Conclusions drawn from retrospective observational work have been shown often to be misleading after randomized trials are performed.

One of the best examples of this is the current controversy over hormone replacement therapy (HRT) in postmenopausal women. For over 30 years, supplemental estrogen and progesterone were recommended to these women. Based on retrospective, observational studies, estrogen supplementation was thought to both make the woman feel better and to prevent heart disease (Stampfer & Colditz, 1991), hip fractures (Weiss, Ure, Ballard, Williams, & Daling, 1980), and potentially to prolong life (Grodstein et al., 1997). A few observational studies suggested that there might be an increased risk of breast cancer (Steinberg et al., 1991). Nonetheless, decision analyses suggested that, given the large benefit against

Figure 9.2
Medical evidence is derived from many types of studies. The strength of inferences
that can be drawn from different study types varies. Case reports are the least useful
for deriving conclusions; randomized trials are the most widely accepted source of
rigorous evidence.

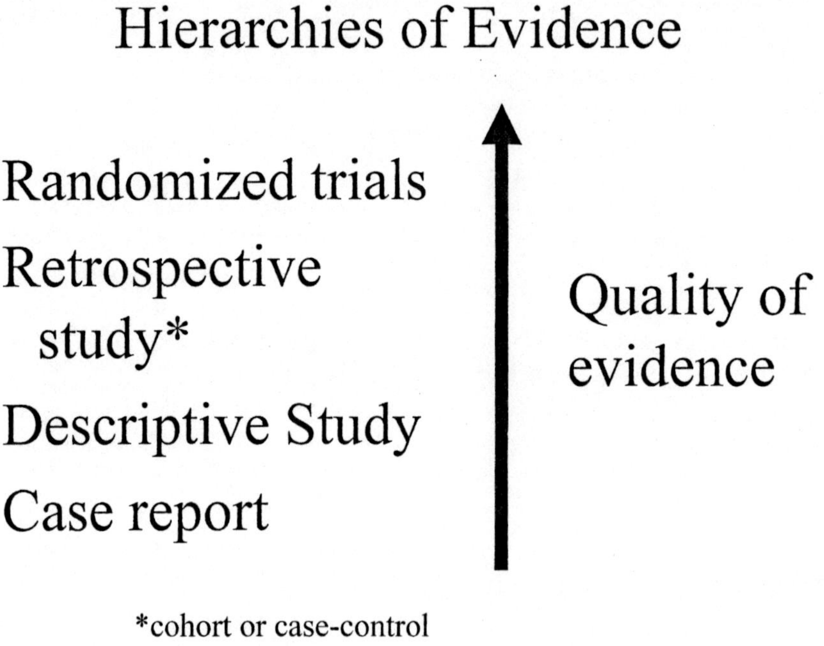

Hierarchies of Evidence

Randomized trials

Retrospective
study*

Quality of
evidence

Descriptive Study

Case report

*cohort or case-control

heart disease, it was still beneficial to take HRT (Col et al., 1997). Early studies all suggested an approximate 50 percent reduction in coronary artery disease for women on HRT. These estimates were based on retrospective cohort studies and were further supported by meta-analyses summarizing these data (Stampfer & Colditz, 1991).

In 2002, the Women's Health Initiative Study (WHI) (Writing Group for the Women's Health Initiative Investigators, 2002) closed early because of a 32 percent increased risk of coronary events. The WHI was a randomized, blinded trial, and the demonstration of an effect opposite to what was previously thought true clearly reflects the limitations of cohort studies. It is very likely that the women in the earlier retrospective studies who were placed on hormones were actually healthier than women from which it was withheld. It was this underlying greater degree of health that probably led to their decreased incidence of coronary events, not any effect of the estrogen.

A similar effect has been noted with other treatments where the same topic was studied by both RCTs and nonrandomized, usually retrospective studies. Ioannidis et al. (2001) studied 45 topics that had been previously studied with both nonrandomized and randomized study designs. In all instances, the cohort studies showed a greater treatment effect than the RCTs. In a number of studies, statistically significant differences were noted in the cohort studies but not in the RCTs. The WHI study is particularly interesting, because it seems to be the first important example where the RCT not only failed to find a benefit but rather identified a risk to the therapy.

Unfortunately, many important issues cannot be studied with RCTs. Notably, uncommon complications of treatments and health consequences of risky behaviors are not appropriate. For example, it would not be ethical to study the ill effects of smoking by randomizing patients to smoking and not smoking. Thus, public health problems and outcomes need to be studied observationally. The large number of subjects required to have statistical power to detect differences of outcomes that occur uncommonly also make randomized trials prohibitively large and expensive. Only the magnitude of the question regarding HRT, something that applied to every woman over age 50, allowed a trial to be performed that was able to study small increments in adverse outcomes like incidence of breast cancer, blood clots, and cardiac events.

INTEGRATING THE EVIDENCE

EBM relies heavily on published evidence. With the use of microcomputers and the Internet, it is now possible to access a huge number of journal article abstracts, and a significant number of entire journal articles, quickly. Many journals put their entire contents on-line so that accessing huge amounts of information no longer requires a visit to the medical library. Several computerized indexes allow easy searching of this information by keyword or title word. The U.S. federal government provides free access to MEDLINE, the most commonly used literature-searching tool, through the National Library of Medicine (http://www.ncbi.nlm.nih.gov/entrez/query.fcgi).

This information is both a blessing and a burden. In order to attempt to bring order to the huge amount of evidence that is suddenly at the practitioner's fingertips, efforts have been made to develop methods of preprocessing and organizing the information. Authorities (Guyatt, Meade, Jaeschke, Cook, & Haynes, 2000) have suggested that it would be unwieldy for every provider to devote the time and energy to develop the epidemiologic skills necessary to do evidence-based synthesis for medical decisions, and the effort at present is to optimize preprocessed and pre-assimilated medical information. This is done in a number of ways.

Meta-Analysis

One of the most important tools is meta-analysis. This is a technique for pooling data from multiple studies on the same subject. Usually, specific search criteria are developed to find the published literature on a specific clinical question. Attempts are often made to access unpublished data. The studies are then critically evaluated first to be certain that they meet acceptable methodologic criteria and then to make sure that they are adequately similar. If so, they can be pooled using statistical techniques to estimate the combined effect measure over multiple studies. This has a number of advantages. Sometimes when studies have conflicting results, by using objective techniques that pool the studies based on weighting, it is easier to determine the actual effect of the treatment. Other times, information can be gained by systematically comparing studies with different results to look at the differences and thus gain insight into the factors responsible for the differences in observed outcomes (Cooper & Hedges, 1994; Mulrow & Cook, 1998).

In addition, for an uncommon outcome, pooling multiple, smaller studies may be able to show a statistically significant effect that had been previously hard to detect. For example, we performed a meta-analysis (Chelmow, Ruehli, & Huang, 2001) looking at the effect of antibiotic prophylaxis to prevent infection after cesarean delivery in women with a low risk of infectious complications. In these women, antibiotic prophylaxis had previously been thought to be of no help. Seven prior studies had been performed, and none showed a statistically significant decrease in infection with prophylactic antibiotics. We pooled the data from these seven published studies and detected a large, statistically significant decrease in infection with the use of prophylactic antibiotics (Figure 9.3).

Decision Analysis

Decision analysis is a technique that allows pooling of data regarding different treatments or diagnostic techniques from multiple studies, to ascertain the optimal choice as measured by an outcome, such as minimizing cost or maximizing quality adjusted years of life saved (Drummond, O'Brien, Stoddart, & Torrance, 1997; Haddix, Teutsch, Shaffer, & Dunet, 1996; Petitti, 2000). Often multiple treatments or diagnostic techniques can be used for a given medical problem. One must then determine which is the most appropriate. Sometimes it is clear that different treatments apply better to different groups of patients. For example, there are several methods for evaluating minimally abnormal Pap smears. These include repeating the Pap smear in 4–6 months, performing colposcopy (viewing the cervix with magnification) and performing biopsies of suspicious areas, or performing a test for human papillomavirus (HPV probe). Each of these techniques differs in cost, convenience, and accuracy for detecting precursors of cervical cancer.

A decision analysis of the Pap smear problem above was performed (Kim, Wright, & Goldie, 2002), suggesting that the newer technique, the HPV probe, was an acceptable alternative, having a comparable cost without decreasing life expectancy and being a faster way to resolve a question of great worry to patients.

In the prophylactic antibiotic example used in the meta-analysis section, one argument against using prophylactic antibiotics in low-risk women is that, given the rarity with which the outcome occurs, it may be less expensive to not give the antibiotic prophylaxis and to treat infections as they occur instead. Formal decision analysis methodology suggests that, despite the rarity of infectious complications, given the low cost of antibiotics, it is still cost effective to use prophylaxis even given the low-risk cesarean deliveries (Chelmow, Hennesy, & Evantash, in press).

Guidelines

Guidelines are meant to be the highest level of preprocessed evidence. They are a combination of literature review, meta-analysis, and decision analysis. If adequate evidence is not available, expert opinion is included to give providers complete suggestions for management. The U.S. government maintains a guidelines clearinghouse (http://www.guidelines.gov) that now includes over 1,000 guidelines on medical topics.

Guidelines do suffer a number of limitations. They are expensive and difficult to develop. They also are only current on the day they are written. Because information changes rapidly, they are out of date quickly. A number of attempts have been made to develop systems for continuously updating guidelines. The *British Medical Journal* maintains a Web site called Clinical Evidence (http://www.clinicalevidence.com) that includes similar guidelines and topic reviews, but that are updated on an ongoing basis. The updates become available instantaneously over the Internet.

General Limitations of Evidence Synthesis

All of these methods for synthesizing evidence are limited by issues of publication bias. Unfortunately, much medical research is done that is never published. Some of it is presented at meetings and is available in abstract form. Other unpublished data can sometimes be obtained from pharmaceutical companies. There is now an attempt at maintaining a controlled trials register (http://www.controlled-trials.com) that tracks all ongoing clinical trials whether or not they are ultimately published. Publication bias becomes an issue in attempting to do meta-analysis or other synthesis because it is clear that unpublished studies are more likely to have negative results than published studies. In addition, studies that showed no effect that are published take longer to be published than studies in which patients showed a treatment benefit or adverse outcome (Montori, Smieja, & Guyatt, 2000).

Another important issue is that the same evidence can sometimes be synthesized in more than one way. Pooling information is somewhat subjective, and different methods exist for pooling it. Hopayian (2001) illustrates this in a report of three systematic reviews of epidural steroid injections for sciatica, where two showed no evidence for effectiveness and the third showed benefit.

OTHER DECISION-MAKING PARADIGMS

EBM seems to be the ultimate in rationality. One might then ask, what other alternatives are there (Figure 9.1)? Prior to the widespread availability of the Internet and easy access to medical journals and published studies, medical decision making was traditionally based on a number of informal paradigms. Initially, it was based on the provider's clinical experience and expert opinion. The growth of basic science research in the last century led to treatment recommendations based on the understanding of the pathophysiology of the disease. Both paradigms seemed to be reasonable approaches. Medical providers tend to be good observers, and in most instances their observations of treatment effects, particularly when the effect is large, are correct.

However, a large number of examples demonstrate the perils of relying strictly on these paradigms. Lacchetti and Guyatt (2002) present a long list of examples. The HRT example we previously presented was based both on the observations of physicians and on pathophysiology. Numerous published retrospective studies showed decreased cardiac events and even a prolongation of life in these patients. Studies of pathophysiology showed that estrogen improved lipid profiles, and other studies showed that lowering blood lipid levels decreased the risk of myocardial infarction. Similarly, there seemed to be beneficial effects on brachial artery reactivity, which is a measure of coronary artery spasm. Nonetheless, the WHI (Writing Group for the Women's Health Initiative Investigators, 2002) provided clear RCT-based evidence that the opposite effect, through unknown mechanisms, seems to be the case.

SUPPORT FOR EBM

EBM has developed a host of proponents. The Agency for Health Care Research and Quality (AHRQ) is an agency of the U.S. federal government that gives as one of its main functions to sponsor and conduct "research that provides evidence-based information on health care outcomes; quality; and cost, use, and access" (http://www.ahrq.gov/about/profile.htm). It disseminates grant money specifically for synthesizing evidence, developing guidelines, and disseminating the results of the guidelines. Similarly, the National Health Service in the United Kingdom has added similar priorities. The U.S. government's commitment to outcomes research and evidence-based medicine is well demonstrated by the AHQR's budget, where an appropriation of $306 million was requested in fiscal year 2002 (http://www.ahrq.gov/about/cj2002/ budbrf02.htm). Through their patient outcomes research teams ("PORTS") and evidence-based practice centers, they have developed a large number of evidence-based reviews and guidelines.

More importantly, EBM is now required in medical school and residency training curricula. This requirement has been made by both the American Association of Medical Colleges (AAMC), the accrediting body for U.S. medical schools, and the American College of Graduate Medical Education (ACGME), the accrediting body for specialty training programs. The ACGME requires EBM to be one of the "core competencies" that all residents in all specialty training programs learn.

Although the ultimate aspiration of having all practitioners comfortable evaluating evidence critically seems worthy, more realistically it seems that most providers will become users of preprocessed evidence.

British general practitioners have been extensively surveyed (McColl, Smith, White, & Field, 1998) and have specifically stated this. In their survey, only 5 percent of 302 general practitioners stated that the best way to move from opinion-based to evidence-based practice was by "identifying and appraising the primary literature or systematic reviews" while the other 95 percent stated they preferred use of preprocessed guidelines or evidence-based summaries.

EBM has also become attractive at other levels. Other groups who are looking at EBM with close scrutiny are insurers and the U.S. government. Managed care organizations are attempting to minimize cost, and one powerful argument, given irrational use of services, is that only services with well-substantiated effectiveness should be paid for. Some are incorporating requirements for evidence in their decision of what procedures to reimburse. EBM is being used by the U.S. government for policy decisions with similar rationale. It will be interesting to see whether patients begin to incorporate EBM into their decision process. Although most patients do not have the same sophistication as trained medical providers, much of this information can be summarized and presented in ways that are clear to patients.

IMPLEMENTING EBM

The greatest difficulty now is implementing EBM. Although it is difficult to make estimates for what fraction of decisions we currently make with EBM, even optimistic providers seldom cite numbers over 20 percent. Specific barriers to widespread EBM use will be discussed in a separate section. In an attempt to make EBM easier to practice, the largest efforts have been directed at making preprocessed evidence-based reviews and guidelines widely available.

Processing the Evidence

At the lowest level, a number of journals have been developed, for example the *ACP Journal Club,* which extract the most important studies from among a large number of journals, abstract them, and give brief summaries, in an effort to allow providers quicker access to individual new studies. Of special note is the Cochrane Controlled Trials Register. This is an ambitious attempt to create a computerized library of all published, high-quality RCTs. The Cochrane Database staff reviews the literature on an ongoing basis and includes trials meeting rigid criteria. Where multiple trials of a single topic have been done, the Cochrane staff attempts to maintain up-to-date meta-analyses, incorporating new studies as they are published. These meta-analyses, the Cochrane Database of Systematic Reviews, are done with rigid criteria and uniform standards to make them easy to interpret. These evidence-based summaries are available for free over the Internet and cover many common medical and primary-care topics.

Disseminating the Preprocessed Evidence

Dissemination was initially attempted in print form; in 1997, the U.S. Preventative Services Task Force (U.S. Preventative Task Force Staff, 1997) printed a summary of their primary-care recommendations in book form. The *British Medical Journal* publishes *Clinical Evidence* as a book biannually. This appeals to many providers who like to read books and find books easy to access but does not take into account the rapidity with which information changes. Many of the guidelines in the U.S. Preventative Task Force book were out of date within one year. *Clinical Evidence* gets around this difficulty by publishing more frequently.

Many providers now rely on the Internet to be able to get current evidence. The content of *Clinical Evidence* is available on-line, and topics are updated on an ongoing basis. The Cochrane Database of Systematic Reviews are available online for free, and their entire controlled trials register is accessible over the World Wide Web for a subscription fee. MEDLINE is available through many medical libraries, medical societies, and specialty groups, and it is also provided for free through the National Library of Medicine (http://www.ncbi.nlm.nih.gov/entrez/query.fcgi). Many journals have created e-journals, where recent articles can be obtained over the World Wide Web, frequently without charge.

BARRIERS TO EVIDENCE-BASED MEDICINE

Despite the many attractive aspects about EBM, a number of significant barriers and obstacles stand in the way of universal acceptance. Some of these are quite serious.

Time

One major issue is time. This was the primary obstacle noted by clinicians in several qualitative studies (Ely et al., 2002; McColl et al., 1998). The vision of a provider going to primary medical journals or even the Internet for every clinical decision to ensure that they have reviewed the proper studies, synthesized them, and applied the information properly is far too time consuming. Many providers now see patients as often as every 10–15 minutes. Within each of those patient interactions, a number of clinical questions and management decisions arise. Under normal circumstances, providers rely on their clinical experience and memory to answer these questions and make decisions as they arise. Even when a presynthesized source is available, to attempt to look up the answer in a book or in a readily available on-line source would likely take at least several minutes, prohibitively long in the pace of clinical encounters, and disruptive to the flow of the provider–patient encounter. When presynthesized information is not available, it would take at least an hour to synthesize information for providers comfortable with the required skills. Ely et al. (2002) recorded the time necessary for providers to research two typical clinical questions encountered in their study and noted median times of 45 and 95 minutes.

Training

To answer evidence-based questions requiring a literature search, critical evaluation of studies, synthesis of evidence, and deciding whether it applies to an individual patient requires skill in interpreting studies and epidemiology that most providers do not currently have. Even adding these skills to the requirements for medical and graduate medical education is unlikely to universally prepare practitioners, given that the time commitment necessary is unlikely to be available. McColl et al. (1998) surveyed British general practitioners and noted that 90 percent did not believe it a priority to learn these skills. However, it is realistic to expect that adequate training could be provided to have individual practitioners able to search for previously prepared, presynthesized evidence, to critically evaluate it, and to apply it properly to their patients. McColl noted that 72 percent of the providers surveyed did use evidence that had been prepared by others. This seems to be the current focus of most medical education regarding EBM.

Proper curricula for teaching EBM to medical students, residents, and the continuing education of established providers have not been worked out. Opportunities for teaching students and residents occur during didactic sessions and journal clubs as well as in formalized teaching sessions, such as teaching rounds and morning report. However, Ghali, Lesky, and Hershman (1998) reviewed these opportunities and concluded that "isolated teaching interventions in critical appraisal and literature searching are not sufficient for promoting EBM" but rather "a longitudinally integrated curriculum targeting each of the component skills of EBM needs to be implemented." Bazarian, Davis, Spillane, Blumstein, and Schneider (1999) performed a randomized trial of teaching critical appraisal skills to emergency medicine residents by randomizing trainees to a structured journal club focusing on teaching these skills and a traditional unstructured journal club. They did not note any improvement in these skills with the structured approach. Hatala (1999) in an accompanying editorial raised the question of whether EBM is a teachable skill; more recently, Hatala and Guyatt (2002) reviewed the continued lack of evidence on teaching EBM but concluded that, given the rising number of providers with skills, it must be a learnable skill. They also stated that "there is a universal agreement that such material is teachable." It is interesting that EBM providers who usually insist on the highest quality of evidence for implementing new techniques are so accepting of a lack of true evidence for EBM itself, but the statement is generally accepted.

Lack of Evidence

While there is a huge body of evidence available, with thousands of medical journals and estimates of 6,000 medical articles published each day, nonetheless, many medical questions and management decisions do not have evidence to support them. One vision of EBM would be similar to mathematics, where individual theorems are based on previously proven theorems. This will never be the situation in medicine. Much of what we already do is based on things that will never be studied formally, some because they seem so obvious that a study could not be adequately performed (e.g., treating diabetes with insulin or severe infection with antibiotics). Far more are obscure enough that they would be difficult to perform. Many individual patients differ in significant ways from those enrolled in randomized trials, and the applicability of the study results to the individual patient is not clear. Estimates of the fraction of treatment decisions based on evidence are derived from a study of 109 patients hospitalized on a university medical service, where 53 percent of primary treatments were found to be supported by RCT data (Ellis, Mulligan, Rowe, & Sackett, 1995). Another estimate comes from a suburban training general practice, where 30 percent of 101 therapeutic decisions were supported by randomized trials (Gill et al., 1996).

Application of Generic Evidence to Individual Patients

Attempting to apply published evidence based on populations of patients to an individual patient in the office is one of the most significant issues in using EBM as a tool to move from the universals of general medical knowledge to the particulars of decision making for an individual patient. RCTs often enroll patients who are substantially different from patients encountered in usual practice. Also, most analyses report average effects for average patients, and they are unable specifically to look for the implications of individual differences, which may be important for individual patients. Many procedures are used in the community for indications for which effectiveness data do not exist. One of the most difficult issues is for the provider who has evaluated the evidence to decide if the evidence actually clearly applies to this patient, who may or may not be similar to the initial study population. Further, the individual patient is not interested in the average effect but rather the effect it will have on them (Welch, 2000). The patient does not so much care that about a 5 percent chance of dying from the disease but rather whether they will be one of the 5 percent to die. EBM does not provide answers to such questions. This limitation is not restricted to EBM but applies to all medical decision-making paradigms.

The effect of use of EBM and communicating the EBM process in an individual physician–patient relationship has not been well studied. The ability for the provider to be able to tell the patient that recommendations are supported by well-performed scientific studies is probably comforting to the patient, especially if presented in addition to the traditional comments of "in my experience" or "we usually." It would be hard to envision a situation where this additional information would be unwelcome, except perhaps in the situation where a treatment desired by the patient is withheld because of evidence suggesting its ineffectiveness. Patients clearly do pay attention to the results of major randomized trials with important findings. For example, the early stopping of the WHI study (Writing Group for the Women's Health Initiative Investigators, 2002) was carried on the front pages of most major newspapers and television news. This was clearly noted by patients, as physicians were immediately inundated with phone calls from worried patients. Interestingly, it is not as clear that patients actively seek out this type of evidence as they seek information. Many people search for health information on the Internet, and many health-related Web sites have been started. A qualitative study of patients' use of the Internet (Eysenbach & Köhler, 2002) found that none of the subjects observed inquired into the sources of information or how the information on health Web sites had been compiled. A single study (Freeman & Sweeney, 2001) used focus groups on 19 general practitioners in the U.K. The focus groups noted several instances of how the provider's relationship with the patient caused them to alter how they implemented guidelines on individual patients and that physicians perceived that the extra manipulations they were performing to achieve targets suggested by guidelines potentially raised anxiety in patients.

Potential for Abuse

It is easy to envision payers and insurance companies, who like to limit their costs, restricting reimbursement to procedures and treatments that have been proven beneficial with sound scientific evidence. Unfortunately, many things have not been studied. Just because something has not been studied does not necessarily mean it does not work. Requirements for strict evidence for allowing a treatment option may unnecessarily restrict patients from beneficial but not yet proven therapies.

Summary of Limitations

Despite high expectations, EBM has several limitations, some making it difficult to universally implement and others making it inadequate for many clinical circumstances. One approach to the implementation issues has been to divide providers into two types (Guyatt et al., 2000). Some providers truly have the skills to answer evidence-based questions by integrating primary sources and have the time to do it for a limited number of questions. Others cannot do this, nor do they have the time or desire, but are able to apply presynthesized evidence. This is why much of the current focus is on the development of evidence-based reviews of topics, such as the Cochrane Database, as well as guidelines whose development is often government sponsored, both by the AHQR in the United States and the National Health Service in the United Kingdom. Libraries of guidelines are frequently maintained in easy-to-access places, such as the U.S. federal government Guidelines Clearinghouse (http://www.guidelines.gov). However, even frequent referral to guidelines is more time consuming than can routinely be done in a busy practice.

It is also important to note that several of the criticisms of EBM, particularly the shortage of consistent, coherent scientific evidence and the difficulty in applying the evidence to the care of individual patients, are not truly limitations of EBM but are actually limitations of any paradigm for medical decision making (Straus & McAlister, 2000).

REFERENCES

Bazarian, J. J., Davis, C. O., Spillane, L. L., Blumstein, H., & Schneider, S. M. (1999). Teaching emergency medicine residents evidence-based critical appraisal skills: A controlled trial. *Annals of Emergency Medicine, 34,* 148–154.

Chelmow, D., Hennesy, M, & Evantash, E. (2004). Cost effectiveness of prophylactic antibiotics for low risk cesarean delivery. *American Journal of Obstetrics and Gynecology,* in press.

Chelmow, D., Ruehli, M. S., & Huang, E. (2001). Prophylactic use of antibiotics for nonlaboring patients undergoing cesarean delivery with intact membranes: A meta-analysis. *American Journal of Obstetrics Gynecology, 184,* 656–661.

Col, N. F., Eckman, M. H., Karas, R. H., Pauker, S. G., Goldberg, R. J., Ross, E. M., et al. (1997). Patient-specific decisions about hormone replacement therapy in postmenopausal women. *JAMA, 277,* 1140–1147.

Cooper, H., & Hedges, L. V. (1994). *The handbook of research synthesis.* New York: Russell Sage Foundation.

Drummond, M. F., O'Brien, B., Stoddart, G. L., & Torrance, G. W. (1997). *Methods for the economic evaluation of health care programmes* (2nd ed.). New York: Oxford University Press.

Egger, M., & Smith, G. D. (1998). Bias in location and selection of studies. *BMJ, 316,* 61–66.

Ellis, J., Mulligan, I., Rowe, J., & Sackett, D. L. (1995). Inpatient general medicine is evidence based. A-Team, Nuffield Department of Clinical Medicine. *Lancet, 346,* 407–410.

Ely, J. W., Osheroff, J. A., Ebell, M. H., Chambliss, M. L., Vinson, D. C., Stevermer, J. J., et al. (2002). Obstacles to answering doctor's questions about patient care with evidence: Qualitative study. *BMJ, 324,* 1–7.

Eysenbach, G., & Köhler, C. (2002). How do consumers search for and appraise health information on the World Wide Web? Qualitative study using focus groups, usability tests, and in-depth interviews. *BMJ, 324,* 573–577.

Freeman, A. C., & Sweeney, K. (2001). Why general practitioners do not implement evidence: Qualitative study. *BMJ, 323,* 1–5.

Ghali, W. A., Lesky, L. G., & Hershman, W. Y. (1998). The missing curriculum. *Academic Medicine, 73,* 734–736.

Gill, P., Dowell, A. C., Neal, R. D., Smith, N., Heywood, P., & Wilson, A. E. (1996). Evidence based general practice: A retrospective study of interventions in one training practice. *BMJ, 312,* 819–821.

Grodstein, F., Stampfer, M. J., Colditz, G. A., Willett, W. C., Manson, J. E., Joffe, M., et al. (1997). Postmenopausal hormone replacement therapy and mortality. *New England Journal of Medicine, 336,* 1769–1775.

Guyatt, G. (1991). Evidence-based medicine. *ACP Journal Club, 114,* A-16.

Guyatt, G. H., Meade, M. O., Jaeschke, R. Z., Cook, D. J., & Haynes, R. B. (2000). Practitioners of evidence based care: Not all clinicians need to appraise evidence from scratch but all need some skills. *BMJ, 320,* 954–955.

Guyatt, G., & Rennie, D. (2002). *User's guides to the medical literature.* Chicago, IL: AMA Press.

Haddix, A. C., Teutsch, S. M., Shaffer, P. A., & Dunet, D. O. (1996). *Prevention effectiveness: A guide to decision analysis and economic evaluation.* New York: Oxford University Press.

Hatala, R. (1999). Is evidence-based medicine a teachable skill? *Ann. Emerg. Med.,* 34: 226–8.

Hatala, R., & Guyatt, G. (2002). Evaluating the teaching of evidence-based medicine. *JAMA, 288,* 1110–1112.

Hopayian, K. (2001). The need for caution in interpreting high quality systematic reviews. *BMJ, 323,* 681–684.

Hulley, S. B., Cummings, S. R., & Browner, W. S. (2001). *Designing clinical research: An epidemiologic approach* (2nd ed.). Baltimore: Lippincott Williams and Wilkins.

Ioannidis, J. P., Haidich, A. B., Pappa, M., Pantazis, N., Kokori, S. I., Tektonidou, M. G., et al. (2001). Comparison of evidence of treatment effects in randomized and nonrandomized studies. *JAMA, 286,* 821–830.

Kessler, R. C., Frank, R. G., Edlund, M., Katz, S. J., Lin, E., & Leaf, P. (1997). Differences in the use of psychiatric outpatient services between the United States and Ontario. *New England Journal of Medicine, 336,* 551–557.

Kim, J. J., Wright, T. C., & Goldie, S. J. (2002). Cost-effectiveness of alternative triage strategies for atypical squamous cells of undetermined significance. *JAMA, 287,* 2382–2390.

Lacchetti, C., & Guyatt, G. (2002). Therapy and validity: Surprising results of randomized controlled trials. In G. Guyatt & D. Rennie (Eds.), *User's guides to the medical literature.* Chicago: AMA Press.

McColl, A., Smith, H., White, P., & Field, J. (1998). General practitioner's perceptions of the route to evidence based medicine: A questionnaire survey. *BMJ, 316,* 361–365.

Montori, V. M., Smieja, M., & Guyatt, G. H. (2000). Publication bias: A brief review for clinicians. *Mayo Clinic Proceedings, 75,* 1284–1288.

Mulrow, C., & Cook, D. (1998). *Systematic reviews: Synthesis of best evidence for health care decisions.* Philadelphia: American College of Physicians.

Petitti, D. B. (2000). *Meta-analysis, decision analysis, and cost-effectiveness analysis: Methods for quantitative synthesis in medicine* (2nd ed.). New York: Oxford University Press.

Pilote, L., Califf, R. M., Sapp, S., Miller, D. P., Mark, D. B., Weaver, W. D., et al. (1995). Regional variation across the United States in the management of acute myocardial infarction. *New England Journal of Medicine, 333,* 565–572.

Stampfer, M., & Colditz, G. (1991). Estrogen replacement therapy and coronary heart disease: A quantitative assessment of the epidemiologic evidence. *Preventive Medicine, 20,* 47–63.

Steinberg, K. A., Thacker, S. B., Smith, S. J., Stroup, D. F., Zack, M. M., Flanders, W. D., et al. (1991). A meta-analysis of the effect of estrogen replacement therapy on the risk of breast cancer. *JAMA, 265,* 1985–1990.

Straus, S. E., & McAlister, F. A. (2000). Evidence-based medicine: a commentary on common criticisms. *CMAJ, 163,* 837–841.

U.S. Preventative Task Force Staff. (1997). *The guide to clinical preventive services: Report of the United States Preventive Services Task Force.* Alexandria, VA: International Medical Publishing, Inc.

Weiss, N. S., Ure, C. L., Ballard, J. H., Williams, A. R., & Daling, J. R. (1980). Decreased risk of fractures of the hip and lower forearm with postmenopausal use of estrogen. *New England Journal of Medicine, 303,* 1195–1198.

Welch, H. G., Lurie, J. D. (2000). Teaching evidence-based medicine: Caveats and challenges. *Acad. Med.,* 75: 235–40.

Wennberg, D. E., Lucas, F. L., Birkmeyer, J. D., Bredenberg, C. D., & Fisher, E. S. (1998). Variation in carotid endarterectomy mortality in the Medicare population: Trial hospitals, volume, and patient characteristics. *JAMA, 279,* 1278–1281.

Wennberg, J., & Gittelsohn, A. (1973). Small area variations in health care delivery. *Science, 182,* 1102–1108.

Writing Group for the Women's Health Initiative Investigators. (2002). Risks and benefits of estrogen plus progestin in healthy postmenopausal women: Principal results from the women's health initiative randomized controlled trial. *JAMA, 288,* 321–333.

EDITORIAL COMMENTARY

It is somewhat rare for a paper in gynecology to become one of the most important issues in the entire field of medicine, but that's exactly what happened a few months ago. A prospective randomized trial (RCT) of postmenopausal hormone therapy versus placebo found that not only was hormone replacement therapy not helpful for several endpoints but also that it increased the occurrence of some diseases! As Chelmow points out, an RCT represents the highest level (i.e., most believable) of evidenced-based medicine.

The finding of this trial was unexpected and upsetting to both clinicians and patients, as the medication was widely used. Many physicians found it very difficult to accept the results of the trial, even though the design and execution were "pretty good." The result is that there remains a great deal of controversy about the use of hormone replacement therapy. On one side, the skeptics point out inconsistencies in the recruitment and retention of the study participants. On the other, the researchers stand by their publications (which seem to occur at weekly intervals) mostly based on the strength of their study design. The bottom line seems to be that there is no type of study, no plan of design, and no strictness of execution that can prevent a study from being criticized.

—Kenneth L. Noller

Part III

LAYPERSONS ENCOUNTERING MEDICAL PRACTICE: PERSONAL DECISIONS UNDER UNCERTAINTY

Chapter 10

SEEKING HEALTH CARE: PRACTICAL STEPS TAKEN BY A WOMAN IN AN IMMIGRATION CONTEXT

Sofie Bäärnhielm

In this chapter I will discuss the case of a Turkish-born immigrant woman, living in Sweden, who, upon seeking medical care for physical symptoms, encountered clinicians who interpreted her symptoms within a psychological and psychiatric framework. This particular case illustrates some aspects of the general phenomena of health seeking and medical decision making when lay and professional meanings differ with regard to illness.

Seeking health care is a complex process that can be broken down into several components. It ranges from experiencing distress and cognitive labeling that something might be wrong, to the decision and action of seeking medical help. For the help-seeker, it includes handling the responses of the health care system and its professionals. For an immigrant seeking health care in a new society, the encounter may include unfamiliar ways of looking upon and expressing distress as well as new ways of viewing socially acceptable communication of distress. It may also include new treatments and models of organizing medical care.

Immigration in itself includes a stressful and disruptive life situation and may affect health. Patterns of seeking health care among immigrant groups can be different from those of the majority population (Kirmayer, Galbaud du Fort, Young, Weinfeldt, & Lasry, 1996; Stuart, Klimidis, & Minas, 1998). In Sweden there is a paucity of studies regarding immigration and cultural background and the utilization of mental health care in general. This is despite the fact that Sweden has an increasingly more culturally diverse population. Sweden is one of many countries being transformed into a multicultural society through the migration of many refugees and other immigrants. Eleven percent of the population is foreign-born (Statistics Sweden, 2001). In Sweden there is a lower psychiatric care utilization rate for non-Scandinavian immigrants (Diderichsen & Varde, 1996), and in Stockholm there are diverse patterns of utilizing psychiatric mental health care (Oxenstierna, 1998). Health care in Sweden is delivered by a comprehensive, universal, and mainly tax-funded public health care system available to all official residents (Ekblad, 2004).

Individuals express their distress through expressions both peculiar to cultural worlds and constrained by shared human conditions (Kleinman, 1988). Avoidance of the open expression of emotions can be one normative ideal (White, 1982). Culture affects and participates in the transformation of experiences to symptoms and how people express emotional distress, which can be expressed in many ways. Analyzing the role of culture in the transformation of affects, Obeyesekere states,

> The *work of culture* is the process whereby painful motives and affects such as those occurring in depression are transformed into publicly accepted sets of meanings and symbols. (Obeyesekere, 1985, p. 147)

For an immigrant seeking health care, traditions of expressing and communicating distress may fit poorly with the medical traditions in the new society. Angel and Thoits (1987) hypothesize the existence of learned cognitive structures, through which physical experiences are filtered and influence the interpretation of deviations from culturally defined physical and mental health norms. Discussing this in relation to migration, they propose that the specific situation for immigrants is one of having to restructure cognitive categorizations, to reorder their cognitive structures to conform with those that are consensually validated in the new society.

Somatic symptoms are a common global way of clinically presenting emotional distress (Isaac, Janca, & Orley, 1996; Kirmayer, 1984). For a patient using a bodily idiom of expressing emotional distress, encountering clinicians who interpret their suffering in a psychiatric or psychological framework can be a problematic experience. Psychiatric and psychological attributions of distress can be difficult to accept, and psychiatric treatment can be stigmatizing. Kirmayer and Young (1998) suggest that to introduce a psychological language as a way of understanding a problem is to introduce a culture-specific concept to the person, which may conflict with the values and perspectives of the patient's culture of origin.

Health seeking in practice will be discussed here by reference to the case of Havva, a woman I met during my Ph.D. work at the Karolinska Institutet in Stockholm, Sweden (2003).

CASE PRESENTATION: HAVVA, A WOMAN IN PAIN

Havva participated in a qualitative research project in which I was interviewing ten Turkish-born women, assessed by their caregivers as somatizing, about experiences and meanings given to illness. The definition of somatization adopted in the study was a tendency to experience and communicate psychological and social distress in the form of physical symptoms and to seek medical help for them (Lipowski, 1987). After some years, I met each research participant again and conducted new interviews. This time I wanted to find out about the restructuring of illness meaning. This opportunity presented itself as the participants had encountered professional caregivers imposing a message of a "psychological language"[1] for understanding their physical symptoms and distress.

The first time I met Havva was in the spring of 1998. Her primary-care physician had recommended that she participate in the research project. I interviewed Havva four times between 1998 and 2001. Except for the first encounter, the interviews were conducted in Havva's home. I interviewed Havva about her illness experiences, meanings given to illness, clinical encounters, and restructuring of illness meaning. Havva spoke fluent Swedish. The interviews were tape-recorded and transcribed verbatim. In the interviews, Havva was encouraged to respond in a narrative format. In relating her story of suffering, she focused to a great extent on her health-seeking actions. Some parts of the interviews with Havva have been published elsewhere (Bäärnhielm, 2004; Bäärnhielm & Ekblad, 2000). The quotes that appear in this chapter have not been used in other texts.

Context and Suffering

Havva was 45 years old when we first met. She lived in a multicultural low-status suburb of Stockholm, where a great majority of the inhabitants are immigrants and refugees and many are socially and culturally marginalized.

Havva had grown up in a village in a rural area in the Kulu district of Turkey. She was the second child, and oldest daughter, of ten siblings. Her parents were farmers. She started to help her parents with the day-to-day work on their farm at the age of seven. By the age of ten she took great responsibility for the family, younger siblings, and the household. Her family and those in her surroundings used traditional medical folk remedies. Havva had five years of education in Turkey. When she was twenty-three years old, in 1976, she emigrated from Turkey to Sweden together with her husband.

On her arrival in Sweden Havva immediately started to work. Her first job was as janitor. Later, she had diverse service jobs. For many years she had two full-time jobs. Within six years, Havva had four children, first three sons and finally a daughter. The children were all born in Sweden. At the time of our interviews, they were schoolchildren. Havva continued to work after becoming a mother. After giving birth, she was at home for six months with each son. When she started to work again she had two jobs. When her fourth child was born, she was at home for a year. When she started back to work, she reduced her hours to one full-time job.

Havva and her husband had immigrated to Sweden with the intention of returning to Turkey after saving enough money. For many years, Havva lived with this dream. She had two homes: one in Sweden and one in Turkey. Finally, she found two homes to be too demanding and decided to stay in Sweden. Every other summer she visited her family in Turkey. She felt more and more like a stranger to her family in Turkey. Her children considered themselves Swedish. About her current social situation and about where to live, Havva said:

> . . . I have lived for many years with two thoughts, or with two homes. Now I am tired of living that way. I have put that behind me. My home country will be Sweden. When I said to my oldest son that he was an immigrant here in Sweden. He said to me 'You might be mum, but not me. I am born here, I have grown up here, I am Swedish although my parents are immigrants.' That's how it is in reality.

In the interviews Havva talked about her distress and suffering. She suffered from fatigue and experienced pain day and night. She felt angry and hopeless, and that she was a bad mother and wife. She avoided doing demanding things and felt restricted in her daily life. Havva had a bad conscience regarding her children. Havva described her situation like this:

I have no bed, no pillow, no cover, no mattress that fits me. Days and nights are hell. I live. I live, but I live physically. One can see that I am alive but I am not alive inside myself. As I said, I am not a good mother. I am not a good wife. I do not know how many more years my husband will put up with me. And what hurts is when I shout at my children. When I hurl abuse at them it hurts afterwards. I get a bad conscience. When I don't have the strength to make breakfast for my children I regret it the whole day afterwards.

Havva described shortcomings in relation to her family:

I am sulky. I am almost always sulky. The kids ask "Why are you sulky?" I tell them I'm not sulky. Yes you are sulky they say. My husband says the same thing. He says, "When I see you when I come in the door I want to go out again."

Havva was worried about her suffering and future and said:

How long will it go on, how long will it go on? I am 45 now. If I live another twenty years? How will I stand living with this?

Havva had stopped working prior to the interviews and was on sick leave. She felt shame and worthlessness for not being able to work. She said:

In some way I feel outside of society. I am used to work. I want to work. But I can't do it.

Becoming Aware of Suffering and Starting to Seek Help

Havva had started to notice her physical pain some years before her oldest son was born. She did not pay any attention to it until several years later, when she was at home taking care of her fourth child. She discussed her symptoms and suffering with her husband and close family in Sweden, but avoided talking about it with others.

During the years between the onset of her pain and seeking the help of a physician, Havva had tried folk remedies that were familiar to her. She had tried cupping,[2] and she visited hot springs in Turkey (see Bäärnhielm & Ekblad, 2000). Her husband suggested that she should seek the help of a physician in Sweden. Her relatives in Turkey recommended that she visit a Hoca (traditional healer). Havva rejected their advice and said:

. . . I do not believe in them. I believe in God. I believe in our prophet. I believe that you have a destiny. But I do not believe in that way [a traditional healer].

For a long time Havva tried to manage and cope with her suffering. It took six years from becoming aware of her pain until Havva decided to seek medical care. Havva said that she started to seek care when was no longer able to stand her pain:

I decided to seek care. I could not stand the pain. It was impossible to say that it'll pass. I did not have any free time. I did not have a minute without pain. It did not matter what I did. I got more and more pain. It got worse and worse until I was forced to seek a doctor.

I asked Havva why she had waited so long. She told me that people from her country of origin had a tradition of not seeking medical care until there were "real" problems. Havva said:

We don't bother about it (referring to distress).

About her own situation she said:

Now I feel like a disabled person. It is true but no one believes it. This pain, this fatigue. I did not seek help until it was a crisis.

Havva had put off seeking care until she found her distress to be unbearable. Until then, she had the idea that her pain was connected with her long work hours. When she was at home with her newborn daughter, the pain continued and increased even though she was not engaged in physically hard work. She concluded that the pain was not related to work. Havva could no longer understand her distress:

At that time I noticed that I had pain. I'd worn myself down to the bone. When things were quiet the pain increased.

Additionally, Havva found that her strategies for handling her distress no longer provided relief. She decided to seek medical attention when she was no longer able to make sense of the suffering and traditional treatments no longer worked.

Encountering Medical Care

Havva started seeking medical care by contacting a clinic close to her home in Sweden. After a few appointments the physician told her that she was suffering from anxiety. She was referred to a local psychiatric outpatient clinic. Havva commented on her primary-care physician's referral:

> Not the first time but the second or third I think, she [primary-care physician] sent a referral to psychiatry. I told her that I wasn't crazy, that I actually had pain. 'When the soul is not well the body is not well either' she said. OK, I went there [psychiatric outpatient clinic]. I did not get any medication. I don't need a psychologist. I have pain. It doesn't matter if they believe me or not. I have pain and I know my body. I did not have the sort of problems the psychologist could help with.

Havva associated the word "anxiety" with mental illness. She took the primary-care physician's statement about mental attribution of her physical pain as an indication of not being trusted (Bäärnhielm, 2004). She tried to understand the idea of a psychiatric basis for her pain but could not (Bäärnhielm, 2004). She did not accept the idea behind the referral to psychiatry, and said of her psychiatrist:

> She (the psychiatrist) said that I had pain in my soul. I said that I did not have pain in my soul. She spoke my language (Turkish). It became a real conflict between us. I told her that she knew how we lived and how we worked and that it did not have anything to do with the soul. If it had been because of the soul I would have gone to Beckomberga (name of a local mental hospital). She asked me whether I heard voices, if I thought, if I did this and that.

When Havva had started to seek health care, she had no idea that her physical distress could or should be attributed to a mental illness. She felt she was being accused of malingering and started to doubt herself. She found that her husband believed her and supported her. She said:

> I asked my husband many times "Do you think I have pain in my soul? Do you think I am stupid in some way? No, he said." He supported me in some way.

During my four interview sessions, Havva often asserted a body/mind split and said that it was important that her mind was intact. Weakness of the body was, on the other hand, acceptable. Havva often talked in

terms of the mind/brain and the body fighting each other, and described
how she was sometimes able to do things. She explained:

> The brain works and the body doesn't keep up. Sometimes the brain wins
> over the body. There is strength coming from somewhere and I go out. It
> is like I make a firm decision that I am going to do this.

Havva tried the suggested psychiatric treatment but did not limit herself to it. She initiated a period of "medical shopping." She visited several different physicians, clinics, and rehabilitation clinics. She arranged
an appointment at a prestigious private clinic in the city of Stockholm.
After several visits, Havva was no longer welcome at the private clinic
and was informed that "no surgery was necessary." She was put on the
sick list and was referred to a rehabilitation clinic. During this period of
"medical shopping," Havva received several treatments and medications,
including antidepressants. Havva said:

> I was like pushed back and forth. No one believed that I had pain. They
> said that I imagined having pain. For a while I thought that I had imagined
> having pain. One starts to doubt whether one has pain or not.

Finally, she was again referred to the local psychiatric clinic. This time
the referral was made by a rehabilitation clinic.

Before starting to seek medical health care, Havva had used various
forms of traditional treatment. She stopped using folk treatment strategies
after visiting the local primary-care clinic. Now and then she thought
about starting cupping again, as it had given her some comfort. She asked
a physiotherapist and a physician about cupping. She was told that it
was not dangerous but could not help. Talking about her previous experiences of cupping, Havva said:

> In some way it gave me comfort.

Havva had stopped visiting hot springs in Turkey during vacations.
Sometimes she went to a sauna in the public baths close to her home in
Sweden. It gave her some pain relief and reminded her of the hot springs
in Turkey. In the interviews, it never became clear why she stopped using
the traditional treatment strategies. Except for the sauna, there were no
links between the medical remedies that she tried before seeking primary
care and the treatments she tried afterward.

Discussion

For Havva, seeking health care became a long and complicated process. Her first search for a cure involved trying medical remedies within her private sphere of familiar folk remedies. She tried cupping and hot springs in Turkey but rejected her relatives' suggestion of visiting a traditional healer. She sought medical health care at the local primary-care clinic where she lived. Havva took this step when her symptoms became severe, her lay remedies had failed to work, and when she felt that she could no longer understand her distress.

The primary-care clinician she met quickly attributed her pain to anxiety and referred her to a psychiatric outpatient clinic. The psychiatric referral and attribution of her pain were not comprehensible, meaningful, or acceptable to her. Havva, and her family members, did not understand that her distress could be attributed to mental illness. For Havva, and her family, psychiatric treatment was stigmatizing as it inferred losing control and undesirable behavior toward others, although a somatic language of distress (Heilman, 1998, p. 235) was acceptable. Rogler (1996, p. 148) suggests significant others' evaluation of distress shapes the person's pathways to mental health care. For Havva, her pain had nothing to do with mental illness. She could not accept a psychiatric cause for her pain.

Havva's third action was a period of "medical shopping." She turned to several different clinicians and clinics. She received diverse and sometimes opposing information and suggestions about investigations and treatment. The period of "medical shopping" ended with being referred to psychiatric care, which she found difficult to accept.

There were many years between Havva's first symptoms and when she began to seek medical care. Her encounters with medical care introduced her to new concepts, treatments, and to a psychiatric and psychological attribution of her physical symptoms (Bäärnhielm & Ekblad, 2000). Seeking health resulted in Havva needing to try to reorient herself regarding her suffering and its treatment. She struggled with trying to understand the clinicians' meanings and the treatments they suggested. She accepted some new ideas and rejected others. Seeking health care involved Havva giving up the traditional treatment strategies that she had tried earlier. She was not asked to do so; she did this on her own initiative. Havva's account did not include anything about her clinicians being interested in the meanings she gave to illness or her ideas about healing.

Havva spoke of clinicians trying to convey their messages and meanings. She never reported clinicians paying attention to her views and values or bothering about how she made sense of their messages and ideas. Havva once asked about cupping. Except for this, she did not tell her clinicians about her use of traditional folk medicine and no one asked her about it. Havva never complained about the clinicians not being interested in her meanings and treatment traditions. This situation was taken for granted.

The process of seeking health care and encountering clinicians with diverse and opposing or unfamiliar views and meanings was complicated for Havva. As little or no attention was paid to Havva's perspectives, she did not receive much help in her process of restructuring the meaning given to illness. This lack of support for reorientation and restructuring should be seen in the context of Havva also enjoying little support from her family. Havva avoided speaking about her distress outside her immediate family. It was difficult for Havva to create coherence between her clinicians' messages and her own experiences and meanings. Seeking medical help became quite a disruptive experience for her.

General versus Particular

Havva's decisions, actions, and experiences cannot be generalized to others. However, her story illustrates the general issue of seeking medical care and medical decision making when lay and professional meanings of illness differ. Seeking health care is an interactive process between the individual and the health care system and its professionals. Havva was never locked out of the health care system.

Difficulties understanding and accepting professional meanings given to illness may easily put a person on the margin of the health care system. Immigrants, especially those recently arrived, with poor knowledge of the health care system of the new host society may be at risk of becoming marginalized.

Havva's case underscores the view that people seeking health care need support in order to be able to construct coherence between lay and professional meanings. This can be of special significance for immigrants. An individual's process of creating coherence between frames of meaning can be facilitated in many ways. It can be supported at public health levels, by adapting local health care organizations to local populations, and in the individual interaction between patient and clinician. Mental health care, especially in multicultural milieus, must include openness and acceptance for working with diversity and pluralism of meanings and realities.

ACKNOWLEDGMENT

I thank Associate Professor Solvig Ekblad at the IPM (National Institute for Psychosocial Factors and Health) and Karolinska Institutet for constructive comments and supervision of the research project, and Steve Wicks for help with English.

NOTES

1. Helman (1998) uses the expression *language of distress* to describe how different social and cultural groups communicate their suffering to others, including doctors. Helman describes how different social and cultural groups may utilize different languages of distress, verbal or nonverbal, and the problems that arise when clinicians fail in decoding them.

2. For Havva, cupping had been carried out by burning a piece of paper inside a glass. The warm glass was then attached to the skin. Havva had the idea that fluid was drawn from the flesh of the back and that this was helpful (Bäärnhielm & Ekblad, 2000).

REFERENCES

Angel, R., & Thoits, P. (1997). The impact of culture on the cognitive structures of illness. *Culture, Medicine and Psychiatry, 11,* 465–494.

Bäärnhielm, S. (2003). Clinical encounters with different illness realities: Qualitative studies of illness meaning and restructuring of illness meaning among two cultural groups of female patients in a multicultural area of Stockholm. Doctoral dissertation, Division of Psychiatry, Neurotec Department, Karolinska Institutet, Stockholm, Sweden.

Bäärnhielm, S. (2004). Restructuring illness meaning through the clinical encounter: A process of disruption and coherence. *Culture, Medicine and Psychiatry, 28,* 41–65.

Bäärnhielm, S., & Ekblad, S. (2000). Turkish migrant women encountering health care in Stockholm: A qualitative study of somatization and illness meaning. *Culture, Medicine and Psychiatry, 24*(4), 431–452.

Diderichsen, F., & Varde, E. (1996). Konsten att fördela resurser efter behov. Stockholmsmodelens kriterier [The art of allocating resources according to need. The Stockholm model's criteria]. *Läkartidningen, 93,* 3677–3683 (Swedish).

Ekblad, S. (2004). Migrants: Universal health services in Sweden. In J. Healy & M. McKee (Eds.), *Health care: Responding to diversity* (pp. 159–181). Oxford, England: Oxford University Press.

Helman, C. (1998). *Culture, health and illness* (3rd ed.). Oxford, England: Butterworth-Heinemann.

Isaac, M., Janca, M., & Orley, J. (1996). Somatization—a cultural-bound or universal syndrome? *Journal of Mental Health, 5*(3), 219–222.

Kirmayer, L. J. (1984). Culture, affect and somatization. Part I. *Transcultural Psychiatric Research Review, 21*(4), 159–188.

Kirmayer, L. J., Galbaud du Fort, G., Young, A., Weinfeld, M., & Lasry, J-C. (1996). *Pathways and barriers to mental health care in an urban multi-cultural milieu: An epidemiological and ethnographic study* (Report No. 6, Part 1, Culture & Mental Health Research Unit, Sir Mortimer B. Davis—Jewish General Hospital). Montreal, Canada: McGill University.

Kirmayer, L. J., & Young, A. (1998). Culture and somatization: Clinical, epidemiological, and ethnographic perspectives. *Psychosomatic Medicine, 60,* 420–430.

Kleinman, A. (1988). *Illness narratives: Suffering, healing and the human condition.* New York: Basic Books.

Lipowski, Z. J. (1987). Somatization: The experience and communication of psychological distress as somatic symptoms. *Psychotherapy and Psychosomatics, 47,* 160–167.

Obeysekere, G. (1985). Depression, Buddhism, and the work of culture in Sri Lanka. In A. Kleinman & B. Good (Eds.), *Culture and depression: Studies in the anthropology and cross-cultural psychiatry of affect and disorder* (pp. 134–152). Berkeley, CA: University of California Press.

Oxenstierna, G. (1998). Invandrare, sjukvård och socialförsäkring [Immigrants, health care and social insurance]. In S. Ekblad, G. Oxenstierna, & A. Akpinar (Eds.). *Invandrarbakgrundens betydelse för sjukvård och socialförsäkring. En folkhälsorapport för Stockholms län 1998* (pp. 23–48). Stockholm: Stockholm County Council. (Swedish)

Rogler, L. H. (1996). Framing research on culture in psychiatric diagnosis: The case of the DSM-IV. *Psychiatry, 59,* 145–155.

Statistics Sweden (2001). Population statistics. Retrieved from http://www.eu2001.se/static/eng/facts/kort_befolking.asp.

Stuart, G. W., Klimidis, S., & Minas, I. H. (1998). The treatment prevalence of mental disorder amongst immigrants and the Australian born: Community and primary care rates. *International Journal of Social Psychiatry, 44*(1), 22–34.

White, G. M. (1982). The role of cultural explanations in 'somatization' and 'psychologization.' *Social Science and Medicine, 16,* 1519–1530.

EDITORIAL COMMENTARY

Many, perhaps most, researchers are skeptical of reliance on single case studies as a source of knowledge. There are, however, distinctive contributions to be gained from such an approach. There are very different genres that attempt to unite particulars and universals—genres that will vary when the label is "research" compared to "teaching." Traditional approaches to research, articulated by Isaac and Michael (1982, p. 43), in the planning and conduct of research include identifying the problem area, surveying the literature relating to it, defining the actual problem for investigation in clear, specific terms, and forming testable hypotheses that define the basic concepts and variables. Variables are defined in four categories: independent, dependent, control, and intervening variables.

A drawback from my perspective is that the basic steps in research are all initiated and determined by the researcher. This is in sharp contrast to teaching and preparing professionals for the world of practice. The world of practice requires professionals to deal with particulars, and such particulars will vary from a person to an institution. Many professional schools in varied disciplines all adhere to the case method for uniting particulars to generalizations. Historically, the Law School at Harvard led the way in 1870, followed by the Business School in 1920. The Medical School began using cases in 1985. "All were designed to cement students' understanding of basic science by linking it immediately to practical problems—typically, the case histories of individual patients" (Garvin, D. A., *Harvard Magazine*, 9/17/2003).

Explanations throughout the ages that have attempted to understand behavior have vacillated, and continue to alternate, between explanations that focus on nature and nurture, on the person, or on the environment. Further, social psychologists remind us that "the cause we often hypothesize to explain behavior can be quite different when applied to others from the ones we attribute to ourselves" (*House of Cards,* Dawes, 1994, p. 209). Dawes goes on to remind us of a fundamental "attribution error or bias to attribute the behavior of others to personality factors and that of ourselves to situational factors" (Dawes, 1994, p. 209).

Importantly, underlining both the basis for the distinction between these two genres generally and how individuals behave in all interactions with the environment, "we are biased to attribute causality to the focus of our attention" (Dawes, 1994, p. 209).

The attention of researchers is directed to generating principles from groups so that these basic principles can then be applied by others to understanding differences between groups and types of individuals with groups.

A distinctive value to a case history is that the history of an individual, as in the chapters by Micheline de Souza Silva and Sofie Bäärnhielm, addresses change over time. This issue of *intra-individual variability* is not addressed in most mainstream approaches to research. Rather, "at-

tention in psychological research is almost exclusively restricted to variation between individuals . . . To the neglect of time-dependent variation
within a single subject's time series" (Paper presented, "A manifesto on
psychology as idiographic science: Bringing the person back into scientific psychology–this time forever," page 1, Molenaar, 2003). Granted,
a case history is not a time-dependent time series, but these chapters do
address major changes in a person throughout the course of his or her
life or, in the case by Micheline de Souza Silva, the life and death of a
child.

A second major difference relates to the assumptions being made by
both researchers and clinicians regarding the relationship between a researcher and a researcher participant or the relationship between a clinician and a patient. Commonly accepted labels such as "researcher" or
"clinician" do not describe (see chapter 6 by Noller and Bibace; chapter
7 by Bibace and Noller; and chapter 8 by Bibace, Leeman, and Noller)
the actual relationship and the specific interactions between the people
involved. Rather, such labels are relied upon to justify some practices
and condemn others. Thus, the "researcher" label assumes that the same
researcher will behave in identical, standardized ways with all the people
who are recruited as researcher participants. The psychological boundaries between the researcher and the researcher participant are presumed
to be "the same" especially in the United States. Yet the very selection
of the particular person(s) studied in these two chapters, required for the
collection of data, and the relationship between such researcher and researcher participants, changed over time. A limitation of both chapters
is that the private thoughts and feelings of both researcher and researcher
participant in such interactions are not reported. For instance, a third
professional did not interview both sets of participants to elicit such
private, subjective reactions from both the researcher and researcher
participant.

Information obtained from these two genres should be included in an
attempt to depict how different professionals relate to universals. The
actual content, referring to what is to be included in a case study or how
such contents should be organized, is not standardized. There is no single
accepted form for a case presentation. Yet the distinctive knowledge that
can be obtained from these two genres is a justification for including
these two examples of how different professions attempt to relate the
particulars of the people they relate to as "cases" to more generally
recognized issues.

—Roger Bibace

Chapter 11

MEANING AND DECISION MAKING PROCESSES ABOUT HEALTH ISSUES: TOWARD A QUALITATIVE METHODOLOGY OF INVESTIGATION

Katia S. Amorim and Maria Clotilde Rossetti-Ferreira

Ordinary people, as well as physicians and scientists, must deal with diseases and make decisions concerning them. In this chapter, we will discuss how making sense of health and disease issues is embedded in a complex *network of meanings,* and how those issues acquire meanings through personal interactions, by the articulation of personal components, and interactional and contextual aspects. To facilitate the discussion, a study of children's health and illness at a day-care center will be presented.

This setting was chosen because in Brazil medical providers believe that day-care centers are not adequate environments for care, pointing to the high prevalence of infectious diseases. During the last three decades, this issue has been a prominent health topic, inspiring a large body of research (Marbury, Maldonado, & Waller, 1997). This research stresses that children in collective care are at a high risk for infection (Fuchs, Maynart, Costa, Cardozo, & Schierholt, 1996; Nafstad, Hagen, Botten, & Jaakkola, 1996; Schwartz et al., 1994; Victora, Fuchs, Flores, Fonseca, & Kirkwood, 1994), greater severity (Schwartz et al., 1994), and longer duration of illness episodes (Fuchs et al., 1996; Simpson, Jones, Davies, & Cushing, 1995). Furthermore, it is generally stated that the illness rate is highest among those in their first two years of life (Louhiala, Jaakkola, Puotsalainen, & Jaakkola, 1995; Marbury et al., 1995; Nafstad et al., 1996). As such, many consider day-care centers as an "epidemiological focus of diseases" (Schwartz et al., 1994) and a source of economic damage, either from the treatment expenses or by the parent's absence from work (Denny, 1995; Simpson et al., 1995).

Our investigation was inspired by the thought that babies at day care get sick more frequently as a result of anxiety due to mother–baby separation plus the difficult adaptation to the day-care center routine and new relationships. Those thoughts are closely related to widespread social conceptions about maternity, the importance of the mother concerning health, and early child development (Ainsworth, Blehar, Waters, & Wall, 1978; Belsky, 1990; Bowlby, 1969).

However, we understand that these ideas are inconsistent with modern society in which women increasingly participate in the labor market and share the care of their children with others (Roberts & McGovern, 1993; Roberts, 1996; Rosemberg, 1995; Ministère de la Famille et de l'Enfance, Canada, 2000). Some parents go through deep feelings of ambivalence and guilt.

An extensive analysis of the literature concerning day-care centers was performed. The prevalence of infectious diseases was determined mainly by comparison of infectious disease rates of children at home with those in collective environments.

As Osterholm (1994) stresses, accurate rates require accurate numerators and denominators. Sacks (1993) mentions that a numerator should not contain conceptual differences but rather should highlight significant and comparable episodes. The denominator should include all children in a given setting and comparable conditions. Only with such information can an accurate illness rate be calculated (Osterholm, 1994).

Nevertheless, the review of the literature revealed that, more often than not, there were inadequacies and even discrepancies in the criteria. For example, comparisons and generalizations were carried out between children with diverse socioeconomic statuses and who were attending very different types of day-care institutions (Fuchs et al., 1996; Marbury et al., 1995; Nafstad et al., 1996; Takala et al., 1995; Turner, Stewart, & Freeman, 1995).

Researchers and their investigations often seemed to be guided by implicit assumptions that were embedded in cultural conceptions about the best way to raise children (Amorim & Rossetti-Ferreira, 1999). Disease was most frequently not investigated as a process but as an isolated event that had occurred months to years before the study was performed. Longitudinal studies, searching for developmental aspects under specific conditions of raising children, were very rare (McCutcheon & Woodward, 1996; Vives et al., 1997; Yagupsky, Landau, Beck, & Dagan, 1995).

Finally, most studies required a massive investment of funding and expensive and complex statistical procedures (Arnold et al., 1996; Brieman et al., 1996; Gessner, Ussery, Parkinson, & Brieman, 1995; Takala et al., 1995).

As Heyman, Henriksen, and Maughan (1998) and Spink, Medrado, and Mello (2002) affirm, risk assessment occupies a central place in contemporary culture and provides a tool that can be used to foresee and control the future. It involves a concept of adversity, which projects negative value judgments onto an event. These judgments are usually implicit and sometimes contested. Yet, the negativity rests in the eye of the beholder. That implicit negativity is encoded into numbers. Observed frequencies of events in the past are employed as guides to predicting events in the future. This, however, requires the assumption that the future will repeat the past.

Our literature review found that that the results of most studies would require a reorientation of the family toward home care by the mother, since collective care resulted in a higher rate of illness. This evaluation of risk could result in a disruption of current social systems and in re-defining and remodeling the modern family's way of life (Amorim, 2002).

What became clear from the review is that what remains out of focus in many of these investigations is the actual process by which health and illness occur in the child-care setting. Challenged by this perspective, our research center in Brazil has, for two decades, concentrated on the actual social and interactional processes that mediate children's care in day-care centers (Rossetti-Ferreira, Amorim, & Vitória, 1997; Rossetti-Ferreira, Ramon, & Barreto, 2002)

In this chapter, some empirical data will be presented and analyzed through the theoretical–methodological *Network of Meanings* perspective (Amorim, Vitória, & Rossetti-Ferreira, 2000; Rossetti-Ferreira, Amorim, & Silva, 2000; Rossetti-Ferreira, Amorim, & Vitória, 1996).

THE *NETWORK OF MEANINGS* PERSPECTIVE

The theoretical–methodological *Network of Meanings* perspective is the result of the work of our research group (CINDEDI[1]) on developmental processes and on early childhood education. This perspective was initially developed to analyze processes that occurred among babies, families, and caregivers during the infants' entry into a day-care center (Rossetti-Ferreira, Amorim, & Vitória, 1994). Later, its scope was broadened, and it was proposed as a tool for the investigation and understanding of the complex processes of human development in a variety of situations. Presently, it is being also used for the analysis of diverse social circumstances (Rossetti-Ferreira, Amorim, & Silva, 1999).

Its theoretical assumptions are sociohistorical, based on Wallon (in Werebe & Nadel-Brulfert, 1986), Vygotsky (1991, 1993), and Bakhtin (1981, 1997, 1999). The *Network of Meanings* presupposes that development is a time-irreversible coconstruction of an active person (Valsiner, 1994), through the interactions he/she establishes, in specific situations, all of which are socially and culturally organized.

The Person and His or Her Personal Components

A person is considered to develop throughout their whole life. Many features such as age, health, abilities, and education are considered relevant, but such elements only acquire meaning when considered within the interactions established with other persons, in specific environments, and when impregnated with the rules and values present in their culture.

The Interactive Fields

Interactive fields are established between persons, through dialogical intersubjectivity, in everyday life events. Within such fields, each person has his/her behavioral flow continuously framed and interpreted by others' and his/her own actions, through the attribution to one another of reciprocal roles and counter-roles (Oliveira & Rossetti-Ferreira, 1994). In this role-coordination process, the interacting persons take on, deny, confront, and negotiate these roles and counter-roles, depending on one another's conduct and expectations as well as on the situation and the scenarios in which they are inserted.

The Scenarios

Scenarios are conceived as being culturally organized and socially regulated, guided by specific functions and routines. They define and are defined by the participants' social roles and by affective and power relationships, which lead into varied behavioral pathways. In such scenarios, persons simultaneously have to negotiate their social roles and their positions, one in relation to the other (Oliveira & Rossetti-Ferreira, 1994).

In the here-and-now situation, concrete semiotic evidence of the past, present, and future can be perceived, revealing the multi-temporal characteristics of the situation. Thus, it is possible to apprehend the visible signs of different time periods, the diversity of superimposed epochs, and the peculiarities of the ongoing time, always as a whole in continuous development (Bakhtin, 1997).

For the *Network of Meanings* perspective, four intertwined times scales were defined to make this temporal perspective explicit: *present time, life time, historical time* (Spink, 1996), and *future-oriented time* (Rossetti-Ferreira, Amorim, & Silva, 1999). This has allowed us to identify its *temporal* completeness, the presence of the past that is active in the present, creatively binding it together, dimensioning the future, all dynamically interrelated, each sustaining and transforming the other.

The Sociohistorical Matrix

Persons, interactions, and scenarios are considered as impregnated by a sociohistorical matrix, which is composed of social, economical, political, historical, and cultural elements.

The matrix is conceived as being composed of two intimately and dialectically interrelated parts:

1. **The socioeconomic and political structure** represents the conditions in which the person is born, inserted, and developing. It encompasses the social context, which is constituted by the life-set conditions of the specific community, and the more stable social pressures on people.

2. **The ideological structure** encompasses profound differences, as this is the domain of representations, religious symbols, scientific formulae, and so on, through which a phenomenon is materialized as a picture, music, a ritual, a word, or a human behavior. Despite all their differences, what holds the various manifestations together is their semiotic character, being the sign in a miniature arena where the intersection and struggle of social values with contradictory orientations occur. Each sign is linked to different historical periods and social processes, revealing different weights and power hierarchies in each society, culture, subgroup, context, situation, and relationship.

The *Network* Configuration, Which Constrains Persons' Meaning Making, Social Practices, and Development

The dialogical and dialectical interrelations between all these elements create what we are metaphorically calling the *Network of Meanings*. The acquired network configuration structures, signifies, and canalizes a set of possible actions, emotions, and conceptions, acting as a constraint on the situation, providing possibilities and limits to the person's behaviors and development.

Various persons participate in a given scenario, each occupying different social roles and carrying diverse life histories and varied future expectations. They are related to others by different power statuses, and they are also linked to other scenarios. There are many superimposed and transforming nets, which are structured in a mesh with a variety of intersecting points, continuously constraining the person's development.

The Study of Developmental Processes

The *Network of Meanings* perspective is proposed for the analysis of the developmental processes, but it requires a methodology able to capture the course of those processes throughout time and across situations.

Based on Vygotsky (1991), it is understood that the basic goal of the analysis is the reconstruction of each stage, analyzing the dynamics of the process, in a search for the origins of the transformations, through a historical view. This means an investigation of the process of transformation, comprising all its phases, from birth to death, a history of the behavior.

Our proposal is, therefore, to study the phenomenon in development, which implies capturing the movement while preserving the time in the global construction and retaining the information about the observed dynamics. Thus, one seeks to apprehend new and old behaviors, emotions, and conceptions as well as the coconstruction and mutual transformations through which persons, relationships, and contexts pass.

Within a diverse set of investigations, conducted using the *Network of Meanings* perspective, we will present our efforts to investigate the contextualized processes of meaning making and decision making concerning health and disease situations. In the following case, the main goal was to analyze babies' illness events that occurred in day care, seeking to apprehend the adults' meaning construction and care practices related to some babies' illness episodes, during the children's attendance at a day-care center.

Procedures

Our empirical investigation was based on the Research Project database *Babies' Adaptation Processes at a Day Care Center* (Rossetti-Ferreira, Amorim, & Vitoria, 1994). This project has followed 21 infants (4–14 months of age), their families, and caregivers from the time of the babies' admission to a university day-care center in Brazil throughout the entire year of 1994. Among the goals of this project was examining the health and disease occurrences of the children.

Several procedures were used to record the situation, including enrollment interviews and a set of observational records. In addition, 72 interviews were carried out with the six caregivers, three day-care center technicians, and six of the 21 babies' mothers. Finally, subjects were videotaped during their three first months in day care.

For our specific project, which focused on health and disease topics, a file for each of the 21 infants based on the enrollment interview and on the observational records was created initially. Each file contains general information about the baby and his/her family as well as a record of all illness episodes during his/her attendance at day care.

Among all identified episodes, six were selected for analysis. Selection criteria restricted analysis to episodes that occurred during the first semester of attendance and that involved acute episodes of illness and/or if the illness led to the child's withdrawal from the day-care center.

For each of the six cases, the data set was based on the interviews and video records. All interviews were read, searching for and recording information related to the baby as well as the way adults usually took care of him/her. In the videos, all the appearances of the main subjects were identified and chronologically marked. Subsequently, the tapes were transcribed, focusing on the interactive episodes, with special attention to gaze, posture, vocalization, emotional expression, and body movement, within the overall situation and context.

A detailed account of each episode was organized from the interview and videotape-obtained data. The aim was to follow the adults' and baby's behavior and development throughout the illness episode, analyzing the meaning making at each moment and its transformation throughout the processes. Analysis was limited to the weeks before, during, and after the illness episode.

Histories of Particular Cases

Two of the analyzed cases were selected for this chapter presentation—Vera's and Linda's cases.[2] Both children were being cared for by the same caregivers, Branca and Mirtes. These two cases were selected to present how medical and scientific discourses are concretely present in nonmedical settings, constraining the layperson's meanings and attitudes. Furthermore, the cases were selected because of the evidence of multiple and contradictory health and disease discourse voices and

knowledge, leading the meaning-making and decision-making procedures to follow diverse and even contradictory pathways.

VERA'Ş CASE

Vera's Flu and Conjunctivitis Episodes

Vera was 10 months old when she began attending day care. Her
parents were university health students. At the enrollment interview, the
mother mentioned that Vera had already had the flu, diarrhea, and otitis
at home.

One week later, Vera developed the "flu," which lasted for 10 days.
Branca, the afternoon caregiver, commented how the parents reacted to
Vera's disease: *"It seems that the father does not admit that the child is
sick. . . . Each time the little girl gets sick, the father almost has a
breakdown."*[3]

Concurrently, Vera had conjunctivitis. The rule for that specific day-
care center was that children with conjunctivitis had to be withdrawn
from the center until they recovered. Thus, according to the afternoon
caregiver, after the conjunctivitis was diagnosed *"when the mother come
to visit her daughter during lunchtime, we asked her to take the girl
home . . . the day Vera was withdrawn from day care . . . the mother
was very angry. She was bitterly hostile."*

Mirtes, the morning caregiver, reported comments that reveal why the
mother felt so angry. According to the mother, before attending day care,
her *" . . . child was never sick. And once she was infected at the day
care center, there was no reason for her to be removed."* The situation
was further aggravated, because the mother *" . . . was going to have a
test at the university! She couldn't stay at home with her child. She had
to take the girl to her own class. It must have been very hard."*

This part of the episode reveals that, even in a situation external to a
medical setting, medical discourses guide decisions. Day care is ruled
by conceptions about diseases such as conjunctivitis which are considered to be highly contagious, demanding the withdrawal of the sick person from that environment. Despite the absence of a medical doctor, the
medical knowledge constructed within the last two to three centuries is
strongly established in a nonmedical setting (as this setting of early childhood education), constituting not only the discourses but also the day-
care social practices and guidelines.

In the analyzed case, such normalization leaves no possibility for any
kind of negotiation regarding the child's presence in the day-care center.

The rule was no doubt strictly enforced due to the highly contagious nature of the of illness and the fact that the population was composed of babies in their first year of life with immature immune systems. In addition, this day-care facility was organized in such a way that the babies stayed mainly on the floor and on mattresses, thus favoring contact among the children.

This case demonstrates how meaning making and decision making about illnesses cannot be viewed as an isolated problem, as they are embedded in a social network. It was through caregiver–child relationships that the disease was identified, and, with the diagnosis of conjunctivitis, the demand to withdraw the child was communicated to the child's parents.

The decision to withdraw Vera affected not only her life but others' lives as well, chiefly the mother. The mother had the roles of both mother and student. She also had other activities, such as her classes and her tests. The mother had to perform these diverse social activities simultaneously and react appropriately. Vera's illness affected the entire social network within which she was inserted.

This illness changed the way that the mother viewed the day-care setting. First, it led her to question the procedures of the day-care center. Secondly, it set the stage for the mother's meaning making related to day care: "Day care is a place with a high risk of infectious diseases."

Such discourses appear in the mother's speech, when she mentions that, before entering day care, her daughter had never had been ill. Her claim was clearly false, as the mother herself had declared during the enrollment interview that Vera had previously had the flu. Thus, it can be said that the interrelation of diverse and contradictory aspects of the situation determined the way the mother looked at it and at day-care institutions. This caused a rearrangement of the family–day-care relationship.

One Month Later, Vera's Second Fever Episode

One month after, the child had another flu episode. When the girl developed a fever at the day-care center, she was medicated with Dipirona (dipyrone, metamizole). For days after that, the child was not taken to the day-care center. According to the morning caregiver, *"Vera was a bit sick. . . . The mother began Vera's follow-up with a homeopath. Homeopathy is a very slow procedure . . . as long as she has a fever, she is staying at home."*

Two weeks later, the parents informed the day-care center that they were withdrawing Vera from it.

Interviews reveal how the staff interpreted the parents' attitude. According to Mirtes, the morning caregiver, *"The mother began treating her daughter with a homeopath medical doctor. And . . . he is against day care centers. . . . Now, I don't know if there was already an intention of withdrawing the child, and the doctor was just an excuse."*

Branca, the afternoon caregiver, related the mother's motives for leaving the day care. The mother mentions, " . . . *the auxiliary nurse medicated the girl with an analgesic . . . ,"* but should not have done so as *"The girl was using homeopathic medicine."* However, according to the caregiver, the mother *"Forgets that the only person who knew about homeopathy was her* [the mother]. *The day care center couldn't guess. Until then, she hadn't informed us."*

The caregiver also mentions that the father was the person *"who was really insisting on withdrawing the child. . . . The father didn't want her to stay anymore, as she got sick. . . . He even wanted the mother herself to withdraw from her university classes, to take care of her baby girl. . . . Then, she succeeded in finding someone. . . . The child's grandmother gave up her job to care of her granddaughter. . . . Because she got sick . . . there's a revolution within the whole family."*

Finally, the day-care center psychologist says, *"In terms of conditions, it's clear that the child is well sheltered and cared for at the day care center. . . . We believe that children in day care develop more certain things. . . . We believe in day care as an educational project. In this way, I was sad about Vera's withdrawal. But I also think . . . with a father who questions if it's good or not for her all of the time, I don't feel this is a good situation."*

In this particular case, the type of medical care, homeopathy, leads to the unfolding of the process. Homeopathy understands illness to be an unbalanced state in which symptoms are the expression of a disharmony in the person's *vital forces.* Homeopathic treatment attempts to reestablish the girl's equilibrium. As such, day care is understood as leading the child to a state of disequilibrium, thus the child should remain at home (Luz, 1988).

The health and disease meaning making and decision making are social in their roots. Thus, caring for the child at home imposes new perspectives to the resolution of the case and leads to a rearrangement of the child's network of support. In order to reorganize the situation, the father asks the mother to give up her career, at least temporarily, giving priority to their child's care and education.

As such, the father's requests resurrect the traditional ideas related to maternity, which had not been evident until now. However, such ideas confront and compete with others, especially those of a professional woman and mother. Thus, in a contemporary context, Vera's mother does not renounce her professional role, by continuing her classes at the university. Nevertheless, to ensure her daughter's care and education at home, the child's grandmother leaves her job, thus rearranging the family's organization.

Finally, this episode reveals that there are different approaches (allopathic and homeopathic) to health and disease, each with specific theories and explanatory systems and social practice. Allopathic medicine claims to investigate the causes of diseases through scientific investigation. Homeopathy, on the other hand, does not introduce explanations about diseases, but attempts to explain illness as an imbalance of the natural order (Luz, 1988). The two fields often lead to different processes of decision making, although in this specific case, both arrive at the same conclusion: the child's withdrawal from the day-care center.

LINDA'S CASE

First Week of Attendance

Linda is a nine-month-old child who lives with her mother. The mother is a lecturer on a nursing faculty and occasionally works as the day-care center advisor on caregivers' training on health topics.

The father lives in another town but maintains an affectionate relationship with the mother and child. The mother raises Linda by herself and through her work helps to ensure financial support for the family. Linda's mother shares her care with the day-care center.

The mother, however, has her own special way of understanding such care. Mirtes, the morning caregiver, refers to the mother's comments during Linda's enrollment interview, in which the mother says that she expects that " . . . *the care giver will take care of Linda as she* (the mother) *does.*"

The mother's comment upsets the caregiver: "*I felt like . . . My God! How does this woman expect me to take care of her child exactly as she does, if I don't even know her and her child!? . . . I was a little distressed. Then, I told her . . . I tried to be gentle, as I was afraid to hurt her feelings. I said, at home, as far as I know, you only have Linda as a child. . . . So that's going to be somehow hard . . . as this is a collective environment, and I have six children directly under my responsibility!*"

During the first week of attendance the mother stayed for some time with Linda at the day-care center. The caregivers commented that they felt uneasy, as Linda's mother was always watching the caregiver, showing and explaining how care should be provided. For Branca, the afternoon caregiver, such uneasiness was due to the fact that the mother is " . . . *someone who works with us, who knows our work. And I know she is very demanding. Very much, indeed. So, we are not worried about the child, but about the mother's complaints.*"

This caregiver thinks that the mother is too concerned with the child's physical care and attributes it to " . . . *the field in which she works.*"

For the morning caregiver, the mother's attitude was felt as a threat to her professional confidence, evoking irritation, and led her to define Linda's mother as a *"hygienist,"* that is, someone whose worries were mainly focused on the child's physical care.

Describing the child, the morning caregiver referred to Linda as " . . . *very concentrated . . . always alone, on her own. . . . She doesn't cry and is very reserved. . . . You have to observe her frequently, to grasp something about her.*"

For the afternoon caregiver, Linda was " . . . *very quiet. She doesn't cry for anything. . . . I think that for her nothing is strange. . . . It seems that she already knows everybody . . . that she does the routine that we want her to do. . . . She is so calm, that I became frightened.*"

Commenting about the child's neuromotor development, the afternoon caregiver said, *"She doesn't crawl, yet. Only two weeks ago she became able to sit."* Thus, the caregiver believes that Linda " . . . *is a bit . . . delayed"* and attributes it to home care, where *"She is often kept in her cot or pen"* and has little " . . . *opportunity to explore the environment.*"

Thus, the caregiver thinks that, now, *"By being at day care, she will develop more, because we won't leave her in her cot. Thus, she will have to learn the law of survival, because if she wants a toy, she will have to go and get it."*

In the first week of attendance, the interpersonal relationships were developing and being constructed. The most significant relationship was the power dispute between the mother and the caregivers, primarily guided by conflicts and confrontations involving their roles. On one side, mother and caregivers have a similar social function, to take care of and educate the child. Nevertheless, the sociohistorical matrix drew a line between them, setting the mother as the primary caregiver and the most responsible for the child's care and education. Despite being in a different environment, the mother seeks to uphold such power and responsibility.

Even in the enrollment interview, Linda's mother expressed her expectation that the caregiver would care for her child as she herself would.

In the day-care center environment, however, those roles are partially reorganized. Greater responsibility and power over the child's care rests on the caregiver. Hence, an ambiguous and contradictory situation emerges, based on the presence of multiple role conceptions and diverse contextual constraints. One of caregivers refers to the mother's social status due to her professional position. Linda's mother is a senior lecturer, a symbol of high status on a university campus. In the specific cultural setting, this sets her in a higher position than the caregivers. This high position is reinforced during the first week of Linda's attendance, as the mother is given the role of introducing her child and of showing the way she usually cares for her child.

Furthermore, these same persons were already related to each other through the performance of other roles, in the same context. The mother, besides being a mother with a child at day care, also performed a professional role, advising the same caregivers about hygienic procedures. Hence, the "health professional" was superimposed on top of the "mother" role. The relationships between mother and caregivers were regulated by different goals, namely, the health of all of the children attending day care and the care of Linda.

Depending on the interlocutor and their dialogical relations, the effect of all these elements results in the configuration of specific networks for each of those persons. The network configuration constrains their process of meaning construction, leading to a varied set of reactions and negotiations. Mirtes was particularly caught up by the mother's attitudes; she becomes emotionally involved, rejects her expectations, and tries to draw up boundaries to it. This leads her to attribute to the mother the concept of "hygienist." Thus, personal conflicts trigger the emergence of other social meanings related to historical confrontations and disputes between diverse perspectives about children's care.

On the other hand, Branca, the other caregiver, relates with Linda and her mother in a different way. Although she opposes the mother's conception of care at a day-care center, she keeps herself apart from this conflict and sets her focus on Linda. Despite having the same element in a foreground position, this does not mean to Branca that everything in the network is flavored by it. On the contrary, Branca highlights Linda's behavior and development. Those ideas consider the child to be developing "normally" only when she is seen as active. Thus, Linda's ability to adapt and to accommodate to the adult's routine is matched with passiveness. Therefore, her peacefulness is understood as motionless. This results in Branca's worry about a possible neuromotor delay, leading to the emergence of concerns about her amazingly good disposition. Such conceptions lead Branca to stimulate the child, and she is often seen helping Linda toddle around the room.

Linda's Fever Episode

During the second week, the mother left town for three days to participate in a scientific meeting. During this period, care for the child was shared between the day-care center and the grandmother.

The child's morning caregiver reported that, before leaving her child, Linda's mother called her and asked to *"Give her child all her loving care. . . . It was really touching. She began to talk to me and I almost cried. . . . Then, I told her that she could relax, that her child was in good hands. . . . 'Or, you don't trust me!?' I teased her. . . . So, we can see that she is . . . suffering. She suffered to leave Linda."*

The day before the mother's departure, Linda developed a fever (37.8°C). Linda's mother comments: *"It has coincided with her vaccine reaction. . . . So, she has had a fever for three days, something that she has never had in her life."*

For the caregivers, the focus was on the fact that this was the first time Linda had been separated from her mother, and, according to the afternoon caregiver, *"She is feeling it quite a bit. . . . I don't know if she got sick because she misses her mother."*

The day-care auxiliary nurse briefly comments on the episode: *"She (the mother) traveled the day before yesterday. Then, Linda began to have a fever and she still has the fever."*

The psychologist said: *"I believe that all this history makes me think that she is suffering. . . . She has a fever. To me, that is a clear hint."*

However, what draws the attention of the day-care staff is Linda's behavior. The morning caregiver says, *"Poor little girl! But she is all right! . . . She has the right to be in a bad mood . . . cry and do all those things. But no! She is very quiet, playing. She really didn't change her behavior . . . And she would be justified to be upset. . . . But she still is the same."*

Yet, the caregiver states, *"I say: 'I am very concerned about you, supposing you're suffering and you're pretty good!' . . . She demonstrates that she is very well . . . that suffering is my fantasy. . . . "*

On the other hand, the day-care psychologist makes a different sense of Linda's good behavior: *"She doesn't cry. Because crying is more cultural, it is harder to see suffering. . . . Linda is a . . . very different*

child. . . . Her behavior . . . worries me a lot. Because . . . I think it is
better when a child. . . . So, I don't know. We're observing her and let's
see next week, when her mother returns."

During these days, on videotape the caregivers can be seen acting with
the child quite differently from the week before. The child is often seen
in the caregivers' lap, usually being comforted by them. On other occasions, when caregivers just pass by Linda, they stop, kiss, and hug her.

Analysis revealed that the fever episode has led the persons involved
to varied interpretations, pointing again to a diversified set of rationalities dealing with health and disease topics. For example, the mother,
whose logical view is being coconstructed by ideas present within the
field of medical science, interpreted the fever as an organic reaction to
a vaccine. For the day-care staff, however, Linda's fever seemed to be
a reaction induced by psychological suffering due to the mother's absence. The caregivers show ambivalence regarding that interpretation,
which is implicit in the auxiliary nurse's statements and explicit in the
psychologist's.

The use of such psychological "lenses" by the staff is not surprising,
as the day-care center is closely linked with the work of a psychology
faculty. Such views of suffering due to mother–child separation are heard
from different authors and psychological perspectives (Ainsworth et al.,
1978; Bowlby, 1969; Freud, 1969; Klein, 1973, 1981; Spitz, 1979; Werebe & Nadel-Brulfert, 1986). It is also based on an interdisciplinary link
between psychological and medical views, constructed through psychosomatic fields. Such interpretations lead to the expectation of physical
or psychosomatic illness, due to the child's situation.

However, the interpretation of the fever as a result of psychological
suffering contrasts with the child's calm, placid behavior. Such contrast
gives rise to different meaning processes involving the staff. In the morning caregiver's case, it questions her own premises, disrupting some of
her interpretations, leading her to new knowledge. For the psychologist,
it leads to apprehension. Concerns about the child's good behavior
emerge as they are contrasted with the expected behavior of an active
child. This leads to the emergence of notions of normal and abnormal
behavior and the presence or lack of the child's expressiveness. Thus,
specific assumptions of child behavior and child development guided the
way each viewed the child.

As a result, the psychological aspect of "lack of expressiveness" is
taken as being quite relevant, and the fever itself is overlooked. It also
induces concerns about the child's emotional future. This explanation
leads to an emotional feeling of pity or sorrow directed toward the child

that promotes new practices with her, with the staff trying to be more aware of the child, responding to her smallest requests.

It could be questioned why the same caregivers looked differently at similar fever episodes in Linda's and Vera's cases. It could be argued that such meaning making and the practical intervention toward the children were supported by the way their relationships were constructed. In Linda's case, such construction was guided by the conflicts between the mother and the caregivers, which set in motion a conflict between psychological and medical views related to understanding and caring about children. As such, meaning making and decision making related to the fever episode were based on and built within the very specific situation and context in which these participants were involved.

GENERAL DISCUSSION

These studies have made it clear that meaning making and decision making concerning health issues also takes place in ordinary people's lives and that those processes are not restricted to medical settings or involve only medical scientists and/or health professionals. Even without the actual presence of health professionals, medical discourses can be heard, seen, and felt and can contribute to constrain laypersons' understanding of their lives. Medical discourse is not an abstract or cognitive process involving the medical professional, but it is a discursive practice that has concreteness in the here-and-now. As such, it contributes to the functional organization of a whole set of environments and, as is impregnated on ordinary people's ideas, interpretations and interventions related to health and illness, which regulate much of the physical and social phenomena of human life.

By being so, it can be said that general knowledge does not exist abstractly, as something that is "out there." Medical general knowledge and the particular nature of its decisions are linked together, each one helping to construct the other. It is always in the particular cases and events that general thinking emerges, and it is through them that it is preserved, enhanced, disrupted, and/or transformed.

More significantly, this study highlighted that meaning making and decision ,making, as semiotic processes, involve other aspects beyond cognition and that they are always constituted within the specific context in which they are inserted. Thus, research on such issues requires the study of the processes by which specific endpoints are achieved, demanding a qualitative methodology. By that, a researcher can apprehend the mutual coconstruction by which persons pass through the dialogical relations of the various participants under the situation. It enables researchers to contemplate the complexity of those processes, seeking to understand the large set of elements involved in the situation, and the dynamics by which they are articulated, the constraints they set on participants, and their meaning construction processes, as well as the way those relations and meanings are updated.

In this study, through the use of qualitative analysis, it could be seen that decision making concerning illness events occurs based on meaning making about a specific case, to which are attributed specific conceptions of health and disease, normality and pathology, equilibrium and deviance. Despite a prevailing way of understanding body functions, it could be shown that meaning making is derived from a multiplicity of ideas about health.

Each of these rationalities is understood as a socially constructed interpretation, historically produced in our society. Accordingly, it can be stated that a universal nature of scientific knowledge cannot be reached. On the contrary, that there is multiple, diverse, and even contradictory knowledge being continuously constructed and applied, resulting in confrontation, with each idea disputing a place and a high status in the health field and society.

Finally, due to its complexity, research on meaning making and decision making could only be conducted through systemic and process-based methods of qualitative approach. These enable researchers to understand the centrality of the interactions established in the processes of meaning production and transaction.

NOTES

The authors acknowledge FAPESP, CAPES, and CNPq for the financial support of the research project.

1. Brazilian Research Center on Human Development and Early Childhood Education (CINDEDI), University of São Paulo, Campus of Ribeirão Preto, Brazil.

2. Pseudonyms.

3. The texts in italic are the parents' and caregivers' transcribed words obtained from interview and video records.

REFERENCES

Ainsworth, M.D.S., Blehar, M. C., Waters, E., & Wall, S. (1978). *Patterns of attachment.* Hillsdale, NJ: Erlbaum.

Amorim, K. S. (2002). *Concretização de discursos e práticas histórico-sociais, em situações de freqüência de bebês a creche* [Discourses and sociohistorical practices concretizations, during babies' attendance at day care]. Unpublished doctoral dissertation, University of São Paulo, São Paulo, Brazil.

Amorim, K. S., & Rossetti-Ferreira, M. C. (1999). Artigo especial análise crítica de investigações sobre doenças infecciosas respiratórias em crianças que freqüentam creche. *Jornal de Pediatria, 75* (5), 313–320.

Amorim, K. S., Vitória, T., & Rossetti-Ferreira, M. C. (2000). A rede de significações como perspectiva para a análise do processo de inserção de bebês na creche. *Cadernos de Pesquisa, 109,* 115–144.

Arnold, K. E., Leggiadro, R., Breiman , R. F., Lipman, H. B., Schwartz, B., Appleton, M. A., et al. (1996). Risk factors for carriage of drug-resistant *Streptococcus pneumoniae* among children in Memphis, Tennessee. *The Journal of Pediatrics, 128*(6), 757–764.

Bakhtin, M. (1981). *The dialogical imagination.* Austin: University of Texas Press.

Bakhtin, M. (1997). *Estética da criação verbal.* São Paulo: Martins Fontes.

Bakhtin, M. (1999). *Marxismo e filosofia da linguagem.* São Paulo: HUCITEC.

Belsky, J. (1990). The "effects" of infant day care reconsidered. In: N. Fox & G. G. Fein (Eds.), *Infant day care: The current debate.* Norwood, NJ: Ablex.

Bowlby, J. (1969). *Attachment and loss. Vol. 1: Attachment.* New York: Basic Books.

Denny, F. W., Jr. (1995). The clinical impact of human respiratory virus infections. *American Journal of Respiratory and Critical Care Medicine, 152,* S4–S12.

Freud, S. (1969). *Obras psicológicas completas de Sigmund Freud.* Rio de Janeiro: Imago.

Fuchs, S. C., Maynart, R. C., Costa, L. F., Cardozo, A., & Schierholt, R. (1996). Duration of day-care attendance and acute respiratory infection. *Cad Saúde Pública, 12*(3), 291–296.

Gessner, B. D., Ussery, X. T., Parkinson, A. J., & Breiman , R. F. (1995). Risk factors for invasive disease caused by *Streptococcus pneumoniae* among Alaska native children younger than 2 years of age. *Pediatric Infectious Disease Journal, 14,* 123–128.

Heyman, B., Henriksen, M., & Maughan, K. (1998). Probabilities and health risks: A qualitative approach. *Social Science and Medicine, 47*(9), 1295–1306.

Klein, M. (1981). *Psicanálise da criança* (3rd ed.). São Paulo: Mestre Jou.

Klein, M. (1973). *A educação de crianças à luz da investigação psicanalítica* (2nd ed.). Rio de Janeiro: Imago.

Louhiala, P. J., Jaakkola, N., Ruotsalainen, R., & Jaakkola, J.J.K. (1995). Form of day care and respiratory infections among Finnish children. *American Journal of Public Health, 85*(8), 1109–1112.

Luz, M. T. (1988). *Natural, racional, social: Razão médica e racionalidade científica moderna*. Rio de Janeiro: Ed. Campus Ltda.

Marbury, M. C., Maldonado, G., & Waller, L. (1997). Lower respiratory illness, recurrent wheezing, and day care attendance. *American Journal of Critical Care Medicine, 155*, 156–161.

McCutcheon, H., & Woodward, A. (1996). Acute respiratory illness in the first year of primary school related to previous attendance at child care. *Australian and New Zealand Journal of Public Health, 20*, 49–53.

Ministère de la Famille et de l'Enfance, Canada. (2000). Retrieved from http://www.famille-enfance.gouv.qc.ca.

Nafstad, P., Hagen, J., Botten, G., & Jaakkola, J.J.K. (1996). Lower respiratory tract infections among Norwegian infants with siblings in day care. *American Journal of Public Health, 86*(10), 1456–1459.

Oliveira, Z.M.R., & Rossetti-Ferreira, M. C. (1994). Coordination of roles: A theoretical–methodological perspective for studying human interactions. In N. Mercer & C. Coll (Eds.), *Teaching, learning and interaction: Vol. 3. Explorations in socio-cultural studies* (pp. 217–221). Madrid: P. del Rio.

Osterholm, M. T. (1994). Infectious disease in child day care: An overview. *Pediatrics, 94*(6), S987–990.

Roberts, C. R., & McGovern, P. (1993). Working mothers and infant care: A review of the literature. *AAOHN Journal, 41*(11), 541–546.

Roberts, I. (1996). Out-of-home day care and health. *Archives of Disease in Childhood, 74*, 73–76.

Rosemberg, F. (1995). A criação de filhos pequenos: tendências e ambigüidades contemporâneas. In I. Ribeiro & A. C. T. Ribeiro (Eds.), *Família em processos contemporâneos: inovações culturais na sociedade brasileira* (pp. 167–190). Sao Paulo: Loyola.

Rossetti-Ferreira, M. C., Amorim, K. S., & Silva, A. P. S. (1999). The network of meanings which structures and canalizes interactions, interpretations and comments. *Culture and Psychology, 5*(3), 341–353.

Rossetti-Ferreira, M. C., Amorim, K. S., & Silva, A.P.S. (2000). Uma perspectiva teórico-metodológica para análise do desenvolvimento humano e do processo de investigação. *Psicologia: Reflexão e Crítica, 13*(2), 281–293.

Rossetti-Ferreira, M. C., Amorim, K. S., & Vitória, T. (1994). A creche enquanto contexto possível de desenvolvimento da criança pequena. *Revista Brasileira de Crescimento e Desenvolvimento Humano, IV*(2), 35–40.

Rossetti-Ferreira, M. C., Amorim, K. S., & Vitória, T. (1996). Emergência de novos significados durante o processo de adaptação de bebês à creche. *Coletâneas da ANPPEP, 1*(4), 111–143.

Rossetti-Ferreira, M. C., Amorim, K. S., & Vitória, T. (1997). Integração família e creche—o acolhimento é o princípio de tudo. *Estudos em saúde mental* (pp. 107–131). São Paulo: USP Ribeirão.

Rossetti-Ferreira, M. C., Ramon, F., & Barreto, A. R. (2002). Improving early child care and education in developing countries. In C. von Hofsten &

194   SCIENCE AND MEDICINE IN DIALOGUE

L. Bäckman (Eds.), *Psychology at the turn of the millennium: Vol. 2, Social, developmental and clinical perspectives* (pp. 101–132). Hove, England: Psychology Press.

Sacks, J. J. (1993). In rates we trust (editorial). *American Journal of Diseases of Children, 147,* 813.

Schwartz, B., Giebink, G. C., Henderson, F. W., Reichler, M. R., Jereb, J., Collett, J. P., et al. (1994). Respiratory infections in day care. *Pediatrics, 94*(8, Pt. 2), 1018–1020.

Simpson, S. Q., Jones, P. W., Davies, P.D.O., & Cushing, A. (1995). Social impact of respiratory infections. *Chest, 108,* 63S–69S.

Spink, M. J. (1996). O discurso como produção de sentidos. In C. Nascimento-Schulze (Ed.), *Coletâneas da ANPPEP. Novas contribuições para a teorização e pesquisa em representação social* (pp. 37–40). Florianópolis, Brazil: UFSC.

Spink, M.J.P., Medrado, B., & Mello, R. P. (2002). Perigo, probabilidade e oportunidade: a linguagem dos riscos na mídia. *Psicologia reflexão e crítica, 15*(1), 151–164.

Spitz, R. (1979). *O primeiro ano de vida.* São Paulo: Martins Fontes.

Takala, A. K., Jero, J., Kela, E., Rönnberg, P. R., Koskenniemi, E., & Eskola, J. (1995). Risk factors for primary invasive pneumococcal disease among children in Finland. *Journal of the American Medical Association, 273*(15), 859–864.

Turner, A. L., Stewart, M. A., & Freeman, T. R. (1995). Illnesses of one-year-old children: A health diary study. *Canadian Journal of Public Health, 86*(5), 313–316.

Valsiner, J. (1994). Irreversibility of time and the construction of historical developmental psychology. *Mind, Culture and Activity, 1*(1–2), 25–42.

Valsiner, J. (2000). *Culture and human development: An introduction.* London: Sage Publications.

Victora, C. G., Fuchs, S. C., Flores, J., Fonseca, W., & Kirkwood, B. R. (1994). Risk factors for pneumonia among children in a Brazilian metropolitan area. *Pediatrics, 93*(6), Part 1, 977–985.

Vives, M., Garcia, M. E., Saenz, P., Mora, M. D., Mata, L., Sabharwal, H., & Svanborg, C. (1997). Nasopharyngeal colonization in Costa Rican children during the first year of life. *Pediatric Infectious Disease Journal, 16,* 852–858.

Vygotsky, L. (1991). *A formação social da mente.* São Paulo: Martins Fontes.

Vygotsky, L. (1993). *Pensamento e linguagem.* São Paulo: Martins Fontes.

Werebe, M. J., & Nadel-Brulfert, J. (1986). *Henri Wallon.* São Paulo: Ática.

Yagupsky, P., Landau, D., Beck, A., & Dagan, R. (1995). Carriage of *Streptococcus pyogenes* among infants and toddlers attending day-care facilities in closed communities in southern Israel. *European Journal of Clinical Microbiology and Infectious Disease, 14,* 54–58.

EDITORIAL COMMENTARY

This chapter is a great example of the many differences between the disciplines of psychology and medicine in attempting to understand the same problem. If an allopathic physician were studying disease in day-care centers, no doubt the study would include many centers and at least several hundred children. The evaluation would certainly be based on quantitative measures of pooled data.

In sharp contrast, in this chapter we see that these psychologist-investigators spent all of their efforts on a very thorough evaluation of just a few child–family–center interactions at only one day-care center. Although we are presented with only a fraction of the material in the whole study, it is clear that important information was gleaned from this sample of only 21 subjects.

While both medicine and psychology use large samples for many studies, the type of in-depth evaluation that was performed by these authors is virtually never seen in medicine. The use of recorded interviews and video tapes, as well as the time-consuming review of these materials, is virtually absent in clinical research. Large medical studies are very defensible on a statistical basis, but they only provide an "eagle's eye" view, that is, the pooled data never represent any specific individual, and the conclusions might not be appropriate in the particular. "N of 1" studies can be criticized in just the opposite direction, as the sample is so small that the conclusions might not be applicable to any other place or any other group, at any other time. Both techniques are searching for the universal "truth." Neither will find it, but each can come close enough.

—Kenneth L. Noller

Chapter 12

GENERIC DISEASE AND PARTICULAR LIVES: A SYSTEMIC AND DYNAMIC APPROACH TO CHILDHOOD CANCER

Micheline Silva

Health sciences have been primarily oriented to the *disease*—a construct that refers to generic biological processes that take place within the malfunctioning body. However, when any generic disease is actualized within the body of a concrete individual, it is also subjectively experienced by such individual in terms of *illness* (Bibace, Dillon, & Dowds, 1999). As a heart attack and cancer survivor, Arthur Frank (1991) points out:

> Illness is the experience of living through the disease. If disease talk measures the body, illness talk tells of the fear and frustration of being inside a body that is breaking down . . . What happens to my body happens to my life. My life consists of temperature and circulation, but also of hopes and disappointments, joys and sorrows, none of which can be measured. In illness talk there is no such a thing as *the* body, only *my* body as I experience it. Disease talk charts the progression of certain measures. Illness talk is a story about moving from a perfectly comfortable body to one that forces me to ask: What's happening to *me?* Not *it,* but *me.* (p. 13; emphasis from the original)

In this way, illness can be understood as an inherently idiosyncratic and subjective phenomenon, which happens as part of a particular life trajectory, embedded in a specific sociohistorical context. It means that, although individuals might share similar experiences while going through a specific kind of disease and treatment, the way each of them will make sense of his/her situation, and emotionally experience it, is still unique.

Thus, we may observe variability not only in the way different individuals experience the same disease, but also how the same individual experiences a specific disease during different moments along its course. These inter- and intra-individual variations are due to the interaction between diverse factors that are simultaneously at work while an individual is experiencing a specific disease.

Despite the intrinsic subjectivity and variability of the illness experience, diverse studies interested in the impact of certain diseases in the lives of particular populations have searched for generic patterns of coping mechanisms and psychological adjustment, as if the individuals in the population formed a homogeneous group. These studies normally assume causal (and unidirectional) relationships between certain characteristics shared by a group of individuals, patterns of coping mechanisms used by them and/or their families, and types of psychological adjustment used by them.

My goal here is to critically discuss the current body of studies in childhood cancer, pointing to some limitations in the way they approach the process of coping and adjustment. I intend to question their efforts to find general patterns by reducing variability found between and within cases to "noise," "errors of variance," or "deviation from the norm" to be excluded from the data. I believe that the exploration of such variability is important in order to reveal the particularities in the way different individuals experience childhood cancer as well as the fluctuations in the way the same individual experiences it through time.

I will also analyze the adequacy of such studies while searching for the ultimate cause(s) for the use of different coping mechanisms and/or for the attainment of different types of psychological adjustment by the child and/or family. I will show how the experience of coping and adjustment to childhood cancer and its treatment can be understood as a system of multiple interactions between biological, psychological, sociocultural, and situational elements. These diverse elements are constantly coregulating and changing each other in such a way that it is impossible for a researcher to isolate and treat any of them as the ultimate cause(s) of certain types of coping and/or adjustment. Moreover, I claim that coping and adjustment should not be seen as a permanent characteristic of an individual but rather as a dynamic transformative process, inasmuch as the mutual interaction between the elements that constitute this system is constantly changing over time.

I will also discuss the necessity of developing longitudinal and detailed analyses of particular cases as a way of shedding light into the inherent variability and complexity involved in the phenomenon of coping and adjustment to childhood cancer. My ideas are based on the transactional approach to stress and coping developed by Lazarus and colleagues (Folkman & Lazarus, 1980, 1985; Folkman, Lazarus, Gruen, & De-Longis, 1986; Lazarus, 1966; Lazarus & Folkman, 1984). I will illustrate my points using one empirical case study that took place in a Pediatric Bone Marrow Transplant (BMT) Unit in the United States. I will discuss the case of a nine-year-old girl, called Carol, diagnosed with leukemia and undergoing BMT and followed on a weekly basis for a period of eight months.

COPING AND ADJUSTMENT TO CHILDHOOD CANCER: CURRENT STATE OF AFFAIRS

Childhood cancer is an especially traumatic life experience that children and their families have to face. The treatment introduces the child and the family to a new life scenario, which includes the hospital, treatment procedures, and the interruption of regular activities. The possibility of treatment failure and death are especially powerful stressful features (Thompson, 1985; Thompson & Gustafson, 1996).

For the child, the situation normally involves physical discomfort and psychological distress brought about by a variety of problems related to the illness and treatment side effects (Bearison, 1991; Kubler-Ross, 1969; Thompson and Gustafson, 1996). We can also see psychological effects in the organization and dynamics of the family as a whole.

As a consequence, we observe increasing efforts to understand the impact of cancer and its treatment on the lives of the child and his/her family. Particular attention has been given to the use of different coping mechanisms by the child and the family while facing this stressor and to the quality of psychological adjustment attained by them through the use of such coping mechanisms (Docherty, 1999; Moos & Tsu, 1977; Stein & Jessop, 1982; Thompson & Gustafson, 1996). Before we start exploring empirical investigations of this phenomenon, it seems important to first clarify how terms such as "stressors," "coping," and "adjustment" are defined and used within social and health sciences.

THE COGNITIVE–MEDIATIONAL MODEL OF STRESS AND COPING

"Stress" and "coping" are worn-out terms in social and health sciences, and there is no consensus about what each of these terms mean. Despite this fact, these terms have been defined, measured, and used in various ways and contexts. The "cognitive–mediational model of stress and coping" developed by Lazarus and colleagues has been influential (Folkman & Lazarus, 1980, 1985; Folkman, Lazarus, Dunkel-Schetter, DeLongis & Gruen, 1986; Folkman, Lazarus, Gruen & DeLongis, 1986; Lazarus, 1966; Lazarus & Folkman, 1984), becoming the basis for empirical studies in diverse fields, such as childhood cancer.

Lazarus and his collaborators conceive "stress" as a generic term that refers to a dynamic interplay between the environment and the individual who presents the stress reactions, mediated by the appraised level of threat. It means that the environment in itself is not enough to produce stress responses. The cognitive appraisal of the threat by the individual is an essential step for the determination of whether or not a situation will be stressful and the quality of the stress responses.

According to this coping model, the process of threat appraisal is determined by a combination of factors, some of which are situational factors, while others are personal factors. Lazarus and Folkman (1984) highlight that, although immediate and unintentional cognitive–affective responses are triggered by the certain situations, the cognitive appraisal refers to a more complex, meaning-related cognitive activity, serving as an emotional and behavioral regulator. Thus, once a situation is cognitively appraised as threatening, different levels of stress responses can be observed in the individual, such as emotional, motor–behavioral, cognitive, and/or physiological.

The process of "coping" is a consequence of the primary threat appraisal. Coping is basically understood as a strategy for dealing with a threat. While the primary appraisal of threat refers to its recognition, the process of coping refers to the level of actions related to how the individual will manage the stressful situation. In this model, the process of coping involves an evaluation of how the threat will be dealt with (called secondary appraisal) followed by some action toward the appraised threat. As in the case of the primary threat appraisal, the secondary appraisal is also considered to be determined by situational as well as personal factors. Although appraisal is basically a cognitive process, it does not necessarily follow that it is always a conscious, rational, and deliberate process. The individual may not be aware of which internal and/or external factors are contributing to the sense of stress and may sometimes not be aware that a threat has been appraised.

According to this model, two types of coping processes can be identified: Problem-focused coping, which are efforts to eliminate, alter, or control the perceived source of stress; and emotion-focused coping, which are efforts to regulate stressful emotions that emerge as a stress response. Although the authors argue that one or the other form of coping may be predominant depending on the context, they affirm that both forms are simultaneously at work in any stressful situation. They state that problem- and emotion-focused coping processes are dynamically interrelated in such a way that they can mutually facilitate and/or impede each other. Thus, the use of coping mechanisms works by changing the perceived characteristics of the stressful situation through a combination of alterations of the source of stress and/or regulation of the emotional stress responses.

Lazarus and Folkman (1984) define coping as "constantly changing cognitive and behavioral efforts to manage specific external and/or internal demands that are appraised as taxing or exceeding the resources of the person" (p. 141). This means that the perceived stressor will be constantly reappraised, and coping mechanisms will be constantly in use, until the situation is appraised as no longer exceeding the person's resources. It does not necessarily mean that the situation will actually stop being a threat. In life-threatening diseases, even though the situation has the potential always to be reappraised as threatening, no matter which coping mechanisms have been used, the level of stress can increase or decrease over time, depending on the efficiency of the individual's coping mechanisms. Sometimes, individuals can reach such a great level of adjustment to the stressful situation through the use of coping mechanisms that they can maintain a reasonably well-balanced life.

Lazarus and colleagues' coping model seems to describe a spiral dynamic pattern, that starts with a primary threat appraisal leading to stress responses, that lead to coping processes, that may change the perceived characteristics of the stressful situation, leading to a reappraisal of the situation and so on. Figure 12.1 is a schematic view of the cognitive–mediational model.

APPRAISAL OF THE APPRAISAL MODEL

The cognitive–mediational model developed by Lazarus et al. was a major milestone in the study of stress and coping. It broke the old-fashioned separation between individual and environment posed by the behaviorist traditions and by the psychoanalytic traditions.

According to the "transactional" approach (Lazarus & Folkman, 1984) that underlies their model, individual and environment are understood as in a dynamic, mutually reciprocal, bi-directional relationship, in such a way that they cannot be disentangled from each other as two distinct determinants of coping. An analogy can be made with cells working

Figure 12.1
Cognitive–mediational model of stress and coping.

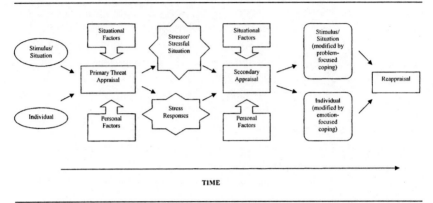

together and forming an organ. The organ integrates these cells so that no one of them can be isolated as the source of the organ's function. In the same way, "an appraisal does not refer to the environment or to the person alone, but to the integration of both in a given transaction" (Lazarus & Folkman, 1984, p. 294).

Another interesting aspect of this transactional approach is that, although there is a clear emphasis on cognition, there is also an effort to not treat it separately from emotion as if they were two independent entities. The authors defend the idea of a "bi-directional causality" between emotion and cognition. Instead of questioning whether emotion or cognition comes first, they understand them as being simultaneously in action, and constantly interacting and regulating each other. Cognitive activity is seen as an essential part of the process of emotionally responding to an encountered situation as it provides the evaluation of meaning that regulates the emotional responses. At the same time, emotions are also an essential part of the process of cognitive evaluation of the situation. Emotional reactions not only constitute the situation that will be cognitively evaluated by the individual as threatening or not, but they also shape the way the individual thinks, perceives, and evaluates such situation.

According to this transactional approach, coping and adjustment are understood as fundamentally fluid and dynamic rather than as static phenomena. In other words, coping and adjustment are seen as processes, instead of unchanging outcomes. The authors affirm that the way an individual appraises and emotionally responds to a specific situation may dramatically change in quality and intensity as a result of how the transactions between this individual and the environment unfold or flow over time. Thus, the encountered situation, as well as the way the individual copes with it, will be constantly changing in an integrated/coordinated manner as the encounter unfolds. Though the use of a certain coping mechanism in one specific situation may have been very effective, in the very next moment the same coping mechanism may be completely ineffective, depending how the encounter with the situation flows over time.

As a follow-up to this process-oriented approach, the authors emphasize the necessity of designing longitudinal studies in which particular individuals can be compared with themselves over time. They argue that the microanalysis of the encounter of a particular individual with a specific stressful situation over time can provide a broader (and more accurate) picture of such phenomena in contrast to a "one-time-only" assessment). In the words of Lazarus and Folkman (1984):

> This interindividual, or normative, perspective therefore fails to take into account the context in which the observations are made. If, for example, the person must function under severe environmental demands or conditions of deprivation, the use of an interindividual standard of comparison may lead to a distorted evaluation of that person's functioning. By ordinary standards he or she might be judged as having inadequate coping skills or resources or a weak ego, or as lacking resilience, or the like, when in fact the person is functioning reasonably well in an environment that is posing extraordinary or novel problems. (p. 299)

The microanalysis of particular cases over time provides us with information about the social context in which the individual is embedded while dealing with a stressful situation. Using the context of illness, the experience of being ill is not experienced by the patient isolated from their social environment. Rather, it happens as part of a whole that includes others, such as family members, negotiating personal values and beliefs within specific sociocultural backgrounds (Waddell, 1983). The longitudinal analysis of particular cases also allows us to observe how an individual develops dynamic patterns of coping and adjustment over time.

The authors emphasize that once we have a detailed and dynamic picture of the process of coping in particular cases, we can then make inter-case comparisons that may allow us to identify common dynamic patterns. In this way, once we build abstract models of coping over time, each newly analyzed case will test the adequacy of the model.

Although the Lazarus model is limited and needs further elaboration, we can consider it as a solid theoretical basis for the empirical exploration of coping and adjustment to childhood cancer. The model seems to reflect a systemic and dynamic view of coping and adjustment to stressful situations, in which feelings are constantly shaping thoughts and actions; thoughts are constantly shaping feelings and actions; actions are constantly shaping thoughts and feelings; environmental and biological processes are constantly shaping thoughts, feelings, and actions; and thoughts, feelings, and actions are constantly shaping these environmental and biological processes as well.

This model has been a conceptual ground for a large number of recent studies dedicated to the investigation of child and adult coping and adjustment to childhood diseases (McKeever, O'Neill, & Miller, 2002; Salmon & Pereira, 2002; Thomsen et al., 2002) and to childhood cancer (Coletti, 1997; Grootenhuis & Last, 2001; Manne, Bakeman, Jacobsen, & Gorfinkle, 1992; Romy, 2002; Saiki-Craighill, 2002; Streisand, Rodrigue, Houck, Graham-Pole, & Berlant, 2000). However, most of these studies seem to apply the Lazarus model in an oversimplified or distorted manner. More specifically, the systemic and dynamic approach that underlies the Lazarus model seems to have been lost in such studies. Coping is therefore treated as a fixed series of procedures that can be used by individuals when facing childhood diseases, which will lead to (or be the cause of) positive or negative outcomes in terms of psychological adjustment. In such studies there is an assumption that specific characteristics shared by groups of individuals will be the reason why different individuals use certain coping mechanisms instead of others. I will describe studies that illustrate how the Lazarus model of stress and coping has been applied in the current body of studies on childhood cancer.

STUDIES ABOUT STRESS AND COPING AND CHILDHOOD CANCER

One illustration of how the cognitive–mediational model has been used to investigate stress and coping in childhood cancer is the study developed by Grootenhuis and Last (2001). These authors examined whether or not children with cancer with different survival perspectives differ in terms of the use of coping strategies as well as psychological adjustment. Forty-three "in remission" and forty-one "in relapse" children between the ages of 8 and 18 years answered a series of questionnaires about depression, trait anxiety, defensiveness, and cognitive control strategy. Their hypothesis that children with less survival perspective would rely less on predictive control and vicarious control, and that they would experience more feelings of anxiety and depression, was not confirmed. No differences were found between gender or time since diagnosis. Older children did use less vicarious control and reported fewer depressive symptoms. The authors concluded that the survival perspective of the children did not seem to be related to their emotional adjustment and that the use of predictive control and defensiveness seems to be the most important predictors.

Another example is the investigation by Romy (2002), which had as a goal to explore factors such as gender, treatment status, reciprocity of parent–child coping, and family functioning in the context of children's psychological adjustment to cancer. Forty children with cancer between the ages of 7 and 16 years completed an inventory about their behavioral style, and their parents completed a series of inventories about the child's personality, anxiety, dynamic of adjustment, and family adaptability. No relationship between gender and psychological adjustment was found. A relationship between the treatment status and the children's score in the personality inventory was identified, with higher scores for children who had completed treatment. Children's adjustment was associated with their coping and the concordance between child and parent coping styles, as well as with family adjustment. The author concluded his study suggesting that the interaction of parent and child coping styles and family adaptability must be examined when considering children's psychological adjustment to cancer.

Coletti (1997) tried to identify cognitive appraisals that precede coping responses to two cancer-related stressors, evaluating the relationship between parent and child appraisals and coping responses and the relationship between coping and psychological adaptation. Forty-five children with leukemia between the ages of 7 and 17 years and their treatment companion parent completed questionnaires on their perceptions about two cancer-related stressors. Results indicated that parents viewed both stressors as more threatening and challenging than the children. Positive internal dialogues were evaluated as effective in terms of adaptation, while "catastrophizing" was more associated with poor adaptation. The author concluded his study by highlighting the importance of the use of cognitive coping strategies rather than coping behaviors to reach better psychological adaptation.

ARE THESE STUDIES SUFFICIENTLY ADEQUATE TO CAPTURE THE COMPLEXITIES AND DYNAMICS OF STRESS, COPING, AND ADAPTATION TO CHILDHOOD CANCER?

We observe that these studies treat childhood cancer as a generic stressor, or they determine beforehand which aspects related to cancer are particular stressors, assuming that it will be a phenomenon common to all children and families in the study. However, although "cancer" refers to a generic disease, the process of appraisal refers to how such a disease is subjectively experienced by an ill person. Therefore, appraisal is an inherently personal and dynamic process. We cannot assume that the experience of childhood cancer is appraised as a stressor in exactly the same way by all of the subjects included in the study, or even by the same subject at different times.

The ill child and his/her family face not only the disease "cancer" but also a multitude of specific events or situations related to it (the unpredictability of the future, success or failure of the treatment, pain, physiological, behavioral and body alterations, financial problems, etc.). The combination of different events or situations that are happening simultaneously over the course of each child's disease and treatment constitute a particular scenario within which the cancer will be appraised and emotionally experienced over time by each ill child and his/her family. Therefore, such studies seem to present a very simplistic picture of the phenomenon of appraising, coping, and adjustment to childhood cancer. They seem to impose pre-established general categories onto the child and family's experiences and in this way miss the perspective of those who are actually experiencing it.

Another problematic aspect of these studies is that they believe it is possible to find the ultimate causal explanation for why different children use different coping mechanisms, as well as why they present different psychological responses, when facing childhood cancer. Their main concern is the identification of certain commonalities among groups of subjects in terms of factors related to the illness and/or to the child, coping mechanisms used by the children/caretakers, and the child's psychological adjustment/responses to the stressor. They then try to discover which of those factors are better predictors of the use of specific coping mechanisms and/or specific patterns of psychological adjustment.

In order to prove the causal relationship between the variables hypothesized as the causes and the final responses or outcomes, they allocate the subjects into specific "homogeneous" groups according to those selected factors. They assume the existence of uniformity among the individuals in those specific groups and between the same individual over time. Therefore, any intra-group variability or intra-individual variability is considered "noise" or "errors of variance" and is excluded from the data set, or, if not excluded, are treated as "personality traits."

If we consider coping and adaptation to childhood cancer as a systemic and dynamic process that is particular to each individual, this search for isolated ultimate cause(s) seems to make no sense.

If we analyze any concrete case carefully, what we will observe is a child, as a whole, struggling to deal with a diversity of events and situations experienced as stressful in the context of childhood cancer. In this way, we must consider those different aspects that constitute the child's life not as simple variables that can be taken apart but rather as parts of a complex and dynamic system in which they coexist and develop over time. In this process, different aspects of the child's life are simultaneously at work and influencing each other. None of these variables can be isolated and used as a predictor of how the child will react to the illness and treatment.

Let me use the case of Carol as an illustration of these points.

A DYNAMIC AND SYSTEMIC APPROACH TO STRESS AND COPING ON CHILDHOOD CANCER: CAROL

Dimensions of Carol's Life

The Familiar Scenario

Carol was a nine-year-old first child of a married couple in their early forties, with a five-year-old brother. Both parents came from Asia to pursue college and graduate studies in the United States. Her parents had met and were married after emigrating. They decided to stay in the United States. Both of their children were born on the West Coast. All of their family members still lived in Asia, but according to the parents, they had a supportive system of friends. Both parents seemed very concerned about promoting intellectual, artistic, and social development for their children. The children, in their turn, seemed to be incorporating such values into their lives. Carol and her brother seemed to have a close relationship. This fact was reported not only by their parents but also by the hospital staff, and by Carol herself (and personally observed by me). Carol and her brother seemed to enjoy each other's company and miss each other when they were apart.

The Disease Scenario

When Carol had just turned eight, she was diagnosed with an aggressive form ofacute myeloblastic leukemia (AML). She underwent chemotherapy and radiation. Unfortunately, in less than a year her leukemia relapsed and her only chance of treatment was a bone marrow transplant

(BMT). According to her parents, the doctors were having a hard time finding a marrow donor who matched her blood type. When they finally found a donor for her, she developed pneumonia due to her poor immunity and had to have the transplant postponed. Just as she was getting better from her pneumonia, her leukemia relapsed again, and she lost the opportunity to have the transplant. Her parents found another donor in a hospital located on the East Coast. That was how the whole family flew from the other side of the country and how I later got to meet them.

Carol spent approximately one month in pre-transplant treatment. During this month, her routine was characterized by frequent visits to the outpatient clinic and BMT Unit. At that time she received radiation to treat her relapsed leukemia, drugs to shrink the scar in her lungs from the pneumonia, and drugs to control infections. During this pre-transplant time, she also had a "central line" surgically implanted in her chest. Her transplant took place almost a month after she had arrived at the hospital and just after she turned nine. According to her parents, the transplant "went very smooth," and Carol's case seemed to be evolving well. While the doctors were waiting for the process of "engraftment" to begin, efforts were made to avoid infection, and to treat the side effects of her medications. I was first introduced to Carol and her family ten days after her transplant.

The Hospital Scenario

Before I actually met Carol, I found a very friendly and "full of life" atmosphere in the BMT Unit. It was decorated with children's themes, and each room was personally decorated to welcome that specific child. Additionally, the staff seemed to treat everyone in a caring and joyful manner.

My first impression of the unit was very positive. During the data collection period, I had the chance to have this first impression constantly reconfirmed.

The Interpersonal Scenario: Carol's Social Network

It seemed that everyone I asked about Carol shared similar perceptions about her and about her family. Two teachers said "Carol is a very bright girl . . . very smart and organized, curious" and "she loves to do the school activities." They also mentioned that she was a "very sweet girl" but that sometimes she acted "a little mean" and she could be "very demanding." They said that they had the impression that "Carol knows she is smart and she enjoys hearing that from people," and "she wants to be liked by everybody." They thought that she was "coping well" with her situation and that she had a "good understanding" of it. They saw her parents as "present" and "supportive," but they thought that Carol was very "independent" and "autonomous."

The child life specialist, said, "Since my first meeting with Carol everything flowed very well between us." She thought of Carol as a "very smart girl, and very aware of her treatment." She saw Carol's family as "supportive," and she thought they had established a "good bond" with her. She said that though Carol was "an easy child to communicate with," she thought that Carol had some "problems expressing her concerns and fears" about her situation, so she sometimes expressed them indirectly, saying that she had "tummy pain" or just being "moody."

Carol's mother said that "Carol was always a very alive girl, smart, curious, with lots of friends in school." Her mother thought that Carol was getting "more mature" by going through this experience. She thought that Carol had a "positive attitude" toward her treatment. She said that Carol was friendly with all the nurses and she found "her way inside the hospital pretty easily." She emphasized that she thought of Carol as a "blessed child": "everybody who meets her loves her," "she fights hard to get better," "she is very well skilled on making friends." She also thought that the fact that she had gotten Carol involved in many activities when she was younger was somehow helping Carol to deal with her current situation, "for example, when she is feeling pain, we do yoga movements together, and it helps alleviating her pain."

Carol's father seemed to concentrate on Carol's intellectual skills and strength to fight against her disease. According to him, "she is very smart," "she fights hard to get cured," "she is very careful about her treatment, she was the one who posted that note outside the door telling the visitors to use mask," "she goes to the nurse station and ask them questions about the drugs she is taking, and she keeps a diary about all the drugs she takes and their side effects." He said that they always tried to think positively and they encouraged this positive attitude in Carol. They explained her situation to her, but they avoid talking about "the negative parts of it," such as treatment failure and death.

Carol's Process of Coping and Adjustment: An
Orchestration of Different Dimensions of Her Life

I had the chance to interact with Carol and her family on an almost weekly basis for a period of eight months. During the first three months, I was audio recording almost all of our meetings.[1] After my official period of data collection had ended, I kept meeting her for five more months by request of her family. Thus, during the remaining months I was not recording our meetings, but I continued to write field notes after each of my visits.

My First Impressions of Carol

Based on my initial interactions with Carol, I got the impression that Carol was coping and adjusting very well to the events that she had been dealing with since the transplant. She seemed to be aware of her medical situation, and her major sources of stress seemed to be the possibility of infection and transplant failure. The strategy used by Carol in order to cope with those stressors seemed to be concentrating all her efforts on getting better. Thus, she tried to follow carefully all of the medical instructions about how to avoid infections. She kept track of all of the details about her medical progress. She tried to focus on the positive aspects of her life, and she tried to avoid anything that directly or indirectly reminded her that negative things could actually happen to her. In this manner, she seemed to manage being in a good mood most of the time, being usually very friendly with everybody around her, always smiling and being talkative.

If we analyze my first impressions of Carol, we notice that the transactions between a series of factors—such as her familiar scenario, hospital environment, course of her disease and treatment, her personal and inter-personal characteristics—seemed to constitute the setting in which Carol's dynamics of appraising, coping, and adjustment took place. The orchestration of these different dimensions of Carol's life seemed to form the grounds on which her social network of interrelationships was created. It was precisely within Carol's engagement in these multiple interactions with others, that she found her particular way of giving meaning to and emotionally experiencing her encounters. I noticed, for example, that Carol's appraisal of potential infections as a particular source of stress seemed to find some of its ground in the course of her disease and treatment.

Was Carol a Classical Example of "Positive" Coping and Adjustment?

Based on the discussion above, it is seems fair to say that Carol's setting constituted a favorable place for her process of appraisal and coping to work quite efficiently. However, the elements that constituted this setting were far from stable. A large number of events were constantly happening in the different dimensions of Carol's life, and the orchestration of these events over time led to a constant reorganization of Carol's experiences. During my eight months of interacting with Carol, I observed many variations in the constitution of this setting, in the ways Carol appraised different situations as sources of stress, and the ways she adjusted to them.

Depending on how the multiple factors that constituted her life setting interacted with each other, the same event or situation sometimes would be treated by Carol as a great source of stress and at other times as a minor problem that could be managed easily. Carol's use of the same coping mechanisms sometimes seemed to be very effective. At other times, however, these coping mechanisms seemed completely ineffective.

Gradually it became clear to me that the fluctuations in her way of dealing with her situations were related to diverse factors that were simultaneously at work during the moment she was facing a specific situation or event. Some of the factors seemed to be related to how she developed as part of a family with particular shared values. Other factors seemed to be related to more circumstantial issues. Furthermore, other factors seemed to be contributing on a more physiological level.

It was impossible for me to isolate any of the factors that seemed to be simultaneously at work while she was facing a stressful situation as the ultimate cause of her process of appraisal, coping, and adjustment under that circumstance. For example, the side effect of a drug she was taking at some point of her treatment was making her emotionally very sensitive so that she seemed to be having a particularly hard time coping with stressful events, such as "tummy pain." Although she was well known to initiate strategies to make her "tummy pain" go away, I recall that during various episodes of "tummy pain" she would not even try any of those strategies.

One particular day when she was experiencing this pain, it was exactly the day that her little brother came back for a week-long visit and she had not seen him in more than a month. Though her first reaction to her episode of pain was crying, she gradually became distracted by and relaxed around him. At first, she was sitting in a seat near her bed, leaning her body over the bed, holding her abdomen, with her eyes closed, and complaining of any sound or noise produced by her brother. As he did not stop talking, she eventually started opening her eyes, as if checking what he was doing. She started making comments about how he should be painting the figures in the activity book and correcting him. Gradually her posture started changing. She started getting closer to him and becoming engaged in the panting activity with him. Thus, at some point she seemed to have completely forgotten about her pain.

This example seems to be a good illustration of how a child's process of experiencing a stressful situation can be understood as a dynamic process of coregulation and mutual transformation among a series of different factors. It seems clear that the effect of the drug on Carol's emotional reactions influenced her experience of pain as well as her reaction to the presence of her brother. But, it seems like the presence of her brother also influenced and altered the effect of the drug on her emotions as well as her experience of pain.

It seemed that, over time, Carol was inventing new ways of dealing with her encountered situations, as well as reinventing the already used ones, as part of her struggle to adjust to the multiplicity of issues that constituted the scenario of her life at the time. In other words, as her life setting changed over time, some of her ways of dealing with her situation became ineffective, so she had to constantly try to find new ways in order to maintain a reasonable quality of life.

During the eight-month period I followed Carol's case, her medical situation presented "ups and downs" to the point that she had been discharged from the hospital at least twice but always had to be re-admitted. She was even admitted to the Pediatric Intensive Care Unit, but she managed to recover from all of these episodes. However, at some point the doctors discovered that her leukemia had relapsed and that there were no more treatments available to her. That was when the family decided to fly home, where she died.

These periods of deterioration of her medical condition, and the eventual failure of the treatment, were experienced as especially stressful events. They seemed to have a huge impact in Carol's whole life setting, and I could witness many changes in her ways of coping and adjustment. First of all, I could notice the physiological effects of the disease and drugs on Carol's physical and psycho-emotional responses to her situation. In addition, there was the fact that her family had always tried to maintain a positive attitude, avoiding talking about negative issues, so that the deterioration of her medical condition and the failure of the treatment became a source of various interaction and communication problems. There were long periods of absence of Carol's father and little brother, and during these periods Carol's mother was responsible for all of Carol's care. This fact, combined with Carol's medical problems, was experienced by her mother as another major source of physical and psycho-emotional exhaustion and stress.

Carol's mother reported that she was constantly struggling with how she could make decisions about what and how to share the negative events with Carol, when she herself was already tired and emotionally overwhelmed. Carol's mother told me on different occasions that she did not know if it was actually the best thing to do, but she preferred not to let Carol know about certain aspects of her treatment. However, since Carol was also stimulated to be in charge of her treatment, every time there was bad news, it was hard to keep it secret as Carol was always eager to know the meaning of everything that was going on with her.

These communication problems became such a major issue in Carol's life that not only did they influence the quality of the relationship between Carol and her mother but they also became one more source of stress for both of them. Her mother told me that on various occasions that Carol had asked her about something related to her condition, and she could not help but be silent, because she just did not know what to say. Carol seemed to be so sensitive to that lack of response from her mother that she actually started hiding certain events from her mother.

Therefore, as the deterioration of her condition became evident, and she actually learned that her leukemia was back, it seemed like some of her old coping strategies (e.g., concentrating on getting better) started to be ineffective. Thus, Carol had to start readjusting her ways of dealing with the new events. For example, I noticed that during the days she was feeling particularly weak and/or moody, she started avoiding arts & crafts and intellectual activities, and she would find some distraction watching TV, children videos, or any other low-key activity. I also noticed that Carol seemed to start to express her concerns about negative issues that were happening to her. Nevertheless, she seemed not to be able to disclose it completely. For example, she would unexpectedly make some comment such as, "I wish I didn't have this cancer," or "I wish I had never been born, I just cause trouble to my family," but as I started answering her, she would immediately change the subject, either by saying things such as "but I'm getting better" or just starting a completely unrelated topic.

One illustration of how Carol efficiently reshaped an old coping strategy in order to cope with a new situation was the episode that happened during my last visit to her, just before she returned home. During the whole time I was there, I noticed that she seemed to be to be trying to give some closure to the various relationships she had built while she had been there, by checking on her "importance" in the lives of these others. In my case, for example, when I first got to her room, I found

her very quiet and not responsive. She seemed particularly worried about
going back home. Then, suddenly, she asked me how I was going to
give her the "Pikachu sleepers" I had promised her if she went back
home. I told her that I could send them by mail as soon as I found them.
As I was answering her, she seemed to relax a little. Then she asked me
why I had chosen her to "hang out" with during her illness. I told her
that, it was because the child life specialist had told me that she was a
great girl, and that I would probably enjoy doing my study with her. I
also said that after I got to know her better and I saw how special she
was, I wanted to keep seeing her, even though my data collection period
was completed. As I was answering her, I noticed that her facial expression and body posture started changing. Then, she just said "OK,"
and changed the subject by making jokes and funny comments. Thus, it
seemed to me that her acknowledgment that she was special to me and
that I would not forget her even when she was not around anymore was
one of her strategies for dealing with the stress of leaving.

Over time, I observed the same girl appraising and emotionally experiencing the same type of event or situation in different ways. I also
observed her using different strategies for coping with her illness that
were more or less effective, depending on various factors that constituted
her life setting at the time. If I had collected other data, like the studies
previously described, Carol could very easily have been included in a
group of children that use certain types of coping strategies instead of
others and be classified as presenting signs of either well or maladjust-
ment, depending on which day and under which circumstances the data
collection took place. However, Carol's experiences cannot be understood as being static. The ways she dealt with her life seemed to vary
greatly over time as part of her constant attempts to adjust to a number
of factors involved in her particular experience with leukemia and its
treatment.

GENERIC DISEASE AND PARTICULAR LIVES: SOME FINAL THOUGHTS ABOUT VARIABILITY

It seems clear that based on the theoretical framework defended in
this chapter, inter- and intra-case variability should not be considered as
"noise" or "errors of variance" and eliminated from the data set. Variability points to the flexible character of human adjustment, which allows
different individuals to find their particular ways of functioning under
diverse and changing environmental conditions. Variability also points

to the dynamic character of self-organization and development. At each new encounter with different events or situations, the individual is challenged by uncertainties, conflicts, and confrontations. Life is an ongoing process of dealing with a multiplicity of internal and external situations, and therefore, we are constantly developing self-experience in the world (Bakhtin, 1973, 1986, 1993; Hermans, 1996, 1999; Hermans & Kempen, 1993).

Instead of seeing a child's way of coping and adjusting to cancer as a generic outcome resulting from factors pre-established by the researchers, it seems preferable to try to explore the interrelations between the various processes involved in the emergence of specific outcomes in the case of each particular child and how those outcomes change and develop over time as part of a dynamic process. In this way, the in-depth exploration of longitudinal data from multiple case studies seems to constitute an adequate methodological tool. The comparison of different children may allow the identification of common processes involved in general outcomes, but more importantly, it will point to the many ways that different children reach the same general outcomes.

NOTE

1. Sometimes I was not able to record the meetings because she did not want me to or because the situation was not appropriate.

REFERENCES

Bakhtin, M. (1973). *Problems of Dostoevsky's poetics* (2nd ed.; R. W. Rotsel, Trans.). Ann Arbor, MI: Ardis.

Bakhtin, M. (1986). *Speech genres and other late essays* (C. Emerson & M. Holquist, Eds.; V. W. McGee, Trans.). Austin: University of Texas Press.

Bakhtin, M. (1993). *Toward a philosophy of the act* (M. Holquist & V. Liapunov, Eds.; V. Liapunov, Trans.). Austin: University of Texas Press.

Bearison, D. (1991). *They never want to tell you: Children talk about cancer.* Cambridge: Harvard University Press.

Bibace, R., Dillon, J. J., & Dowds, B. N. (1999). *Partnership in research, clinical, and educational settings.* Stamford, CT: Ablex.

Coletti, D. J. (1997). Stressful medical procedures in the context of cancer: Patterns of parent and child coping strategies and psychological adaptation. *Dissertation Abstracts International. B: The Sciences and Engineering, 58*(3-B), 1523.

Docherty, S. (1999). *Patterns of symptom distress during the initial treatment period in three children with cancer.* Unpublished doctoral dissertation, University of North Carolina at Chapel Hill, NC.

Folkman, S., & Lazarus, R. S. (1980). An analysis of coping in a middle-aged community sample. *Journal of Health and Social Behavior, 21,* 219–239.

Folkman S., & Lazarus, R. S. (1985). If it changes it must be a process: Study of emotion and coping during three stages of a college examination. *Journal of Personality and Social Psychology, 48,* 150–170.

Folkman, S., Lazarus, R. S., Dunkel-Schetter, C., DeLongis, A. & Gruen, R. J. (1986). Dynamics of a stressful encounter: Cognitive appraisal, coping, and encounter outcomes. *Journal of Personality and Social Psychology, 50,* 992–1003.

Folkman, S., Lazarus, R. S., Gruen, R. J., & DeLongis, A. (1986). Appraisal, coping, health status, and psychological symptoms. *Journal of Personality and Social Psychology, 50,* 571–579.

Frank, A. W. (1991). *At the will of the body: Reflections on illness.* Boston: Houghton Mifflin.

Grootenhuis, M. A., & Last, B. F. (2001). Children with cancer with different survival perspectives: Defensiveness, control strategies, and psychological adjustment. *Psychooncology, 10,* 305–314.

Hermans, H. J. M. (1996). Voicing the self: From information processing to dialogical interchange. *Psychological Bulletin, 1*(119), 31–50.

Hermans, H. J. M. (1999). Dialogical thinking and self-innovation. *Culture & Psychology, 5*(1), 67–87.

Hermans, H. J. M., & Kempen, H. J. G. (1993). *The dialogical self: Meaning as movement.* New York: Academic Press.

Kubler-Ross, E. (1969). *On death and dying.* New York: Touchstone.

Lazarus, R. S. (1966). *Psychological stress and the coping process.* New York: McGraw-Hill.

Lazarus, R. S., & Folkman, S. (1984). *Stress, appraisal, and coping.* New York: Springer.

Manne, S. L., Bakeman, R., Jacobsen, P. B., & Gorfinkle, K. (1992). Adult–child interaction during invasive medical procedures. *Health Psychology, 11,* 241–249.

McKeever, P., O'Neill, S., & Miller, K. (2002). Managing space and marking time: Mothering severely ill infants in hospital isolation. *Qualitative Health Research, 12,* 1020–1032.

Moos, R., & Tsu, V. (1977). The crisis of physical illness: An overview. In R. Moos (Ed.), *Coping with physical illness* (pp. 9–22). New York: Plenum.

Romy, E. (2002). Adjustment to childhood cancer: Parent–child coping and family functioning. *Dissertation Abstracts International. B: The Sciences and Engineering, 63*(1-B), 585.

Saiki-Craighill, S. (2002). The personal development of mothers of terminal cancer patients: How Japanese women change through the experience of caring for and losing their children to cancer. *Qualitative Health Research, 12,* 769–779.

Salmon, K., & Pereira, J. K. (2002). Predicting children's response to an invasive

medical investigation: The influence of effortful control and parent behavior. *Journal of Pediatric Psychology, 27,* 227–233.

Stein, R.E.K., & Jessop, D. J. (1982). A noncategorical approach to chronic
childhood illness. *Public Health Reports, 97,* 354–362.

Streisand, R., Rodrigue, J. R., Houck, C., Graham-Pole, J., & Berlant, N. (2000).
Parents of children undergoing bone marrow transplantation: Document-
ing stress and piloting a psychological intervention program. *Journal of
Pediatric Psychology, 25,* 331–337.

Thompson, R. J., Jr. (1985). Coping with stress of chronic childhood illness. In
A. N. O'Quinn (Ed.), *Management of chronic disorders of childhood* (pp.
11–41). Boston: G. K. Hall.

Thompson, R. J., Jr., & Gustafson, K. E. (1996). *Adaptation to chronic childhood illness.* Washington, DC: American Psychological Association.

Thomsen, A. H., Compas, B. E., Colletti, R. B., Stanger, C., Boyer, M. C., &
Konik, B. S. (2002). Parents report of coping stress responses in children
with recurrent abdominal pain. *Journal of Pediatric Psychology, 27,* 215–
226.

Waddell, C. (1983). *Faith, hope, and luck: A sociological study of children
growing up with a life-threatening illness.* Washington, DC: University
Press of America.

EDITORIAL COMMENTARY

I very much enjoyed this review of the problems confronting the evaluation of disease in the pediatric age group. I suspect that this is the
very hardest of all groups to study for many reasons.

I do think that there are two issues that need to be addressed. First,
does the presence of the researcher/interviewer change the actions of the
child and her family? For example, if the child has a good relationship
with the observer (as in this case), is it more likely that the child will
discuss concerns with the observer than with her family? If so, then the
conclusions may not represent what happens in a similar disease setting
when an observer is not present. Another complication of the presence
of the observer is that the younger sibling might become jealous of the
attention the interviewer gives to the "sick" patient and act out. The
observer might attribute this to some effect of the disease on the family,
whereas it may only be the result of an outside, not-normal influence on
the sibling. All such "*N* of 1" studies must be validated by other
examples.

My second concern is that the researcher continued to have a relationship with the child and her family long after the period of study was
concluded. While it would be very difficult to cut off all contact sud-

denly, there are serious questions about the ethics of continuing contact after the period of study is over. In the United States, such actions could lead to sanctions by the research-oversight committee of the investigator's institution. On the other hand, it does seem cruel to suddenly disappear from the patient's life.

—Kenneth L. Noller

Part IV

FROM THE DIALOGUE BETWEEN UNIVERSALS AND PARTICULARS TO NEW METHODOLOGY

Chapter 13

A MICROGENETIC DEVELOPMENTAL PERSPECTIVE ON STATISTICS AND MEASUREMENT

James D. Laird

A core idea in many stage theories of cognitive development is that increasing experience at a particular level of development or stage is both necessary and perhaps sufficient for movement to the next stage. Experience using the mode of thinking of one stage inevitably confronts the person with internal inconsistencies, inadequacies, or weaknesses in that stage, which are resolved by movement to the mode of thinking which constitutes the next stage. Particularly in coexistence stage theories, the stages seem to represent a collection of intellectual tools that are used for different tasks, where each succeeding stage represents a new, additional ability. This description of intellectual development appears to apply very precisely to two major features of measurement and statistical inference, as will be described below. Recognizing the developmental nature of measurement procedures and statistical tests may go some distance toward resolving what otherwise often seem to be ideological battles within psychology.

In psychological discussions, four different levels of measurement are commonly identified: Nominal, Ordinal, Interval, and Ratio. These four are ordered, from Nominal up to Ratio. These are described as levels because each succeeding level permits new, additional statistical manipulations, while the manipulations of the lower levels always remain possible, if inefficient and weak compared to the higher techniques.

Less obvious is the fact that these levels also appear in sequence as people approach new areas of investigation and measurement. This progression can be seen in individuals and in groups of investigators working on similar problems. At the beginning of study of any area, investigators are characteristically only able to identify the presence or absence of particular properties. That is, they use Nominal measurements. Indeed, at the earliest stages investigators simply describe the objects of their study, identifying what is present in the object but locating absence only tacitly in those objects not studied. For example, when Freud connected Anna O's problem in swallowing with a "forgotten" disgusting experience, he had no interest in describing people who did not have difficulty swallowing, although clearly we understand Anna and Freud's analysis by contrast with other people with different experiences (and different difficulties), including ourselves. Piaget's children who stopped reaching for an object as soon as it was covered were not compared, initially, with children who did not stop, although very shortly, Piaget was comparing the younger, nonreaching, with older children who did not stop their search.

Note that the currently popular "qualitative" approaches are exactly of this sort. That is, the basic intellectual task is to identify the presence of interesting properties in the objects of study. At the very beginnings of the work, describing the objects may be quite enough. With a little more sophistication, however, scholars begin to be explicit, noting that one object has property X, while another object does not. This is actually the point at which we can say that we are explicitly using Nominal measures, which are precisely the recognition of both the presence and the absence of some property, such as these children have "object permanence" while those children do not and these children are good students while those children are not.

At this point, we can also begin to see if some nominal qualities are associated with other nominal qualities. We can ask questions like, "are girls more likely to be in the good student group, or are boys?" and "are collectivist cultures more likely to have been influenced by Chinese thought?"

Once properties with interesting patterns of presence and absence have been identified and studied, inevitably the observer begins to notice that among those with the property present, some objects seem to have more than others. The result is the beginning of Ordinal measurements. Children can be ordered, from those who are bad students, to those who are somewhat better, to those who are the best. Ordinal measurement could not occur without Nominal, but it adds some new observations and information.

Once the objects are ordered by the amount of the critical property they have, we are likely to begin to notice that the differences among the objects are also orderable. That is, we can say that, although Ralph is a better student than Clarence, and Clarence is better than Harold, the difference between Ralph and Clarence is much greater than the difference between Clarence and Harold. Formalizing the ordering of the differences requires a bit more sophistication, but is the step that leads to Interval measurement. In the school-aptitude arena, this step was achieved by Binet, with what became the first intelligence test. Once again, Interval measurement adds something to the preceding level, Ordinal, but it could not exist if we did not first understand the Ordinal measures.

The final step, toward Ratio measurement, is rarely achieved in psychology. We might imagine that, at least to some extent, this is because we have not yet had sufficient experience with the Interval level to be able to identify meaningful zero points for our usual measures. But of course, in historically older sciences like Physics and Chemistry, Ratio measurement is routine. However, one does not have to look very far back in their histories to see Nominal and Ordinal measures.

In summary, it appears that the levels of measurement represent a developmental progression, in which development is dependent on extensive experience at lower levels to provide both the foundation and the motivation for the movement to higher levels. The same kind of experience-based progression can be seen within inferential statistics as well.

Of course, each level of measurement has its appropriate kind of inferential statistic, but that is not the progression I mean here. Rather, there is a progression within those levels toward increasing complexity, and what may be characterized as differentiation and perhaps integration.

This progression is most clearly seen among the interval level inferential statistics which are most familiar to psychologists. As an example, I will use my own research program, because the examples come most easily to hand. (Although I will present it historically, I have taken some liberties with the sequence to make the point clearer.) I began one strand of my research with the suspicion that William James was correct, and facial expressions caused emotional feelings, not the reverse. The first test of this idea was extremely simple: a group of participants was surreptitiously induced to adopt smiles and frowns and then asked how they felt, on a single pleasantness scale. The obvious statistical test was a t-test for repeated measures. There were two means, and the question was, simply, are they different? The answer was yes, and for a few subsequent studies the basic form was exactly the same, and the statistic of choice was a *t*-test. (Note that if I were uncertain about the interval status of my pleasantness scale, I could have used a non-parametric test like a Wilcoxon, but the basic comparison was still between just two groups.)

With a little more experience with my *t*-test design, it occurred to me that I should try some other facial expressions, so there was a study in which people adopted expressions of fear and sadness as well as anger and happiness. Now I had moved from a *t*-test to a one-way ANOVA. The move was a consequence of my increasing understanding of the role of facial expressions and confidence in the results of the first *t*-test design and analysis. The one-way ANOVA design embodied a more sophisticated understanding, namely, that there were more than two possible categories of the independent variable.

Almost simultaneously with this movement I noticed among my participants what appeared to be a pattern, that some people felt happier when smiling and angrier when frowning, and so forth, but others did not. That observation suggested there might be consistent individual differences in the effects of expressions. To explore this possibility, we conducted the same experiment with the same participants on two different days, separated by a week or two. The initial analysis was a two-way ANOVA, in which one factor was expression and the other was replication. We found that, as we predicted, the effects of expressions were significant both the first week and the second week. And most importantly, we found that people who were happier when smiling and angrier when frowning the first week showed the same effects on the second week. (This involved a correlation coefficient, which is part of another story that appears below.) Notice that we now had moved to a significantly more complex conception: that not only did expressions affect feelings, but they did so only for some people. Our statistical test had moved from a complex single dimension to two independent dimensions.

James had been quite clear that facial expressions were only one of the kinds of bodily response that led to emotional feelings. So in a series of studies we manipulated other kinds of behavior, like postures, patterns of eye gaze, and appearance. Since we had also determined that only some people responded to their expressions, we wanted to see if these differences in response were consistent across other behaviors. So, in these studies we would assign participants to groups who were, or were not, responsive to what we call "personal" cues. This was accomplished by running them through the expression manipulation task as a separate procedure before or after the other manipulations, of their postures, gaze, and so on. Again, our basic analytical procedure was a two-way ANOVA, with response to personal cues as one factor and the manipulation of postures or whatever as the other. At this point, the basic design was usually a two-way ANOVA, which represented a significant increase in sophistication over the one-way ANOVA, since it represented a much more complex idea: this affects that, but only depending on a third variable.

After a number of these sorts of studies, it occurred to us that in other research the effect of one's own behavior depended on whether or not one was aware of the nature and reasons for the behavior. So we did some studies in which the subjects were divided into those responsive to personal versus situational cues; part of each group performed some behavior, like an angry posture, while others did fearful postures or sad postures, and finally, half of all the participants were informed about the reasons for their behavior, while half were kept in the dark. In other words, a three-way ANOVA was made, which was yet another degree of complexity and sophistication.

Notice that the three-way ANOVA would have been inconceivable at the beginning of this research but became a rather routine further step after the experience and understanding that had been built up by considerable previous research. It seems to me that the progression from *t*-tests, to one-way ANOVAs, to two-way ANOVAs, and then to three-way ANOVAs is a developmental sequence, that is, the steps up involve increasingly complex integrations of ideas and methods, integrations that are possible only because of extensive experience with earlier, less complex systems.

Of course, the whole analysis of variance paradigm contains an obvious limitation: the independent variables are characteristically treated as nominal categories. When we design experiments, most commonly we choose to administer a treatment and compare it with no treatment, or we administer two or perhaps three amounts of a treatment. In other words, although we think of the dependent variable in more developed, Interval terms, in practice our independent variables have been until recently only Nominal. A more sophisticated approach would sample values of the independent variable in some way and would use statistical techniques that approached more correlational approaches. Such techniques do exist, but as yet psychology does not seem to have acquired sufficient experience to make them common.

The same kind of developmental progression can be seen in the correlational domain as well. Correlation examines the relationship between two interval level measures. Often we speak of correlation as a measure of how well we can predict one variable from knowledge of the other. It is a short step then to actually trying to do the prediction, using regression. Once we know how to predict our target variable from one or another single predictor variable, the next step is to try predicting using combinations of predictor variables, in multiple regression. Path analysis seems to be yet a further step in that direction, toward finding theoretically as well as statistically optimal patterns of prediction.

In summary, three major components of statistical methods seem to represent exactly the same kinds of microgenetic progressions, from early, very simple methods of measuring and analyzing to increasingly complex techniques. Each step represents a supplement to the preceding, increasing the precision of measurements and the intellectual complexity of the available inferences and interpretations. Most importantly, however, we cannot begin at the end. In the early stages of investigations, we must rely on less developed measures and inferential supports until we have mastered the basic beginnings.

A common metaphor for these developmental sequences is "structure." The analogy is to the construction of a building, where one begins at a low level, creating a foundation, and then builds up, adding story after story to the edifice. As in all structures, each succeeding level is built on the lower level and cannot proceed until the lower level is well constructed and stable. In science, these architectural principles all seem to fit the nature of measures and analytic techniques very closely.

So what? Yes, perhaps these arrays of methods and procedures are ordered in a kind of developmental sequence. Why should we care? The most important reason we should and do care is that this view makes clear that the various techniques and measures are not rivals, and none is intrinsically more valuable or superior to the others. Rather, each kind of technique is appropriate to a particular point in the development of our knowledge of a phenomenon. It is tempting, of course, to think that more developed measures and techniques are therefore better, but that belief violates the structural metaphor and, more importantly, the history of our discipline and of all science. A foundation may be the first thing constructed, and be a relatively crude structure of raw concrete, but without a good foundation the higher floors and their elegant woodwork could not be built; if we tried, the structure would collapse. So, at any one moment in a discipline or subdiscipline or research area, some kinds of measurement and some kinds of analytic techniques will be favored and others will seem either impossibly complex and abstract or naively simple. With the passage of time and increasing understanding of the phenomenon, however, all areas of inquiry seem to pass through all of the stages.

The current disagreements between those who favor qualitative, interpretative approaches and those who prefer formal experimental methods seem to me to be just this kind of difference. On the side of the qualitative approaches, they are almost by definition going to be more novel and also closer to our everyday understandings of the phenomena—both exciting and relevant. Their weakness is the strength of the formal experimental methods: that the kinds of inferences and conclusions we can draw about phenomena when we first begin to study them are not very different from our everyday understandings, and not very complex.

The developmental view suggests we all should be modest about our methods. If by chance our favored methods are relatively highly developed, it means only that we are working in an area where much preliminary work has already been done, in all likelihood by others who came before us. On the other hand, we should not dismiss the rarified, abstract measures and methods of other areas and claim special status for our homey, direct, and usually nominal measures, just because they are not too distant from everyday experience. If our measures are direct and familiar, then we probably have little prior work to build upon. But we can expect that, when we do, our measures will also become abstract and distant from everyday experience. And when they do, like all such measures, they will be justified by the amount of previous work that precedes and supports these techniques and measures. This movement toward increasing abstraction and distance is simply a development of precision and a recognition of the complexities of observation.

Some developmental theories assume that later stages replace the earlier, but a more reasonable view seems to be that they add new capacities without replacing the need for the abilities that are characteristic of the lower levels. Certainly that is true in measurement and statistics, where in the midst of complex-path analyses or four-way analyses of variance, we may find ourselves measuring nominally and performing Chi-square tests because they are most useful. Whatever the proper conception of development in other areas, in statistics and measurement, a coexistence model is clearly more appropriate.

In summary, a developmental conception of measurement and statistical inference suggests that all methodological imperialism is narrowly blinkered folly. We should all strive to have available for immediate use the widest possible array of intellectual tools. The old proverb says that to a man with a hammer, everything looks like a nail. The only way to do good carpentry is to own a saw, screwdriver, drill, square, and all the other tools of the trade, so that only nails look like nails.

EDITORIAL COMMENTARY

It is hard to find any fault with a chapter that includes such statements as, "So what?" and, "Why should we care?" and most importantly, " . . . all methodological imperialism is narrowly blinkered folly." The author certainly is not bothered by pride or jealousy. Perhaps the most important thought I took away from this piece is always to remember that all of our work is possible only because of those pioneers who went before us. AIDS was first a small series of cases (case report), then was linked to various high risk behaviors (cohort study), then to a virus (experimental design), and then became treatable (RCTs). Each breakthrough was possible only because of the information learned from the previous step. SARS is the latest "new" disease to begin this progression. I suspect that it will not be the last.

—Kenneth L. Noller

The developmental sequence in methodology outlined here allows us to situate any study—be it in psychology or medicine—in a framework of clearly specifiable assumptions about the phenomena, as those assumptions are reflected in the data. Laird's system makes it possible to detect whether the data—as constructed at any four levels of the scales—adequately represent the phenomena. In psychology, that adequacy of representation is rare because the consumeristic appropriation of standard statistical "packages" has widened the gap between statistical scientists and practitioners of statistics.

This chapter also clarifies the relations between the quantitative and qualitative trajectories in data construction. The qualitative trajectory is undoubtedly historically underdeveloped (in comparison with its quantitative counterpart). New versions of modern mathematics—qualitative mathematics—need to be imported into psychology and medicine.

The quantitative and qualitative data construction trajectories start from the same place: the nominal scale. The qualitative perspective moves from the detection of the "event" ("this phenomenon is X") to its systemic analysis. The first decision made is whether X is unitary or multiple (i.e., contains a duality {X and non-X}, or even a multiplicity). Secondly, a decision is made about the kinds of relationships posited for the multiple-parts system: for instance, are X and non-X in mutually "harmonious" or "complementary" relations, or is their "tension" between them? In case of the latter, is that "tension" equilibrational (meaning it will be reduced over time, and may vanish) or disequilibrational (i.e., it is escalating). If the "tension" is disequilibrational, will it lead to emergence of new form of the "event" or to the demolishing of the old one?

—Jaan Valsiner

Chapter 14

DECISION MAKING WITH INCOMPLETE INFORMATION: SYSTEMIC AND NONSYSTEMIC WAYS OF THINKING IN PSYCHOLOGY AND MEDICINE

Aaro Toomela

For making decisions, relevant information should be gathered and organized in the process of thinking. In general, the quality of a decision depends on both whether all of the important information was taken into account (while ignoring irrelevant information) and how that information is organized. In this chapter, I explore the individual differences in the ways that humans organize knowledge and actions, such as thinking (Vygotsky, 1926). Before addressing that issue, an analysis of the information that is available for any decision is necessary.

All decisions are made on the basis of incomplete information. According to General System Theory, reality can be understood as a hierarchy of organized wholes referred to as "systems." All real systems are open; they can interact with other systems (von Bertalanffy, 1968). It is important to recognize that a system has a potential for many more interactions than are realized at any given moment. There is always a possibility that a system upon which a particular decision is made unexpectedly interacts with some other system. In principle, all systems involved in interactions with other systems change qualitatively. Thus, when a particular system we make a decision about interacts with another system, its properties change. Sometimes such interactions can be predicted and taken into account in decision making. But the number of possible interactions of any given system is theoretically unlimited. Thus, there can never be a guarantee that all possible interactions are taken into consideration. Obviously, the more complex the system being considered, the more possibilities for unexpected factors changing the situation.

The most complex system we know—a human being—is the "object of decisions" in medicine. Correspondingly, decisions made in medicine should *a priori* be considered as being based on incomplete information. In medicine, there is too much information available for any single person. Even if all medical information were available to a doctor, the best decision would still not be guaranteed as the available information may be organized in many ways, some of which are more effective for making a good decision than others.

DIFFERENT WAYS OF THINKING

Much of the psychology of thinking is concerned with the question of whether a problem is solved, or how many different problems a person can solve. The cultural historical school of psychology has dealt with the question of how problems are solved and which ways of thinking are available for individuals as well as for cultures at different stages of development (Vygotsky, 1929–1930/1960, 1934/1996; Vygotsky & Luria, 1930/1994, 1994). Vygotsky differentiated the nonsymbolic or "natural" line of thinking development and the semiotically mediated or "cultural" line of thinking development (Vygotsky, 1934/1996; Toomela, 1996a). Both natural and cultural lines of development can be differentiated into substages. In this context, only semiotically mediated cultural mental operations are relevant because practically all decisions made in medicine are based on symbolic operations. According to Vygotsky's theory, three kinds of symbolic operations can be differentiated, and each is connected to a special set of symbols as tools for mental operations,. The three kinds of symbols are "syncretic," "complex," and "scientific" symbols, and they are given in developmental order. Nevertheless, development of every next level of symbols does not replace the earlier level. Rather, the development of symbols is content specific, and, correspondingly, the human mind is heterogeneous, that is, different kinds of symbols and different kinds of mental operations exist in parallel in the human mind (Vygotsky, 1934/1996; Vygotsky & Luria, 1930/1994).

Vygotsky's theory remained incomplete, perhaps due to his early death, and is still incomplete. Probably the most important missing part in his theory is the lack of understanding exactly how development takes place or why novel stages emerge in the course of development. Analysis of recent developmental data together with proposed specific mechanisms of development allows differentiation between five stages of development of symbol meaning. In developmental order, these are syncretic symbols, prototypical symbols, exemplar symbols, symbols for classically defined categories, and systemic symbols (Toomela, 2003a). Depending on which set of symbols is used for a particular thought operation, there are five ways of thinking that correspond to the kind of symbols used. Different kinds of symbols and corresponding ways of thinking can be described as follows.[1]

First, a *syncretic symbol* is fully constrained by the situation where the symbol is used. Depending on idiosyncratic personal experience, the same symbol form has different meanings in different contexts. It is not possible to understand what actually was meant by a symbol without knowing the external context where a syncretic symbol was used. *Prototypical symbols* refer to prototypical categories (Mervis & Rosch, 1981; Rosch, 1978) of objects available to the senses and to the object-specific properties of objects. *Exemplar symbols* refer to exemplar-based categories of objects, properties of objects, and relationships between objects.

Thinking that uses these three kinds of symbols has two common characteristics. First, all information encoded with such symbols is acquired from personal experience. Abstract and theoretical knowledge can be understood only in the limits of personal experiences. For example, "anti-inflammatory drug" would mean, "a drug, after taking, which makes pain and swelling go away." Correspondingly, thinking leads to decisions that can be understood as extensions of personal experiences. Persons thinking with such symbols would not differentiate theoretical and experiential arguments in making decisions. Theory-based suggestions by a doctor to use a certain drug would have the same or even lower value than suggestions of a neighbor who has personal experience with using some "red tablet" in an "exactly similar situation." Second, symbols refer at these stages of symbol-meaning development to categories that have fuzzy boundaries. In thinking, decisions are always context-dependent. There are no context-independent rules that could apply in every possible real-life situation.

Symbols for *classically defined categories* refer to explicitly defined categories with sharp boundaries. Whereas at earlier stages of symbol-meaning development, there is no awareness why certain objects belong to the same category, at this stage every category can be defined by individually necessary and collectively sufficient attributes. At this stage, it becomes possible to represent abstract theoretical nonpersonal knowledge. Inferences with such symbols are made in a coherent formal–logical way. Thinking is not tied to immediate personal context and can be (but not necessarily is) entirely independent from direct sensory experiences. As the category boundaries referred to by this kind of symbols are sharp, inferences made with such symbols are of the all-or-none type. The answers to questions are either correct or incorrect; there is no context-dependence of answers unless the characteristics of the context are explicitly taken into account in formulating an inference.

Finally, *systemic symbols* refer to categories of all types with an explicit definition of context where, and in what case, a particular categorization should be used. With the development of different abstract theoretical frames of reference in a system of symbols, a qualitatively novel way of categorization is acquired. It becomes possible to categorize things and phenomena into more than one category. With the explicit definition of in what sense and in what system of relationships a thing or phenomenon is classified, the same thing can appear simultaneously in different, mutually exclusive categories, even in the classical sense. Therefore, once again, decisions become context-dependent. At the first three levels of symbol-meaning development, both symbol meaning and decisions made with such symbols are also context-dependent. At the systemic symbol stage, in turn, a person actively represents context in decisions. In the course of development from one stage to the next, the amount of information explicitly taken into account increases both quantitatively and qualitatively. At every next stage, novel information that was not encoded at the previous stage will be represented with symbols. More efficient decisions can be made with more information. Later stages of symbol-meaning development allow better decision making.

The last systemic symbol stage of development allows all relevant information to be taken into account. Systemic thinking is theoretically the most effective way of organizing knowledge for making decisions.

DIFFERENT WAYS OF THINKING IN MEDICINE

Thinking in modern medicine is basically systemic. Doctors are taught to consider all relevant information before making a decision. For example, a surgeon planning an operation on a tumor will gather information not only about tumors but also about the patient. (Limiting information only to the tumor would be an example of thinking with symbols for classically defined categories that do not encode contextual information.)

In theory, all decisions in medicine could be based on systemic thinking. However, it is not necessarily so in real life. The first reason for limitation in thinking is that systemic thinking requires explicit definitions of all relevant information both about the system (human being, in this case) and about context. As I mentioned before, a single physician cannot know all of the information available in medicine. Consequently, doctors who are experts in one field, and who can make systemic decisions in their field of expertise, would not be able to make decisions of similar quality in other fields of medicine where they are not experts. The second reason is as important. Doctors cannot be certain of the effectiveness of any specific treatment for a particular patient. For example, it is up to the patient whether and how the doctor's orders are followed. The patient usually is not an expert in medicine, may not understand what the doctor has said, and may misinterpret the doctor's orders. In other words, patients may use a less efficient way for making their own decisions based on limited information.

In order to facilitate understanding of these decision-making processes, I will next analyze several actual cases that I have observed in my role as a child neurologist.

Case 1: An Allergic Child

I was once approached by a neighbor. The woman asked for my advice regarding a rash on her five-year-old grandson. My first look at the child led me to a question, "Does the boy have an allergy?" The woman answered yes and recited a long list of foods that the boy was not supposed to eat. One of these was chocolate, and my neighbor admitted that she had given her grandson both chocolate and other sweets, despite the recommendation of the child's physician not to do so. When I asked, "Why did you give him chocolate?" her answer was very interesting. "I gave it to him because he wanted it." Unfortunately, the grandmother was not satisfied with my suggestion that she not give the boy foods to which he is allergic.

Case 1 is an example of thinking with persona; experience-based symbols. The symbols that were used by the grandmother were of the "exemplar" kind. Justification for her actions were limited to her personal experience and the influence of the specific context ("My grandson wanted chocolate"). For the grandmother, there was no difference between abstract theoretical and personal experience-based concrete arguments for making her decision. Here was a situation where the behavior of the grandmother undermined the allergist's treatment plan. The grandmother did what she thought was best for the boy. The exaggeration of the allergy was caused not solely by less sophisticated thinking and an inappropriate decision by the grandmother, but also by both the allergist and I not taking into account the role of the grandmother in the treatment plan.

Case 2: A Child with Phenylketonuria

Phenylketonuria is a genetic disorder that prevents the normal use of some foods because of a deficiency in the enzyme, phenylalanine hydroxylase. Without this enzyme, phenylalanine accumulates in the blood and body tissues. Chronically high levels of phenylalanine can cause significant brain damage. The condition can be treated with a high degree of success if diagnosed shortly after birth and the child adheres to a low phenylalanine diet.

The parents of a seven-year-old boy who had been diagnosed with phenylketonuria by my colleague six years earlier came to our child neurology department for treatment of mental retardation the parents discovered when the boy had to go to school. The parents had not visited our department since the diagnosis and a treatment plan were made six years previously. The consequences of not following the treatment plan had been explained to the parents.

The parents admitted that they had not followed the diet. The reason why they ignored the treatment plan was that the grandmother of the boy told them that "Doctors know nothing" and children must eat meat and chocolate to grow strong. The parents, both teachers with a university degree, did what the grandmother told them to do. By the time they finally returned to the clinic irreversible brain damage was present.

Case 2 is another example of thinking with "exemplar" symbols. The parents did not differentiate between theoretically supported reasoning and experience-based reasoning. For them, the grandmother was a stronger authority than the doctor. What makes the case unusual is that both parents were highly educated. One would expect individuals with a university degree to be rational in their decisions. What we observe here is a case of heterogeneity of thinking. To graduate from a university, a person must think at least with symbols for classically defined categories in the field of studies.[2] But it does not follow that such thinking be used for every act of thinking. In the field of knowledge where the parents were not experts—medicine—they supported their decisions on less-developed thinking.

Case 3: Prognosis of a Child with Cerebral Palsy

Cerebral palsy is a collective term for syndromes related to a disorder of movement and posture caused by a nonprogressive lesion or injury that affects the immature brain. Once a mother of a three-year-old boy with cerebral palsy asked me whether her son would be able to walk independently in the future. I told the mother that recent studies had shown that nine children out of ten with a similar form and level of motor disability as her son were not able to walk independently at the age of seven. I also explained that I could not predict which one child out of ten would be able to walk. Two or three years later I accidentally met the mother together with her son. The mother pointed to her son and announced proudly, "He can walk! You told me he would never walk independently." I did not remind her of my actual statement. Only later did I realize that her misunderstanding might have been partly my fault. The mother probably did not understand what I told her. Apparently, in the emotionally charged setting of the medical office, she equated "almost all" to "all" in her mind. Such "all-or-none" thinking is based on thinking with symbols for classically defined categories. I had not taken into account the possibility that my conditional statement could be understood as an absolute yes or no. Inadvertently, I had created a dangerous situation. The mother might have given up hope and not tried to treat the child, and the potential of the child would have been remained unrealized. Fortunately, the mother worked hard with the child and he eventually learned to walk.

Case 4: Usage of Antibiotics by General Practitioners

The medical literature strongly supports the fact that antibiotics should be used with care. Many doctors, however, tend to use antibiotics as "anti-inflammatory" drugs, despite that fact that they have been taught that antibiotics affect only microbes and reduce inflammation only when inflammation is caused by these pathogens. Misuse of antibiotics is a very serious problem because it leads to an increase in the number of microbes that are resistant to any antibiotic (see World Health Organization home page at http://www.who.int/csr/drugresist/en/ for problems related to drug resistance).

How can it be that highly educated medical professionals do not understand the damage they are creating by misusing antibiotics? It is possible, again, that this is a case of inappropriate thinking in symbols for classically defined categories instead of systemic symbols. It seems that doctors who misuse antibiotics follow an all-or-none path in thinking: Microbes cause inflammation → microbes can be suppressed by antibiotics → antibiotics can be used for treating inflammation. Therefore, antibiotics are anti-inflammatory drugs. In such thinking, contextual factors (the reasons why an inflammation develops) are not taken into account in the final decision. It is plausible that the problem lies in an inappropriate way of thinking because all doctors should have been taught in their training (they definitely all are in Estonia) that an antibiotic is really an anti-*microbial,* not an anti-inflammatory. Thus, it is not a question of not having the necessary information but rather, how the information is processed.

Case 5: Drugs—Brand-Name or Generic?

Due to economic considerations, there is pressure in Estonia for physicians to use "generic" rather than "brand-name" drugs. A brand-name drug is produced by the corporation that first synthesized it. Generic drugs are chemically equivalent but are manufactured by another company and are often much less expensive.

I utilized an anonymous questionnaire to obtain data from 29 General Practitioners concerning their use of brand-name and generic drugs. I found that many of the doctors clearly made their decisions systemically. They did not routinely use either generic or brand-name medications but rather took into account many different aspects of patient care. These included such things as the specific disease, the type of drug, the financial status of the patient, and published data. However, some doctors gave answers of the "exemplar" or "classical categories" type. For example, some physicians suggested that the only reason they preferred a brand-name drug is because "I believe it is better," "I had *personal* experience that generic drugs do not work," "it feels right," "because of tradition and personal experience" (italics mine). These are examples of thinking with symbols for exemplars. The answers "because it is a brand-name" or "a brand-name is more trustworthy" are probably examples of thinking with symbols for classically defined categories because the decision is made on the basis of belonging to the classically defined category, brand-name, and that category is thought by some to carry attributes such as "innovative" and "scientifically proven."

SUMMARY: WHEN CAN THINKING ABOUT THINKING BE USEFUL?

The five cases discussed above demonstrate that the way of thinking might be an important factor in making medical decisions in two general situations. First, as exemplified by Cases 1, 2, and 3, it is important to understand that patients or their caretakers may completely misunderstand or ignore the directions given by a physician. The doctor, more experienced and educated in medicine, should be responsible for communicating in a way that can be understood by the patient or caretaker. It is not only a lack of relevant background information that is missing in patients. It is also a way of thinking. If a patient thinks with exemplar symbols, then the doctor's message should be most effective if it is illustrated by real-life examples instead of an unintelligible scientific explanation. If a patient thinks dominantly with symbols for classically defined categories, it should be the function of the doctor to define explicitly in what context, and under what circumstances, the therapy will work. The main limitation of thinking with symbols for classically defined categories is an inability to define explicitly the context where a particular principle or order is effective.

Cases 4 and 5 demonstrate that even doctors do not always support their decisions with systemic symbols. Patients may both lack sufficient relevant information and have a relatively less developed way of thinking, and thus make inappropriate decisions. In doctors, the main problem is related to how the extensive information they possess is used. In general, the field of medicine is organized as with systemic thought. Therefore, it should be expected that doctors make decisions systemically in many cases. What should be taken seriously is the possibility that a specific doctor's thinking can be heterogeneous, even in medicine. That should not be surprising, considering the complexity and sophistication of modern medicine. Being an expert and able to think systemically in one field does not make a person a systemic thinker in every other field of knowledge.

CAN THINKING ABOUT THINKING REALLY BE USEFUL?

Considering the possibility that doctors sometimes make ineffective decisions not because of a lack of information but because of an inability to think systemically in a particular field, it might be possible that insight into one's own thinking may make a difference. I conducted a small field experiment of this hypothesis. I presented a two-hour lecture about different kinds of thinking and how to apply systemic thinking for deciding whether to prescribe a brand-name or a generic drug to a patient. I used the same sample of 29 General Practitioners described in Case 5. They were asked which kind of a drug and why they prescribed it for a given medical situation at the beginning of the lecture. At the end of the lecture the same question was asked again together with the question, "Do you now think differently about how to prescribe a drug after listening to this lecture?" Many doctors reported that they did not change their mind and that they already thought systemically before. However, nine of the doctors said now they would think differently and that they would consider many factors, including how patients may think, how things should be explained to a patient, and how they think by themselves when making a decision. These results do not demonstrate that their way of thinking actually changed. Nevertheless, these data suggest that it might be useful for a medical doctor to be aware of personal thinking processes.

ACKNOWLEDGMENT

This research was supported by the Estonian Science Foundation, Grant No. 5388.

NOTES

1. It should be mentioned that a "symbol" is every object that refers to something else; that has a meaning that is shared by humans; and that can be used either in ways or in contexts that are different from ways or contexts of utilization of symbol referents (Toomela, 1996b). Words are the most common symbols.

2. Symbol-meaning development at the last two stages of development, symbols for classically defined categories and systemic symbols, develop in formal schooling (Cole, 1995; Luria, 1974; Toomela, 2003b). Education at the university level consists of knowledge that can be encoded practically only by these two last kinds of symbols.

REFERENCES

Cole, M. (1995). Culture and cognitive development: From cross-cultural research to creating systems of cultural mediation. *Culture and Psychology, 1,* 25–54.

Luria, A. R. (1974). *Ob istoricheskom razvitii poznavatel'nykh processov. Eksperimental'no-psikhologicheskoje issledovanije.* Moscow: Nauka.

Mervis, C. B., & Rosch, E. (1981). Categorization of natural objects. *Annual Review of Psychology, 32,* 89–115.

Rosch, E. (1978). Principles of categorization. In E. Rosch, & B. B. Lloyd (Eds.), *Cognition and categorization* (pp. 27–48). Hillsdale, NJ: Erlbaum.

Toomela, A. (1996a). How culture transforms mind: A process of internalization. *Culture and Psychology, 2*(3), 285–305.

Toomela, A. (1996b). What characterizes language that can be internalized: A reply to Tomasello. *Culture and Psychology, 2*(3), 319–322.

Toomela, A. (2003a). Culture as a semiosphere: On the role of culture in culture-individual relationship. In I. E. Josephs & J. Valsiner (Eds.), *Dialogicality in development* (pp. 129–163). Westport, CT: Praeger.

Toomela, A. (2003b). Development of symbol meaning and the emergence of the semiotically mediated mind. In A. Toomela (Ed.), *Cultural guidance in the development of the human mind* (pp. 163–209). Westport, CT: Ablex.

von Bertalanffy, L. (1968). *General systems theory. Foundations, development, applications.* New York: George Braziller.

Vygotsky, L. S. (1926). *Pedagogicheskaja psikhologija. Kratkii kurs.* Moscow: Rabotnik Prosveschenija.

Vygotsky, L. S. (1960). Povedenie zhivotnykh i cheloveka. In L. S. Vygotsky (Ed.), *Razvitie vyshikh psikhicheskikh funkcii. Iz neopublikovannykh trudov.* (pp. 395–457). Moscow: Izdatel'stvo Akademii Pedagogicheskih Nauk. (Originally written in 1929–1930)

Vygotsky, L. S. (1996). *Myshlenije i rech.* [Thinking and speech]. Moscow: Labirint. (Originally published in 1934)

Vygotsky, L. S., & Luria, A. (1994). Tool and symbol in child development. In R. van der Veer, & J. Valsiner (Eds.), *The Vygotsky reader* (pp. 99–174). Oxford, England: Blackwell. (Originally written in 1930)

Vygotsky, L. S., & Luria, A. R. (1930). *Etjudy po istorii povedenija. Obezjana. Primitiv. Rebjonok.* Moscow-Leningrad: Gosudarstvennoje Izdatel'stvo.

EDITORIAL COMMENTARY

This chapter on "thinking about thinking" is remarkable for the ease with which it breaches the gap between the theory of thinking and the actual practice of thinking. The examples make clear (at least somewhat so to those like me who have no formal background in this area) that it is possible to understand better why some patients do not follow medical directions if one examines the type of thought process that the patient employed in making the decision to ignore the medical advice. Many times, we clinicians fail to present important treatment plans to patients in ways that will lead to their acceptance. Often we are told that we "used words I didn't understand" by the "noncompliant" patient. This chapter suggests that it is not always just the complexity of the words but rather the context or life experience of the patient that is equally or more important.

—Kenneth L. Noller

Chapter 15

LISTENING IS NOT HEARING: IMPROVING DIAGNOSTIC ACCURACY IN CARDIAC AUSCULTATION

Jeremy Golding, David Stevens, and Roger Bibace

The title of this chapter was chosen to emphasize that listening should not be equated to hearing and to draw the reader's attention to several complex and controversial issues. These are related to inferences drawn by an interpreter from sensory evidence. A major source of past and ongoing controversy is the relative importance of the brain compared to the sense organ with regard to selective attention and perception. Many disciplines, including physics, neuroscience, and psychology, have contributed to this diversity of opinion. One important and consistently divisive issue concerns the roles of *sequence* and *simultaneity* in the assumptions and interpretations made by investigators.

These factors are necessarily involved in many medical procedures, such as colposcopy, mammography, and otoscopy. Auscultation is an even more complicated example because the sounds change over a very short duration of time. Simultaneity is also involved in auscultation because there are concurrent sounds. The sounds are related to one another with respect to saliency much as a figure is to its background. In addition, the sequence of sounds in auscultation requires an accurate assessment of the silent intervals between two sounds. For example, lub-dub/lub-dub is different from lub . . . dub/lub . . . dub. Inferences from such intervals are related to categories such as rhythm that are diagnostically meaningful.

This chapter does not examine distal and controversial scientific issues implicated in auscultation. The focus is on the improvement of diagnostic accuracy, a goal that may be facilitated by the technique of multidimensional scaling as a means to differentiate listening from hearing.

Feinstein (1967) believes that there is a three-step process leading from acquisition of clinical sensory input to the production of diagnostic output:

> The main contemporary impediment to detailed specificity in physical examination is the failure of many clinicians to distinguish the three different intellectual disciplines—description, designation, and diagnosis—used for the whole procedure. In description, the clinician gives an account of the sensation, substance or phenomenon that he has actually observed. In designation, he gives a name or classification to the observed entity. In diagnosis, he indicates the anatomic or other abnormality that is responsible for the observed entity. (p. 322)

The resulting diagnosis includes within its substance an anatomic or pathophysiologic depiction of the abnormality, usually with implications for treatment and prognosis. As an example, consider a young woman presenting with the acute onset of redness, swelling, and warmth of both wrists and multiple finger joints (*description*). The experienced clinician *designates* the findings as a symmetric arthritis and *diagnoses* probable rheumatoid arthritis. Another patient exhibits red, warm, and itchy skin bumps on the trunk. An inexperienced medical student may not yet possess the ability to translate the product of sensory experience (*description*) into the appropriate *designation,* urticaria (hives), so the correct *diagnosis* (allergic reaction) is missed.

The purpose of medical school is to teach the student the correct *designation* based on an astute (scientific) *description,* enabling the clinician to establish a correct *diagnosis.* Feinstein argues that both students and more experienced clinicians sometimes fail to separate accurately and sequence the three cognitive components—description, designation, and diagnosis involved in the diagnostic procedure, resulting in a loss of precision in observation: as examples of this are "I heard pneumonia at the left lung base" and "the exam showed arthritis." Explicit criteria are needed to convert description to designation and then again to convert designation to diagnosis.

Of the various physical examination maneuvers learned by students in medical school, cardiac auscultation is among the most complex to learn to perform. A group of sounds together characterizing a given murmur may, in fact, represent several different pathologic entities. That is, although a murmur may be highly suggestive of a specific diagnosis, it is rarely completely diagnostic. A given pathology may even produce different sounds in the same individual over time, related to the position in which the patient is examined, or to the progression of disease. Finally, the listener is challenged by the potential presence of more than one condition—multiple sounds and murmurs occurring simultaneously. According to Feinstein (1967),

> The clinician's attention to cause instead of character of the noise, or to its conversion from auditory to visual entity, is detrimental not only to the auscultory skill that distinguishes the clinician, but also to the characteristics that distinguish a noise. Like proteins, white cells, and other entities observed in the laboratory, cardiac noises have many different properties. The noises can vary in location; radiation; loudness; pitch; time of onset and of cessation in relation to other noises; duration; thoracic site of maximal loudness; response of loudness and of other properties to procedures that induce changes in heart rate, in blood flow, in pulmonary aeration, and in position of the heart during its own cycle and during excursions of diaphragm or of thoracic wall. Like the phenomena assessed in the laboratory, each of these acoustic properties has its own range of variation, and each property can often vary independently of changes in the others. All the properties must be observed for the noises to be described reproducibly; their range of variation in healthy people must be established to determine physiologic boundaries of normal; and each individual abnormality must be identified in criteria for designating the noise and for diagnosing its pathologic significance. Some of these acoustic properties are distorted or unperceived by existing inanimate devices and are better assessed by a human ear and mind. (p. 324)

Recent studies have reported that doctors' auscultation skills are inadequate (Gaskin, Owens, Talner, Sanders, & Li, 2000; Mangione, 2001; Mangione & Nieman, 1997). These studies focus solely on outcomes. In such studies, the results quantify the number of accurate and inaccurate responses or choices made by participants. The psychological processes that the research participants relied upon to arrive at their diagnostic or treatment decisions/answers are ignored. Therefore, what caused the error was not the concern of these studies. By focusing exclusively on outcomes, these studies have identified a problem in the current system of medical education, but they shed little light on the causes of declining proficiency in cardiac auscultation. Presumably, the decline is due to many factors but is most directly related to a declining prevalence of abnormal heart murmurs in the general population, and to the reliance upon the imaging technique of echocardiography to make the definitive diagnosis. Thus, learners have less practice with true abnormal murmurs and no longer have to commit themselves to a diagnosis based solely on auscultation. As a result, students of cardiac auscultation do not learn to identify the sources of their diagnostic errors—specifically, the psycho-sensory processes that result in an erroneous diagnosis. Recall that accurate description and designation are the two steps in the sequence that lead to diagnosis.

From a psychological perspective, the sounds or noises noted in auscultation correspond to Feinstein's *description*. Although presumably all auscultators are presented with the same auditory data, individuals can differ in the translational process from *description* to *designation*. On the one hand, people often do not use the same terms to represent the same sensory experiences, and on the other hand, the sensory experiences themselves differ from person to person.

Even describing the volume of a heart sound is problematic. Standard textbooks of physical diagnosis describe the loudness of heart murmurs on an imprecise 1 to 6 scale. The inter-observer and intra-observer reliability of such a system is highly questionable.

We again wish to stress that "listening" is not "hearing." Hearing implies a dimension of cognitive processing of auditory input. The problem is yet more complex. Even at the strictly sensory level, it is uncertain whether groups of physicians can discriminate the sounds that correspond to all of the various commonly defined categories and subcategories of heart sounds. Certainly, physicians in training gradually acquire some ability to discriminate and then to render the descriptions of sounds in a common parlance. Unfortunately, the common parlance does not contain within it absolute, neat definitions. In dermatology, a raised "bump" greater than one centimeter in size is no longer a "papule" but rather is termed a "plaque." In lung auscultation, however, there is no uniform definition of "rhonchus" as compared to "wheeze," nor is there a clear distinction between a "snap" and a "click" in cardiac auscultation. Even more confusing, basic terms acquire vague modifiers like "sonorous," "dry," "wet," "musical," and "machine-like." Furthermore, we assume that there will be differences in the ability of individual physicians to discriminate (and hence designate) sounds and that there will also be intra-individual variation.

How can one represent a sound to make it most amenable to recognition and interpretation? We used the analytical tool called *multidimensional scaling* (methodology to be described) to attempt to identify separable domains of described sound and to model spatially the contribution of specific sound descriptors to the pathophysiologic process that results in a given murmur. Multidimensional scaling provides a parsimonious description of the basis for the perceived differences (and similarities) among sounds and thus of what is relevant to accurate designation and diagnosis between given pairs of sounds. Thus, multidimensional scaling potentially provides a tool that will allow learners to focus upon, for example, a specific auditory dimension as part of the larger process of analyzing a particular heart sound. To be able to focus upon a limited number of perceptual dimensions that, taken together, provide an accurate diagnosis should facilitate learning and enhance accuracy. Multidimensional scaling permits one to identify describable dimensions relevant to a sound acquired through auscultation and thus to determine the feedback to be given to a particular physician regarding the auditory dimensions which hinder/facilitate best personal practices for that physician.

For many physicians, the process of making precise a cardiac diagnosis through auscultation has been influenced dramatically by the development of echocardiography, a method of ultrasonographic visualization of the working heart and its valves. Even the most experienced cardiologists now use echocardiography to diagnose murmurs, almost regardless of what the clinical examination reveals. Technology has allowed atrophy of skills previously acquired and explains the diminishing emphasis on the physical examination in medical education.

The student of cardiac auscultation, particularly the student destined for primary care, has a simpler and yet more complex task than heart specialists. S/he must be able to distill the auscultation of a great many possible heart sounds into one of two categories: "normal" and "abnormal." Most patients seen by a cardiologist are highly selected compared with the general population of patients in that they usually have some form of heart disease and many have abnormal heart sounds. Unlike cardiologists, primary-care clinicians may listen to many tens of patients' hearts before encountering an abnormality. The low prevalence of abnormal heart sounds in this unselected group of patients means that primary-care physicians obtain less practice listening to abnormal heart sounds than cardiologists. Nonetheless, the clinician must maintain a high degree of accuracy in selecting the abnormal murmur from common physiologic ("normal") murmurs, because it is not possible to obtain an echocardiogram on everyone with a murmur due to cost, availability, and other issues. Precise diagnosis of murmurs and sounds using only the stethoscope is no longer the goal of practice in the developed world. Rather, clinicians must learn to identify those sounds or combinations of sounds that suggest the probability of an abnormal heart. Although they deal with probabilities, clinicians must still arrive at a concrete decision—to proceed to echocardiogram or not.

Students learn about the formation of normal noises during valve closure, ventricular filling, turbulent currents, and other events of the cardiac cycle; about the formation of abnormal noises by damaged valves, congenital defects, or other lesions; and about the analysis of the visual portraits given to the noises by phonocardiographic tracings. The student is often not taught, however, to develop and standardize himself as a competent instrument for recognizing, describing, designating, and interpreting the noise as a noise.

MULTIDIMENSIONAL SCALING

The absence of a standardized method of representing complex sounds (e.g., murmurs) makes giving specific constructive feedback to a learner difficult. Multidimensional scaling (MDS) is a useful approach to this problem. MDS generates a spatial model, for example, a map, for which the distances between items represent the extent to which the items are judged to be similar. The model is a type of cluster analysis, as those items judged to be similar are grouped together. The model also suggests the number of and nature of the factors that underlie the perception and organization of items. The number of orthogonal dimensions of the model suggests the number of perceptual factors, and they need not be identical. If three dimensions are needed to model well the relationships, then three or more factors are likely to underlie the judgments of the items. Because the psychological factors need not be, and indeed rarely are, independent, there could be more factors than spatial dimensions. The qualities and characteristics of the items that define the factors are suggested by the relationships between individual items in the model. For example, if, as is likely, one's perception of tones is based on the pitch, timbre, and loudness of the tone, MDS would be expected to produce a three-dimensional model, with relationships (distances) between the points representing tones corresponding to differences in pitch, timbre, and loudness. If the investigator did not previously know the bases of tone perception, the analysis would be revealing. As another example, Kruskal and Wish (1978) analyzed perceived similarities between Morse code symbols using MDS. A two-dimensional model accounted for the similarity judgments very well, suggesting that two factors underlie the perception of Morse code. Inspection of the model, specifically, the placement of codes in space, showed the factors to be related to the quality of the components (dots *vs.* dashes), and to the number of components of the signal (one dot or dash to as many as five dots and/or dashes). MDS can be applied to any sensory system. Stevens and Lawless (1981) compared groups of people of about 20, 40, and 60 years of age in flavor perception. Four-dimensional solutions modeled flavor perception well for the three groups, but they differed in the characteristics defining the dimensions. For the two youngest groups, hedonics was important, which was closely related to sweetness for the youngest group only. The intensity of flavor was important for the oldest group, for which sweetness was not a factor.

The data for MDS are ratings of similarity (or figures that reflect similarity, such as frequency of confusion of items, or correlation coefficients for pairs of items). Typically, no guidelines are given to the participants on which to base the judgments; the participants must generate their own criteria for similarity, thus avoiding the biases involved when the investigator provides them. A set of judgments, usually the mean judgments of a group of participants, is then analyzed by the selected MDS algorithm.

Most MDS analyses are nonmetric, that is, the set of ratings is considered to be one of ordinal values (having valid rank order) but not necessarily one of equally spaced intervals. Accordingly, MDS programs transform the ratings to rank orders. Using an iterative scheme, the points are moved about in space until the spatial relations best fit the relations in the data. The goodness of fit is measured by stress, an index that runs from zero (an error-free fit) to 1.0 (complete lack of fit). MDS analyses can be performed utilizing up to $n - 1$ spatial dimensions, but to avoid solutions based on chance, the number of dimensions should be limited to one fourth or fewer of the number of items, and solutions should be selected with both stress and parsimony in mind.

IDENTIFYING ESSENTIAL QUALITIES OF HEART SOUNDS

In order to develop a valid classification scheme of heart sounds, the qualities of the sounds actually utilized by listeners in making judgments had to be identified. We explored the use of MDS for that purpose in the pilot study reported here. Once the identification of principal perceptual dimensions underlying the discrimination of murmurs is accomplished, one can determine a process that might be useful to an individual and to groups in learning to distinguish normal from abnormal heart sounds. It is important to remember that in this study, our focus on helping learners to develop the ability to perform a "normal versus abnormal" categorization influenced the selection of the heart sounds we studied.

Research Participants

Participants were three attending physicians, six second-year residents, four first-year residents, and four third-year medical students ($N = 17$) working on the Family Medicine Inpatient Service, a clinical teaching service of UMass Medical School and the UMass Memorial Health Care system.

Stimuli

Recordings of the sounds of eight abnormal and four normal hearts were selected from those provided by Harvey and Canfield (1997). These are described in the list below.

Heart murmurs evaluated in the pilot study

Physiologic murmurs (4)

Pathologic murmurs

- Midsystolic click–murmur
- Congenital ventriculoseptal defect
- Mitral regurgitation
- Aortic insufficiency
- Mitral regurgitation/atrial fibrillation
- Mitral valve prolapse
- Mitral regurgitation
- Aortic stenosis

Sets of 22 pairs of sounds were randomly drawn without replacement from the full set of 132 possible pairs of sounds. Each participant was given one 22-pair set. Thus, with 17 participants, two-and-5/6 full sets of all possible pairs were utilized.

Procedure

A 22-pair set of sounds was presented to each participant with the instruction to rate the similarity of the sounds on a 100-point scale. They were shown a linear scale, which ranged from 1, labeled "not at all similar—as dissimilar as two recordings could be," to 100, labeled "essentially identical—as similar was two recordings could be." On hearing each pair of sounds, its similarity rating was given to the experimenter. After making all similarity ratings, each participant was asked to list the characteristics used to make the similarity judgments. The twelve recordings were then played again, and each was rated on the characteristics listed by the participant using a scale ranging from 1, representing "unimportant," to 100, representing "a very important characteristic."

Finally, several days later, the twelve recordings were played to the participants and they were asked to judge them to be indicative of normal or abnormal heart murmurs. One attending physician, one second-year resident, and one first-year resident did not participate in this phase.

Results

The mean similarity judgments for each pair of sounds were analyzed by MINISSA, a nonmetric multidimensional scaling program (StatSoft, Inc., 2001). A two-dimensional solution was chosen as the best, parsimonious solution (Stress = .107). This level of stress indicates a reasonably good representation of the data. The model is shown in Figure 15.1.

Multiple regression was employed to identify relations between the model and characteristics utilized by the participants. The quality judgments made for each sound were regressed against the sounds' coordinates. The normalized multiple regression coefficients for the model's coordinates for the characteristics are cosines for vectors representing the relation between the spatial model and the characteristics (Kruskal & Wish, 1978, pp. 36–39). Table 15.1 shows the characteristics most often used and the values of the *multiple r*s and *p*s. Two dimensions, roughly orthogonal, were identified. The first is defined by the auditory characteristics described as systolic onset, blow, holosystolic onset, and harshness; the second, by regularity of rhythm. Vectors for these characteristics are shown in Figure 15.1. The remaining characteristics did not relate sufficiently well to the coordinates of the model to be useful in interpretation (*r* values < .75, *p* values < .01).

Discussion of Results

Based on the MDS and multiple regression, we found that the residents' similarity judgments of the heart sounds were based on two perceptual dimensions or factors. The first was defined by the qualities of holosystolic (lasting throughout the contraction), texture (coarseness of

Figure 15.1

MDS model, with regression lines (vectors) for the reported characteristics of harshness, systolic onset, blowing, holosystolic onset, and rhythm.

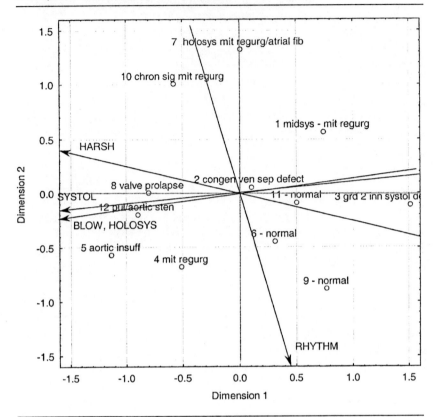

the murmur), and timing with regard to the first and second heart sounds (systolic/diastolic). The second was defined by regular rhythm. Interestingly, rhythm, which is not specifically useful diagnostically, was an important factor in the judgments. This may have been an artifact due to the fact that, in the murmurs chosen for study, all samples of irregular rhythms also had loud, markedly abnormal murmurs. The angles separating the vectors representing the sound qualities described as systolic/diastolic, holosystolic, and texture are small, indicating that the vectors are closely related. That means that they share one and perhaps more auditory characteristics that are critical to the discrimination of murmurs. The search for the auditory cues critical to clinical discrimination is now narrowed to those related to that vector. The participants also utilized

Table 15.1
Auditory Characteristics Most Often Reported and Relationship to MDS Model

Characteristic	Multiple r	p	Normalized coefficient (cosine)
Characteristics highly related to MDS model			
Harshness	.861	.002	-.965
Systolic onset	.829	.005	-.994
Blowing	.823	.006	-.990
Holosystolic	.773	.017	-.991
Regular rhythm	.791	.012	.275
Characteristics not highly related to MDS model			
Click	.695	.051	
Diastolic onset	.564	.177	
Crescendo	.474	.318	
Extra beats	.269	.714	
Decrescendo	.044	.991	

rhythm, a characteristic not well related to abnormality, and that could well have been an important cause of misidentification.

Limitations

There are several limitations to this study. First, the size of the sample of both the numbers of learners analyzing the sounds and the number of somewhat similar heart sounds on which they were tested was small. Second, the majority of those tested were inexperienced (resident physicians). Third, the sound quality of the tape itself was poor, even after reduction of static using a filter. Fourth, the tape did not designate the anatomic landmark at which each sound was acquired (for example, right and left upper sternal borders, left lower sternal border, apex).

SUMMARY AND CONCLUSIONS

It is the sensory interface between doctor and patient during physical examination that results in the description and designation of physical findings. The gap between the underlying words as labels (categories) for describing what a physician sees through the microscope, colposcope, or otoscope and what a physician hears through a stethoscope has yet to be addressed. The bridge between "looking" and "seeing" may be assessed through nonverbal representations. That is, the learner can be asked to represent pictorially what s/he will be looking for. In teaching auscultation, however, it is far more difficult to have learners reproduce the sounds for which they should be listening using oral mimicry. The complexity of simultaneously occurring, multiply pitched sounds of differing durations presents a barrier to the learner trying to reproduce them. Although some physicians may say "I know it when I hear it," it is difficult to establish that they really do "know it" (except by testing). For this reason, multidimensional scaling may, by identifying the auditory dimensions principally used in discrimination, make it easier for physicians to focus on the particular auditory cues that are distinctive for the auditory dimensions underlying discrimination.

Our study suggests that *designation* may be enhanced by the use of multidimensional scaling. The method may be extended to teach concepts other than the categorization of murmurs as "normal" or "abnormal." For example, the duration of a murmur relative to the first and second heart sounds may be highly informative. It is known that the length of some murmurs, and not necessarily the loudness of those murmurs, may relate to the presence of more advanced and clinically significant disease. Learners can be taught this fact and then be asked to focus upon and recognize the relative duration of a murmur.

Electronic stethoscopes hold promise for improving education in cardiac auscultation. These devices amplify sound, filter extraneous noise, and allow multiple listeners to share an identical auscultory experience in real time or digitally slowed to allow emphasis on specific characteristics of a sound or sounds. We propose further studies to test whether these devices improve accuracy of diagnosis compared with traditional stethoscopes and to test whether electronic augmentation will facilitate the description/designation process of learners and experienced clinicians alike. The capability of "beaming" the recorded sound also allows for the possibility of creating a visual representation of the sounds on a computer, allowing learners to correlate auditory input with a more standard "picture."

In conclusion, the use of the stethoscope to make cardiac diagnoses remains a core component of the physical examination. Having learners systematically describe what they hear and then rate the magnitude and relative contributions of each component to the overall sound may help them to improve diagnostic accuracy and, possibly, allow them to make more specific diagnoses. The results of these studies may lead to a new approach to teaching the skill of audition.

REFERENCES

Feinstein, A. R. (1967). *Clinical judgment.* Huntington, NY: Krieger.

Gaskin, P., Owens, S. E., Talner, N. S., Sanders, S. P., & Li, N. S. (2000). Clinical auscultation skills in pediatric residents. *Pediatrics, 105*(6), 1184–1187.

Harvey, W. P., & Canfield, D. (1997). *Clinical auscultation of the cardiovascular system.* Fairfield, NJ: Laennec Publishing.

Kruskal, J. B., & Wish, M. (1978). *Multidimensional scaling.* Beverly Hills, CA: Sage.

Mangione, S. (2001). Cardiac auscultatory skills of physicians-in-training: A comparison of three English-speaking countries. *American Journal of Medicine, 110*(3), 210–216.

Mangione, S., & Nieman, L. (1997). Cardiac auscultatory skills of internal medicine and family practice trainees: A comparison of diagnostic proficiency. *Journal of the American Medical Association, 278*(9), 717–722.

StatSoft, Inc. (2001). STATISTICA for Windows. Tulsa, OK: StatSoft, Inc.

Stevens, D., & Lawless, H. (1981). Age-related changes in flavor perception. *Appetite, 2,* 127–136.

Part V

FROM QUESTIONS TO ANSWERS: THE MICROCOSM OF PARTICIPATION

Chapter 16

RECRUITMENT AND RETENTION: EXAMINING PROCESS IN RESEARCH RELATIONSHIPS

Mary Alston Kerllenevich, Kenneth L. Noller,
and Roger Bibace

When reviewing the ways that researchers and practitioners interact with patients and make decisions regarding their care, the relationship between doctor–practitioner and patient–client is considered essential. Yet relationships in the research process are rarely given much attention, despite the importance of research outcomes in making medical decisions. The relationship between researcher and participant is essential to the research process, from the time the individual hears about the study to the last follow-up, but there are few reflections on how the relationship process may have affected research outcomes, except in the case when a mistake has been made.

As part of this lack of focus on relationships in general, even logistical elements of research procedures are omitted in the literature. Recruitment and retention are essential elements of success in any research endeavor, yet there has been little attention paid to that work. Rather, researchers are left to sort out these issues on their own, with only a few basic ethical guidelines to follow. Depending on the methodology and epistemologies subscribed to by the research project, the value and nature of recruitment and retention strategies may change dramatically. Quantitative research, in particular, treats each individual as one subset of a homogenous whole and often fails to take advantage of the human aspects of participants. Researchers cannot control the participation of human subjects as they can laboratory animals, and yet they set up research designs as if the method is similar. Large numbers of participants are recruited to "cancel out" the variance related to individual differences. Qualitative research seeks the participation of the whole person as a sentient being and often involves extensive communication between researcher and participant. The focus on relationships in qualitative research has had little influence on the lack of focus on relationships in quantitative research.

Once participants are recruited for a prospective project, their retention is essential for the success of the study. When attrition occurs, it introduces error in several ways. First, participant loss may be influenced by the experimental condition, which affects the internal validity of the study. Second, the reason a participant leaves is often unknown, and therefore, the external validity of the study may be undermined (Harway, 1984). Attrition leads to more than mere statistical problems: it means that a great deal of time, energy, money, and potential knowledge has been lost.

The importance of attrition prevention seemingly presents a catch-22 in medical ethics. High-quality medical research is necessary to improve the standard of care, yet we are asking participants to assume a personal risk and to allow that risk to escalate without withdrawing from the study.

The management of risk in medical research occurs through the application of national ethical guidelines that guarantee basic rights for all research participants. However, these guidelines may be difficult to apply to individuals in particular circumstances, may interfere with the relationship between the researcher and the study participant, and may compromise the quality of the results.

FROM "OWNERSHIP" TO ETHICS OF KNOWLEDGE SHARING

We propose that these ethical guidelines will be improved in quality and implementation if researchers begin to focus on the process of research as well as the outcome. We believe that it is imperative to discuss the interpersonal processes and relationships inherent in research practices. However, this idea often meets with resistance. One insight into this resistance came out of the two workshops that were the foundation of this book. Some of the researchers became antagonized and uneasy when presented with the suggestion that participants should be involved as true research partners. One senior researcher said that he would not invite feedback from his research participants because it was *his* project, and he *owned* the data.

This resistance to considering relationships in research may occasionally transfer to the doctor–patient relationship. In another discussion at our workshops, we debated the value of prescribing an antibiotic for a specific patient who did not need but wanted it to the problem of reduced effectiveness of antibiotics (over-prescription of antibiotics contributes to bacterial resistance). In a brainstorming session about values and practicalities, no one thought to ask what our hypothetical patient thought about the situation. What were *her* values and needs? Would we come up with different "best practices" for patients with different values—and do we seek out those values when making decisions about personal care? All of these questions stem from one basic issue: how do we interact with participants in the research and treatment processes, and how much do we allow the participant to have a say in what transpires?

WHAT ARE THE RISKS OF MEDICAL RESEARCH AND HOW DO PARTICIPANTS BECOME INVOLVED?

The first step in relating to the research participant as an individual involves examining the risks of the research. Most experimental research in medicine or psychology asks the participant to engage in a situation knowing that they are being manipulated. The effect of this manipulation on each individual cannot be known or controlled by even the most stringent human research boards.[1] Even more participatory research techniques, designed to level the playing field between researcher and participant, introduce the possibility that the questions asked will have an effect on the individual participants. Even at the most micro level of the research process, principles of quantum mechanics tell us that nothing can be observed without being affected in some way.

Added to the risk of the experimental design are the risks introduced by the societies in which the research takes place. In today's information-rich society, it is increasingly risky for individuals to release personal information. In other cultures, the individual may become vulnerable to risks that depend on the values in that society. For example, in some countries it may be dangerous to sign documents, which may later be falsified by the state and used as evidence in political trials. Research participants are vulnerable when they enter into research relationships. They are releasing control over some information or other aspect of their lives to strangers. Considering the risks, one wonders why individuals would choose to participate in research.

Participants actually fall into two different risk groups. The first have a high level of health (or other) risk and hope participation will reduce that risk in some way. The second group has a low level of risk to start and assumes low levels of risk in participation. Recruitment strategies often play on the needs or desires of these two groups.

Individuals in the first group may be at high risk for various reasons, all of which might be lowered by research participation. Some individuals may be ill, in which the case study offers the hope of finding a cure. Some individuals may be poor and are promised money in return for the inconvenience of participating. Regardless of the potential benefit to the participant, there is a certain degree of risk present in any research project (see chapter 3 herein by Heyman on risk escalators).

The incentives provided to participants have come under ethical scrutiny. For example, too much money may induce some individuals to assume inappropriately high levels of risk (Tishler & Bartholomae, 2002). Nonpaid research participants questioned about compensation thought that compensation for time and travel could be appropriate but felt that too much compensation would be coercive (Russell, Moralejo, & Burgess, 2000). The amount of monetary compensation offered is reviewed by human research boards, but what is "chump change" to one may be wealth to another.

Individuals in the second group participate in research for different reasons. Some feel a spirit of volunteerism and want to contribute to science in a practical way. In this case, the pitch made by the researcher about the value of the research is a big incentive. In other cases, participants volunteer because they have a personal interest in finding a cure or solution to the problem being studied—some close friend or family member is at risk and they hope that the contribution of their time will make a difference. The views of these participants may be reflected by those reported in post-research interviews where participants noted that they were happy with the amount of information they were given about the research, and that researchers should not be afraid of giving too much information. This information gave them motivation to continue, and was used to spark the interest of others, who were referred to the research by word of mouth (van Gelderen, Savelkoul, van Dokkum, & Meulenbelt, 1993). The individuals in this second group often have the education to be able to evaluate the information being given to them by the researchers. In addition, their risk is so low that they can consciously consent to raising their risk in the hopes of lowering the risks of others.

Regardless of the initial group, at the start of the research, once the individual consents to participate, a process is begun in which the participant's risk status is changed. It may be increased or decreased, but the individual cannot be aware whether they are on an upward or downward risk escalator. Instead, individuals are entering into relationships with researchers they hope they can trust, and the researcher has to be their only guide through the research process. They may know only what they are told. In the past, this setup occasionally has led to the abuse of the disempowered. The most famous example in America is the Tuskegee Syphilis Study, in which African Americans were not given an effective treatment for a life-threatening disease. Since that time, guidelines for research ethics have greatly improved. However, the most effective will always be the ethics of the individual researcher and the legitimacy of the researcher–research participant relationship.

It is thus important for us to consider the heuristics and values of research relationships and how those relationships influence the process of our decision making in both research and practice.

USING RELATIONSHIPS TO MANAGE THE RISKS OF RESEARCH

Research relationships can be used as guides in managing the amount of risk an individual is allowed to take on and the amount of risk a researcher proposes. True relationships invite reciprocity, with participants becoming partners in the research endeavor, regardless of their assigned role. However, researchers have very different ideas of what "reciprocity" in research relationships entails. Some interpret it to be only remuneration or some other form of payback. Others interpret reciprocity as allowing the participant to be involved in reciprocal interactions within the research process, the "I'll ask my questions and you ask yours, because both of our perspectives are important in finding a solution" version of reciprocity. The essential difference lies in the amount of ownership or control over the nature and type of reciprocity the researcher will allow. Focusing on research relationships may include some of the former version of reciprocity, but to make partners out of participants, the latter version is required.

To focus on the relationship as a guide through risk management allows for two important safeguards: a focus on process over outcomes and on flexibility over rigidity. When these are maintained, the nature of research ethics subtly changes. Informed consent becomes a process rather than a piece of paper, and more distancing strategies can be engaged to maintain participation. To explore these possibilities, each relational framework will be taken up in turn, and case vignettes will be used to exemplify the processes involved in research relationships.

Participatory Models: Focusing on Process over Outcome

There ,are new models of research that attempt to shift the focus of investigations from hypothesis-confirming outcomes to learning through mutual exploration. In the social sciences, new research methods attempt to diminish the power differential between the researcher and the participant. The researcher is no longer presented as the expert who manipulates the experimental situation but as an investigator who seeks to learn from the experiences of the participants. This model of research embraces individuality (otherwise known as variability) rather than seeking to treat everyone in the exact same manner:

> Researchers using (participatory) methods reject the possibility of a neutral stance; thus, rather than attempting to eliminate bias, we explore and embrace the role of subjectivity in psychological research. Embedded in these methods is the importance of trust and relationship between researcher and participants; such work is anchored by the goals of understanding the experiences of others and working collaboratively with them to generate social change and knowledge that is useful to the participants as well as to psychologists. (Tolman & Brydon-Miller, 2001, p. 5)

Participatory models have gained a modicum of popularity in some fields of psychology, but have made few inroads on transforming other power-laden relationships outside of the research context. One model that seeks to manage relationships in research, clinic, and education situations is the partnership model of Bibace, Dillon, and Dowds (1999). As the name suggests, the physician/therapist and the participant/patient/student seek to have a relationship characterized by partnership rather than expert status. In this model, the researcher does not start out as an expert attempting to prove a hypothesis and nothing else. Rather, the participant and researcher jointly determine what the questions will be, and both individuals answer each other's questions. The participant also provides the researcher with feedback about the conclusions drawn from the study. Throughout the process the researcher asks, "Is what I heard you say, what you wanted me to hear?" Through the triadic process of questions, answers, and feedback, the researcher attempts to appreciate the participant's experiences and knowledge regarding the research question. While in traditional research the participant is only a "subject" to be observed, in the partnership model every aspect of the researcher–participant interaction is a process of mutual discovery.

This process serves as a guide for other interactions in that it is a two-way process of action and reaction. It makes apparent the implicit property of relationships whereby the actions of one person have an effect on the other, and vice versa. The participant is thus explicitly given power in the research process and has increased capability to manage the amount of risk taken on. By embracing the subjectivity involved in the research process, the researcher becomes aware of how the process of the interactions is influencing the outcome of the study and, therefore, the likelihood that the participant, or even groups of participants, will continue.

The subjectivity involved in "data collection" is explored by Günther (1998), as she recounts the various experiences she had interviewing families from different cultures. She found that what was foreign to some groups was commonplace to others. For example, to gain access to a Saudi Arabian group for recruitment, her husband had to call the contact person because an unchaperoned woman cannot speak to a man. When it came time for interviews, she was not allowed to use a tape recorder because "the voice contains the soul" and therefore cannot be registered. In contrast, when she entered one Japanese house and asked if she could tape record, the mother replied that this was not a problem. In fact, *she* had been tape recording since Günther arrived.

Understanding these cultural differences can have a large impact on the retention of participants. While Günther had some ideas about the appropriate manners in the cultures she was working with, she could not know how all of her behaviors would affect the research participants. She had to invite participants' feedback regarding the process of the research. Focusing on the relationship, and being certain that it is one where each person's values, questions, and responses are really heard, can subsume the need to focus on retention strategies.

Flexibility versus Rigidity in Carrying Out Research

The other shift in focus inherent in relationships is that of flexibility over rigidity when interacting with research participants. This was explained in detail to us when we investigated the overwhelming success of five research coordinators in a longitudinal epidemiological study with an overwhelming 77 percent retention rate over 25 years (Kerllenevich, Noller, Bibace, Strohsnitter, & Titus, 2003). The research coordinators appeared to be successful because they were highly flexible in meeting the needs of participants while still following the research protocols with a high degree of standardization. Their primary means of success appeared to be due to forming relationships with their participants over the years. These relationships invited more symmetrical interactions and a

SCIENCE AND MEDICINE IN DIALOGUE

high degree of versatility in order to react genuinely to the research participants. In order to retain participants, they had focused on their individuality and avoided the extreme rigidity suggested in the highly standardized protocols.

Without knowing it, these highly skilled research coordinators used two principles only recently reported in the literature on retention and research ethics. In particular, they turned informed consent into a process that lasted over 25 years and was constantly being renegotiated. In addition, they engaged in processes of psychological distancing with the research participants and principle investigators involved in the research. Examples of their actions, and other vignettes taken from the literature, illustrate how relationships can serve as a guide without charting out the most ethical response. They also illustrate how even the most brief and goal-oriented interactions can be guided by a relationship-focused framework.

Informed Consent as a Process

Recent literature on healthcare ethics suggests that it is not sufficient to make informed consent a one-step procedure in research (or treatment). Rather, it needs to be a process that continues throughout the research. Kuczewski and McCruden (2001) argue that values are not private aspects of the individual but are formed and interpreted during interpersonal relationships and transactions. Thus, they maintain that ethical research procedures, such as informed consent, should be process-oriented rather than preset through the use of forms or protocols:

> This interpersonal determination of values is a kind of "discovery" or "mutual self-discovery." Values are not just arbitrarily chosen but have something of a life of their own as part of the narrative of people involved. These narratives will, of course, be influenced and shaped by many forces including the culture of the persons involved. As a result, informed consent must necessarily be a process that involves the social group. (p. 36)

The Kuczewkski and McCruden argument is based on the idea that as the self emerges through narrative, so values emerge within a relationship rather than outside of it. Ethics are thus considered relative to research participants. While we create protocols based on a notion of universal ethics, research coordinators must integrate these ethical procedures with the values and cultures encountered in the participants.

While this model may at first seem to be a minefield of contradiction between universals and particulars, the process-oriented approach allows for flexibility to meet individual needs. Kuczewski and McCruden call for a conversational approach to informed consent, where the values and wishes of those giving consent are respected. This means that, similar to the partnership model, during the course of research clinicians must seek to understand not only what patients say, but also what they mean. The focus is on understanding one another rather than completing a required transaction. Such understanding has reciprocal effects. Both the researcher and research participant run the risk of being changed by their interactions. Kuczewski and McCruden argue that in these types of interactions between clinician and patient, the clinician will come to better understand herself. "Informed consent is, ideally, not just a process of discovery by the patient; it also holds the promise of being one of mutual self-discovery" (p. 45). We believe that this process of understanding does not just take place in the clinician–patient relationship but may be present anytime a researcher interacts with a research participant (Bibace et al., 1999; Kerllenevich et al., 2003).

The research coordinators we interviewed illustrated the transformation of informed consent into a process. They stressed the "information" aspect of informed consent. They tried their best to explain the research procedures in every interaction and to answer honestly any question put to them by the research participants. They then separated participants' access to information from their participation in the study. Even if a participant refused to remain in the study, the research coordinator would ask if the individual would like to continue receiving the newsletter, or, sometimes, if the participant would be interested in receiving upcoming articles published on the results of the study.

Second, rather than attempting to manipulate individuals into staying in the research project, the research coordinators reported that they sometimes appeared to invite refusals by reminding hesitant participants that they could withdraw from the study at any time. Some research coordinators also reminded participants of their right to skip a question as a preface to highly personal interview questions, and reported that they felt people were actually more likely to answer the questions when they knew they did not have to. Finally, refusals, just like consent, were not a one-step or final process for these research coordinators. When they encountered a refusal to continue participation, they asked if the research participant would like to be contacted in the future and reminded participants that they could always participate in the future.

These negotiations were always done within the rubric of a relationship. As part of the nature of the research, the research coordinators had been interviewing participants about their health concerns over a period of years. After listening to the concerns of the research participants over time, various participants began to stand out from the crowd and became memorable individuals to the research coordinators, despite having never met them. Each research coordinator had examples of real relationships formed with participants, where the participants acted as if the relationship were symmetrical. In one case, a research participant who had trouble conceiving sent a picture of her newborn baby to the research coordinator with a note saying she had finally had a child. Not only was the research coordinator touched, but the next time she was scheduled to call that participant she began the conversation with "What a beautiful baby boy!" (Kerllenevich et al., 2003).

You cannot create these situations without a genuine research relationship. While it is often suggested in the retention literature that researchers send out birthday or holiday cards in order to appear warm or thoughtful, the chances that such contrived strategies will be successful are slim. Participants regularly receive such messages from their banks and other local businesses. They feel as genuine as any other computer-generated mass-mailing. The attributes of a genuine relationship cannot be replaced by such strategies, just as ethical guidelines cannot replace the safeguards built into genuine, symmetrical, reciprocal partnerships. If a researcher or physician is going to be the guide through the continued process of informed consent, it cannot be done without making sure that each person, doctor and patient, genuinely understands the other. To accomplish this goal, the researcher must necessarily put an emphasis on flexibility rather than use universal protocols that appear not only rigid but contrived.

Dynamic Distancing

Maintaining flexibility in responding to the needs of participants may require a process of dynamic distancing, whereby appropriate solutions to individual problems may be found. The process of psychological distancing (Sigel, 2002) involves moving one's thoughts away from the concrete circumstances of people's lives to an evaluation of the task at hand. This process is essential to the retention of research participants. Research coordinators have to be able to understand a concrete problem, keep their emotions in check while remaining empathic, understand the obstacles to continued participation, evaluate possible solutions, and choose one solution that will overcome the obstacle without compromising the design of the study. The process of dynamic distancing entails moving from one's own perspective to that of the research participant, then returning to their own perspective as managers of the research process, and perhaps even joining in the perspective of the principal investigator, and then moving back again.

Hong (1998) refers to this process when discussing Günther's report of her experiences working with participants from various cultures:

> It appeared to me that researchers who successfully surmounted their obstacles were the ones who utilized themselves not only as scientific researchers, but also as research instruments. In this capacity, they facilitated the problem-solving process by actively immersing themselves in the problem, collecting a variety of local perspectives on the difficulty, and participating in its locally appropriate, culturally sensitive resolution by modifying procedures or materials as needed. (p. 82)

To find such locally appropriate solutions, the research coordinator has to be aware of global standards as well as individual needs and to be able to engage in dynamic distancing such that the seeming duality of purpose between research relationships with both participant and principle investigator can be clarified.

In many cases, the research coordinators we interviewed reported a need to see events and procedures from their participants' perspectives. For example, when explaining the protection of the confidentiality of research files, one research coordinator reported that she thought of every way that she might be uncomfortable with her private information being located in a file under someone else's guard. She then worked out an explanation that entailed the location of the file cabinets, the number of locks between a prying person and the file in question, and the number of people who had access to the key. This answer was not part of the protocol suggested by the principal investigator, who did not generally interact with participants and engage with them from their perspective. In another poignant example, a research coordinator described calling a participant shortly after her only daughter had passed away. When she finally reached the participant on the phone, the research coordinator began the conversation with her condolences and a long conversation ensued about the daughter. At the end of the call, the research coordinator asked if the participant would like to complete the interview this year. The participant replied that this year was not going to work out but to give her a call next year. Indeed, the following year the questionnaire was completed (Kerllenevich et al., 2003). The coordinator did not ask about the participant's daughter as a strategy for retention—she asked because the woman was a real person to her, even if she only spoke to her on the phone once every few years.

Research coordinators may take into account the needs of the individual participant that are not necessarily pertinent to the framework of the study (such as needs for privacy, confidentiality, convenience, etc.). Good and Schuler (1997) describe vignettes from a clinical trial where nurses carried out the research. In one example, a patient was in a lot of pain and found it inconvenient to participate in the study. The nurses recognized that this individual was an assertive, self-directed businessman who was used to having much more control than that offered by the hospital setting. Their retention strategies included recognizing his autonomous background and allowing him to share in the decision-making process regarding treatment times. This small inconvenience to the research nurse made a big difference to the research participant and could not have been devised without dynamic distancing between the two individuals' points of view.

In other cases, the research coordinator must step back to the view of the principle investigator or other research manager. For example, the research coordinators reported that if it felt like a participant might not stick it out through an entire interview, they would jump to the most important questions first, so that the answers to the main questions in the study could be obtained. In other cases, when coordinators sensed that participants were growing weary of responding to annual and often monotonous interviews, they would sometimes share their own excitement over the research with the participants. This too, was not a contrived strategy. These research coordinators were sincerely excited about the research they were doing and were willing to share their own perspective with participants when it was appropriate.

It also may be necessary for principal investigators to engage in dynamic distancing with research coordinators as well as participants. Good and Schuler (1997) report a vignette where one research nurse was too pushy and was causing higher attrition rates. As a retention strategy, the nurse was retrained in research protocols and the rights of human subjects as well as encouraging her to share any job-related concerns. The appropriateness of research relationships between research coordinators and principle investigators is important to the success of research.

The process of dynamic distancing is thus a natural part of most human relationships but serves as an important safeguard for participants' risks as well as a tool in increasing retention. Such dynamic distancing necessarily promotes a focus on flexibility rather than rigidity and on process over outcome. Yet the outcome is undoubtedly improved.

Implications for Physicians and Researchers

Managing the universals and particulars in research and clinical ethics can be challenging. It is difficult to know what it means to be "at risk" for a patient or participant. Physicians and researchers play a special role in navigating through a minefield of potential risks—the information and counsel they provide helps guide individuals through their choices to embark on upward or downward risk elevators.

We argue that the best way to manage risk, ethics, and the assumed role of counselor is to maintain a relationship-based approach toward working with individuals in multiple settings. The idea of forming relationships with patients may at first seem ridiculous, yet the research coordinators we interviewed were able to achieve this goal in semi-annual interviews. If we focus more on a triadic process of reaction—one of questions, answers, and feedback—rather than on the outcome of the interaction, our goals of interactions may actually be better met. Relationships in medical settings may be formed in a *pars pro toto* process that fits with brief interactions. Introducing one quality of a reciprocal relationship may automatically call other aspects into play.

To take on such a process of interaction is not simple. It first requires giving up the role of expert for the role of helper. Patients cannot be allowed to follow the advice of physicians or to enroll in clinical trials without first being allowed into the process of medical decision making by invitation from the physician. Informed consent as a process is designed to do just that by enhancing the ability of the individual to make his or her own healthcare decisions. But the information that will empower individuals to be involved in these decisions will come from their physicians, and thus it is the physician who must make the invitation. The quality of the invitation is thus essential to the quality of care.

If a relationship emerges, the essential ethical issues will naturally come into play. The values of each individual will be manifest, and the rights of all will be better protected. In addition, the process of dynamic distancing under the rubric of a relationship will afford the flexibility to find multiple means to meet the ultimate goals of the partnership. This relationship-oriented approach affects medical decision making by influencing the quality of interactions where risks are managed and treatment courses are begun.

However, despite the many advantages of relating to participants as fully cognizant human individuals who should be constantly informed in order to make decisions about their bodies and their lives, many researchers react to the ideas proposed in this chapter as impractical or

idealistic. This may be the typical interaction from independent professionals when asked to seek the input of others. In organizational consulting, the invitation to form teams is often considered an effort to
"make nice." Yet forming relationships in the research process is infi-
nitely more than "making nice" with participants. It is learning to treat
them with respect. It invites a dialogue into the formerly isolated
thought-process of the researcher. We believe that this input, when sought
out, will prove to be invaluable to both researchers and participants and
will ultimately provide feedback that will improve the quality of our
research endeavors and the medical decisions they influence.

NOTE

1. All research on human subjects within the United States must be approved
by human research boards or internal review boards (IRBs) before a researcher
is allowed to collect data on the research project. This is done to ensure that
national ethical guidelines are being met and to protect the safety and rights of
the individual as well as limit institutional liability for the potential dangers of
research participation.

REFERENCES

Bibace, R., Dillon, J., & Dowds, B. N. (Eds.). (1999). Partnerships in research,
    clinical and education settings. Stamford, CT: Ablex.
Good, M., & Schuler, L. (1997). Subject retention in a controlled clinical trial.
    Journal of Advanced Nursing, 26, 351–355.
Günther, I. (1998). Contacting subjects: The untold story. *Culture & Psychology,*
    4(1), 65–74.
Harway, M. (1984). Some practical suggestions for minimizing subject attrition.
    In S. A. Mednick, M. Harway, & K. M. Finello (Eds.), *Handbook of
    longitudinal retention: Vol. I* (pp. 133–137). New York: Praeger.
Hong, G. (1998). Logistics and researchers as legitimate tools for 'doing' inter-
    cultural research: A rejoinder to Günther. *Culture & Psychology, 4*(1),
    81–90.
Kerllenevich, M. A., Noller, K., Bibace, R., Strohsnitter, W., & Titus, L. (2003).
    Implementing research protocols: The pros and cons of flexibility. Un-
    published paper.
Kuczewski, M., & McCruden, J. (2001). Informed consent: Does it take a vil-
    lage? The problem of culture and truth telling. *Cambridge Quarterly of
    Healthcare Ethics, 10,* 34–46.
Russell, M. L., Moralejo, D. G., & Burgess, E. D. (2000). Paying research
    subjects: participants' perspectives. *Journal of Medical Ethics, 26,* 126–
    130.

Sigel, I. (2002). The psychological distancing model: A study of the socialization of cognition. *Culture & Psychology, 8*(2), 189–214.

Tolman, D. L., & Brydon-Miller, M. (2001). *From subjects to subjectivities: A handbook of interpretive and participatory methods.* New York: New York University Press.

Tishler, C. L., & Bartholomae, S. (2002). The recruitment of normal healthy volunteers: A review of the literature on the use of financial incentives. *Journal of Clinical Pharmacology, 42,* 365–375.

van Gelderen, C. E., Savelkoul, T. J., van Dokkum, W., & Meulenbelt, J. (1993). Motives and perception of healthy volunteers who participate in experiments. *European Journal of Clinical Pharmacology, 45*(1), 15–21.

Chapter 17

WHAT HAPPENS WHEN A RESEARCHER ASKS A QUESTION?

Jaan Valsiner, Roger Bibace, and Talia LaPushin

The key issue is whether the respondent's understanding of the question matches what the researcher had in mind: Is the attitude object, or the behavior, that the respondent identifies as the referent of the question the one that the researcher intended? Does the respondent's understanding tap the same facet of the issue and the same evaluative dimension?

N. Schwartz, "Self-reports: How the Questions Shape the Answers"

Traditionally, psychology has done much to persuade itself that answers to the questions raised by Schwartz are in the affirmative—with the possible exception of delusional or strategic answering patterns. However, at best, such a state of affairs of full intersubjectivity between researcher and the research participant can at most be an ideal toward which the communication partners strive (Rommetveit, 1992). It follows from the basics of interpersonal communication that the match between the question asked (by the communicator) is not the same as the question answered (by the recipient). Instead, the asker and the answerer are involved in an act of cooperative encounter of mutually making sense of the other (Bühler, 1934/1990). In that process—a kind of temporary relationship that may qualify as a partnership—both the researcher and the researchee create new understandings of each other.

TWO MODELS OF COMMUNICATION: UNIDIRECTIONAL AND BIDIRECTIONAL

The problem that the questionnaire method uses is the appropriation of one of the two general models of communication—the misfitting one. It is assumed that the *unidirectional* model of communication, where the message as given is received basically as the communicator has intended it, fits the research situations in psychology and medicine. Historically, this model has dominated most of psychology's, medicine's, and education's reliance upon question asking and answering. Its background is down-to-earth pragmatism of the "if you want to know, ask" variety. It assumes that the respondent has complete access to the facts and is willing and able to reveal them when questioned. Yet this need not be so; consider the following example:

Nurse to patient: How tall are you?

Patient: 1 meter 89 centimeters

Nurse: How much is this in feet and inches?

Patient: I have no idea

Even simple differences in different measurement systems—no doubt that the person's height can be objectively measured both in the metric and the imperial system—can lead to a confusion. Here the nurse and patient are mutually ignorant of each other's measurement system—applicable to the same object. The respondent answers the question in factual terms—in his (or her) measurement system. The nurse fails to understand it in her (or his) system.

A frequent event in the course of interviews or questionnaires is the joint construction of illusion of concreteness through the use of fuzzy quantifiers, as in the following example:

Physician: *How often* do you have headaches?

Patient: Very often

Both partners rely on a word that implies the applicability of a framework of frequency—rather than that of form or quality. This example constitutes a case of pseudoquantification—the researcher's question suggests that the issue at stake ("having a headache") can be considered within the quantified frame of OFTEN ↔ NOT OFTEN. Yet the only concrete aspect of the communication effort is the reference to the patient ("you")—all the other aspects of the question/answer sequence remain unclear. There is no referent object available for both interaction partners—outside of the patient's subjective domain of what constitutes a headache. There is illusory intersubjectivity presumed through the notion of "often," with the fuzzy quantifiers (e.g., *very often*) maintained as different from *often* only within the subjective domain of the respondent. The physician has asked the question—and received an answer that is unambiguously recordable ("the patient claims that headaches occur very often")—yet the meanings constructed by both in this sequence remain grossly unspecified.

In the following example, we can see a more complex challenge to the unidirectional communication model—the respondent's diverging counterinterpretation of the question asked:

Physician to an adolescent girl: *Are you sexually active?*

The girl: No . . . I just lie there

Social norms of public discourse about sexuality lead the physician to translate the intended question ("are you having sex with somebody") into the socially sensitized form ("are you sexually active?").

Such "mismatches" between questions and answers are not anecdotal errors from the viewpoint on communication as personal construction of understanding on the basis of different personal perspectives. They all point to the inappropriateness of assuming that the unidirectional communication model is applicable to human communication.

In contrast, research on human communication and metacommunication has rejected the notion of unidirectional message transfer in communication (Branco & Valsiner, 2004). Instead, the participants in any act of communication create the meanings of the communicated messages together—the question asked by A becomes a complex object of meaning making by B. Much of that meaning making may remain hidden in the intrapsychological domain of the responder, especially if the latter is asked to choose between pre-given responses ("yes" or "no"). Human communication systems operate by the principles of a *bidirectional* communication model (Valsiner, 1989, chap. 3). That model is an outgrowth from Bühler's Organon Model (Bühler, 1934/1990) and leads into the domain of partnership model in doctor–patient and researcher–researchee relations (Bibace, Dillon, & Dowds, 1999). The partnership model treats the process of interaction between the "experts"—researchers or medical doctors—and the "laypersons" (subjects, participants, or patients) as an encounter that entails mutual entrance into one another's psychological worlds.

Any research encounter is a process that entails establishing the contact between the researcher and participant, the actual joint interaction in the course of carrying out the tasks (and maintaining cooperation over time; see Kerllenevich et al., chapter 16 this book), and, finally, end of the encounter. Within that process, different tasks, such as items in a questionnaire, sequence of questions in an interview, repeated trials in an experimental task, or persisting encouragement by a clinician to the hesitant client on the couch, all have their microlevel "subevents" within the encounter. Thus, an interpersonally motivated research participant whose goal is to help the researcher get the project done may tolerate all kinds, of questions asked, while a low-motivated participant can be intolerant of even a repetition of a simple question ("but I answered that already before"). However, in the actual clinical and research, these encounters lead to pertinent outcomes, namely, to diagnoses and to responses interpreted as "data" by the researcher (Valsiner, 2000).

THEORETICAL BACKGROUND:PROCESS–OUTCOME RELATIONSHIPS

The focus on the researcher's side can equally well concentrate on either the process, or the outcome, of any task included in the research process. Piaget's revolutionary role in psychology consisted of replacing the focus on aggregation of outcomes—of items in ability tests—to investigating the processes that led to these outcomes. A test item may end up being answered in a "wrong" way while still using a process that could generate also the "right" answer. In contrast, an inferior process cannot generate outcomes at higher levels. The process can determine a variety of outcomes but not vice versa (Werner, 1937).

Four relationships between processes and outcomes can be considered:

One-to-one relation. Here, a single process always generates an outcome—the latter may vary as to specific circumstances. This kind of relationship has been assumed in most of psychology—a posited causal entity (e.g., "g factor" or "social introversion") is assumed to regularly and systematically generate responses on the outcome side. The responses vary only quantitatively, depending upon their conditions of generation.

One-to-many relation. Here a single process generates more than one (at least two) qualitatively different outcomes. This relation is central for *transfer* of existing psychological functions from one context to another. Any procedure—as a means to some end—can be transposed to new ends under the conditions of changing conditions. The immediate adaptability of the organism depends upon that possibility (cases where there exists a one-to-one relation between a process and an outcome are minimally adaptive to new challenges).

Many-to-one relation. In this case a number of qualitatively different processes can lead to the same outcome. This is the case of *equifinality,* a major feature of all adaptive systems. This form of relation leads to *redundancy,* the presence of mechanisms that can take over the generation of an outcome if the primary procedure malfunctions. Redundancy is the basis for all living systems that operate under uncertainty.

Many-to-many relation. This relation is obviously a combination of the two relations mentioned above. The whole pattern of process/outcome relationships is characterized by that form, since the fully functioning person is constantly moving toward a number of outcomes simultaneously and there are parallel processes involved.

Outcomes can be explained only through the analysis of processes that lead to them, but not vice versa. It is possible to explain some outcome measures of a system, for example, a car's performance on the road, by way of pointing to the way the engine is designed. Different versions of engine design can lead to the same outcome result (many-to-one relation). Yet it is impossible to deduce the way in which any of these car engines is built from the outcome results.

However, there is a certain mutuality in the process/outcome distinction itself: an outcome of some developmental process is a new process that leads to new outcomes. The establishment of syllogistic reasoning frames in the cognitive domain of schooled children is a long process of teaching and learning. Once it has arrived in its outcome, that outcome itself becomes a new process of cognitive functioning. In a similar vein, teaching physicians new thinking patterns in making medical decisions (Gigerenzer & Kurzenhäuser, chapter 1, this volume) leads to the establishment of new ways of how to reach decisions, hence outcomes (of previous processes) become new processes.

This outcome-to-process transition should be nothing new for anybody well versed in a consistently developmental theoretical outlook (Werner, 1948). Werner, following Goethe, described through the orthogenetic principle (OP). The OP entails the development of any system to take place through differentiation: emergence of the parts and their hierarchical integration. In that emergence process, development takes place in the form of a spiral (Werner, 1957) or helix: every new curve supersedes the previous one yet analogically shows some similarity to it.

QUESTIONNAIRES AND THEIR USE: NEW POSSIBILITIES

The fact that questionnaires are usually applied to register outcomes need not undermine their potential usefulness for other purposes. For instance, consider the abstract one ↔ many relationship as previously described. This relationship can be seen to guide the respondent in a questionnaire, but it can also be applied to the researcher or clinician who is interested in how many patients view their relationships with one health-care provider. Bibace et al. (1999) have used a questionnaire consisting of 20 questions that was filled out immediately after the patient saw the doctor. The first question, for instance, suggested to the respondent to answer on a five-point scale (strongly agree—agree—unsure—disagree—strongly disagree, or "does not apply") to the question:

The doctor goes straight to my medical problem without first greeting me.

The behavior identified here is specific and refers to how the doctor has actually initiated the interaction with this patient some 15–30 minutes before. Here the interpretation of the researcher who carries out the questionnaire is irrelevant, and the role of the respondent's construction of meaning is reduced to deciding what "agree" means (e.g., does the person agree *with such practice*—whether it happened or not—or agrees *that it did happen*). The data obtained this way proved valuable for the physician—yet under conditions of anonymity. The physician would resist having such information available if it is to be used in actual formal evaluations of him (or her). Obtaining such evidence allows the physician to know how frequently patients are in agreement regarding his (or her) specific ways of their everyday interactions with patients. Doctors, like any busy role-based actors in other professions, are often unaware of how some automatized habits of theirs are perceived by their clients. Some of these habits can themselves lead to extra tension; an extreme example is that of a physician who did not greet his patients before going to their medical problem. The first utterance by the specialist in hypertension was the rendering of the latest blood pressure measurements the nurse had taken before the patient met with the doctor! Yet it is easy to see how such pattern of interaction comes into being: a busy specialist who rushes from one patient to another and gets no feedback from the viewpoint of the people he (or she) treats enters into a routine similar to that of a factory conveyer belt.

A simple questionnaire-based set of answers may prove an eye-opener to the doctor here. The doctor needs feedback that includes all of the variability of patients' views. Yet such feedback minimizes the significance of the psychological processes and intentions of particular patients in checking off that behavior on a rating scale. The doctor may speculate as to "why" a particular patient or a small percentage of the patients "strongly agree" that their doctor goes "straight to my medical problem without first greeting me." The doctor may see that result as a positive endorsement of his (or her) professionalism or as the opposite: a critical evaluation of the dehumanization that goes on in the doctor–patient interaction. The doctor may get the results and decide to change nothing in the way in which things are done, or the doctor may try to modify the routine toward more humane treatment of the patients. All of these particular ways the doctor constructs one's complement to the outcome data obtained from the questionnaires (one ↔ many relation) remain within the domain of personal construction, which involves modulation of the psychological distance in the medical encounter.

QUESTIONING AND ANSWERING IN RESEARCH AS DISTANCING PROCEDURES

A similar one ↔ many relation applies in the researcher's relating with the researchees. Every encounter between researcher and participant includes simultaneous creation of distance and elimination of it. This tension is present everywhere—from the psychology laboratory to anthropological fieldwork (Abu Lughod, 1988; Shami, 1988; see also Kerllenevich et al., chapter 16, this volume).

At times the researcher's closeness to the background of the researchees is an obstacle to be overcome (Abu-Lughod, 1988; Shami, 1988), as it creates a confusion at the border of ingroup/outgroup relation ("you are one of us . . . but you are not one of us . . . "—an attitude toward a returning other-educated Ph.D. researcher to a home village). On other occasions, however, the belonging to the "us" as projected onto the researcher by the researchees makes it possible to access the issues under investigation. Thus, a female researcher studying childbirth experiences in Tamil Nadu changes her distanced position after having a child herself:

> The fact that I had a child myself made an enormous difference in the nature of our discussions. When I talked with women about childbirth during my trip in 1993 I did not have a child of my own. And just as women were reluctant to discuss the details of their birth experiences with

their daughters or daughters-in-law who had not yet had their first child, they were hesitant to speak freely with me about this subject. In part there was a sense that it was a taboo to do so, and in part there was a sense that I simply would not or could not understand. When I began my research in 1995, however, and explained to women that I had a child myself and told them about my own birth experience, they were much more at ease talking with me. The difference did not only lie with their attitude toward me but also with my attitude toward them. Having been through childbirth myself I did feel as though I could understand their experiences more fully, despite the social and cultural factors that made our birth experiences vastly different. (Van Hollen, 2003, p. 32)

The analogical experiences of the researcher and the researchees can create a basis if a wider field intersubjectivity on the basis of which the researcher builds the construction of her data. The creative flow of the interviewer and interviewee (Sigel & Kim, 1996) while "floating" in between the question generated and the answer-to-be-constructed is a deeply intimate process of interpersonal kind. Here the distances between the object of investigation (content field of the question and answer) and the agents (question asker and answerer) are minimal. Yet, simultaneously, from that field of minimal distancing the researcher and the participant are in the process of "moving out" by distancing their personal positions. The researcher abstracts specific features of knowledge out of the shared researching encounter. That generalized knowledge is neither shared (nor sharable) with the researchee. At the same time, the researchee creates new meaning of the encounter in terms of his or her personal lay understanding. That particular knowledge is crucial for the continuing encounter, but in itself it is not part of scientific knowledge.

The unity of immediacy and distance is an example of the unity of the universals (abstracted knowledge) and particulars (context from where the knowledge was abstracted). Distancing dynamics is the core of human psychological processes (Cupchik, 2002; Sigel, 2002) and forms the basis for establishing relations of intersubjectivity or partnerships.

THE PARTNERSHIP MODEL

The partnership model emphasizes the process of mutual meaning construction (Bibace et al., 1999) being the central stage of knowing and decision making. The process of answering a given question is that of joint construction of knowledge by the asker and the answerer. It is through that joint activity that research and medical encounters are characterized by the partnership model.

When viewed from the standpoint of Bibace's partnership model, it is the relationship between questioning-and-answering people that is in our focus of attention. The relationship starts from partners assuming different complementary social roles—those of doctor and patient (in medicine), researcher and *subject* (previously *observer* and currently *research participant,* in psychology), anthropologist and *informant,* epidemiologist and *host,* and so on. These differentiated roles set up an asymmetric role relation based on difference of expertise (or social power). However, behind the asymmetry of roles is the symmetry in meaning construction in the case of partnership; both partners depend upon the participation by the other to achieve their goals.

Bibace's Partnership Model leads to the need to adjust our usual research methodology. In most general terms, partnership-based research methodology entails inquiry into the questioning and answering processes, from one cycle (question → answer → interpretation of the question *and* answer) to many (CYCLE 1: question → answer → interpretation of the question *and* answer → CYCLE 2: question *based on previous interpretation* → answer → interpretation of the question *and* answer → . . . CYCLE *N*). The spiral movement in knowledge construction here is the core of methodological depth (rather than a "nuisance").

In its fullest version, this kind of methodology can be put to practice in interviews or in different kinds of feedback-based learning programs (see the chapters on No-Fault Learning Programs, this volume). In a limited version, the same methodological focus can be taken toward explicating the answering process of any single question (LaPushin, 2002). In the latter case, it entails the investigation of the following minimal subunit of the partnership process:

> **Question** (set by the Researcher) →
> → Participant {**process of answering**
> (based on interpretation of the question
> by the Respondent) → **Answer**} →
> → **Interpretation** (by the Researcher)

Psychology is filled with methods that merely record answers or, at most, look at question/answer correspondences (e.g., "lie scales" in personality tests such as MMPI). What has been downplayed in the past decades is the process analysis of an answer.

In a preliminary study of answering process, LaPushin (2002) investigated 50 college students (25 male, 25 female) whose ages ranged between 18 and 23 years. All participants were given a questionnaire of 15 questions (selected from various Web sites for personality "testing") with the response format TRUE, FALSE, or HARD TO SAY per item. Immediately after they gave their answers, they were asked to give specific details of their "stream of consciousness" while answering the questionnaire. Finally, the participants were asked to rate the certainty of their initially selected response on a scale from –3 (less certain) to + 3 (more certain).

In Figure 17.1 are presented the data from one of the questions—"*I am easily bothered by people making demands on me.*" As can be seen, each of the eight participants who responded to this item utilized his or her unique trail of thought while arriving at one of the three preset response option.

The analysis of the explanations that were provided immediately after the answer entailed a focus on *psychological processes* (reports on the immediate ways used by the person in the decision making) and *personal experiences* (retrospects upon some facets of personal conduct in the past that illuminated the decision process in the course of answering).

This distinction makes it possible to analyze the ways in which general statements about oneself become linked—within the person's self-reflection—with particulars from one's past. Such "meaning excursions" can lead to a dialogue with oneself—"*in general I am X*", and there are sets of particular situations {X} that fit with "*my idea that I am X*" but there are also other occasions {non-X} that contradict the idea that "*I am X.*" The question asked triggers a process that at some moments brings out from the person's intimate history occasions of both kinds.

We reach an interesting point concerning the outcomes here; the only realistic (which means true to particulars) answer to most of psychologists' questions needs to be HARD TO SAY. All the opposing examples, triggered from the past, create a meaning opposition of the posited characteristic and its counter-examples. The answering process is thus an act of differentiation of the field of HARD TO SAY into TRUE or FALSE. Different persons—and different item contents—allow that differentiation process to proceed with greater or smaller ease (as is seen in Figure 17.1). Nevertheless, the process remains universal for each and every person—a question triggers the actualization of a field that triggers different tensions between opposed meanings. A glimpse into the process of how these tensions are handled is the researchers' window into the wonderfully complex world of human subjectivity. The partnership approach allows both researchers and practitioners to bear this in mind.

Figure 17.1
Meanings of responses as explained by the participants.

Question: "I am not easily bothered by people making demands of me"
(Boldface = psychological processes; lightface, personal experiences)

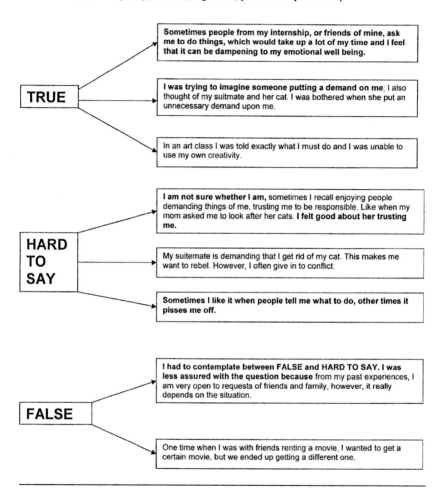

GENERAL CONCLUSION: THE MIRACLE OF ANSWERS

Following the treatment of the questioning and answering process above, it should be almost a miracle that any complex question about a person can be answered at all—be it in simple (TRUE or FALSE) terms or in the form of ratings on some scale (see Valsiner, Diriwächter, &

Sauck, chapter 18, this volume). Yet this is not the case: many questions are unambiguous while others are tolerably ambiguous. Such ambiguity is the basis for adaptation to new ways of thinking in new contexts.

Asking a question entails participation in the answering of the question, and answering the question is being led by the question asked. The asker and the answerer are involved in a mutual relation—a partnership—at least for the sake of arriving at an answer. A number of interesting issues follow from this look at questioning and answering from the standpoint of the partnership model.

First, it becomes clear that, in research and clinical practices, all questions are necessarily "leading questions." Even if the clinician or researcher does the utmost to avoid any "leads," these are constructed and projected by the respondent to any "neutral-looking" question. This is a basic feature of all communication processes (Bühler, 1934/1990). Hence, there are no objective questions that stand on their own. Even if the "input material" that the researcher brings to the participant is admittedly of nondirective origin—such as a set of nonsense syllables in memory experiments or inkblot stimuli—the respondent actively constructs these objects as meaningful.

Secondly, the central issue relevant for both researchers and practitioners is the process of answering rather than its outcome. It is the active psychological process that leads to the outcome, whether the latter is about some generalization from one's past or about development of a new worry about impending future (e.g., elective surgery, etc.). The internalized images, feelings, and meanings play a crucial role. The person imports those into the process of generating a psychological outcome, such as a TRUE or FALSE verdict. In the course of reaching such a verdict, some episode from one's past may remain reverberating in one's mind after a particular question is answered long before. In retrospect to data (in Figure 17.1), a person may keep asking oneself, *"why did they ask me whether I am bothered about people making demands on me?"* It is some version of such reverberating materials that is used by the person's further conduct—perhaps long after the asker had confronted the answerer with the specific item from a standard questionnaire. In a similar vein—the role of writing this chapter is a message that is hoped to initiate the questions in the readers—why are they writing about the partnership in the questioning/answering process?

Perhaps there is basic human dignity involved in the motivation of patients and research participants that their active contributions be given adequate recognition in the complex process of scientific knowledge construction as well as in the course of medical cure in any society.

REFERENCES

Abu-Lughod, L. (1988). Fieldwork of a dutiful daughter. In S. Altorki & C. F. El-Solh (Eds.), *Arab women in the field: Studying your own society* (pp. 139–161). Syracuse, NY: Syracuse University Press.

Bibace, R., Dillon, J., & Dowds, B. N. (Eds.). (1999). *Partnerships in research, clinical, and educational settings.* Stamford, CT: Ablex.

Branco, A. U., & Valsiner, J. (Eds.). (2004). *Communication and metacommunication in human development.* Westport, CT: InfoAge Publishers.

Bühler, K. (1934/1990). *Sprachtheorie* [Theory of language]. Jena-Stuttgart: Gustav Fischer.

Cupchik, G. (2002). The evolution of psychical distance as an aesthetic concept. *Culture & Psychology, 8*(2), 155–187.

LaPushin, T. (2002). *Questionnaires: true, false, or hard to say.* Unpublished Honors Thesis, Department of Psychology, Clark University, Worcester, MA.

Rommetveit, R. (1992). Outlines of a dialogically based social-cognitive approach to human cognition and communication. In A. H. Wold (Ed.), *The dialogical alternative: Towards a theory of language and mind* (pp. 19–44). Oslo: Scandinavian University Press.

Schwartz, N. (1999). Self-reports: How the questions shape the answers. *American Psychologist, 54*(2), 93–105.

Shami, S. (1988). Studying your own: the complexities of a shared culture. In S. Altorki & C. F. El-Solh (Eds.), *Arab women in the field: Studying your own society* (pp. 115–138). Syracuse, NY: Syracuse University Press.

Sigel, I. (2002). The psychological distancing model: A study of the socialization of cognition. *Culture & Psychology, 8*(2), 189–214.

Sigel, I. E., & Kim, M-I. (1996). The answer depends on the question. In S. Harkness & C. M. Super (Eds.), *Parents' cultural belief systems* (pp. 83–120). New York: Guilford.

Valsiner, J. (1989). *Human development and culture.* Lexington, MA: D.C. Heath & Co.

Valsiner, J. (2000). Data as representations: contextualizing qualitative and quantitative research strategies. *Social Science Information, 39*(1), 99–113.

Van Hollen, C. (2003). *Birth on the threshold: Childbirth and modernity in South India.* Berkeley: University of California Press.

Werner, H. (1937). Process and achievement. *Harvard Educational Review, 7,* 353–368.

Werner, H. (1948). *Comparative psychology of mental development.* New York: International University Press.

Werner, H. (1957). The concept of development from a comparative and organismic point of view. In D. B. Harris (Ed.), *The concept of development* (pp. 125–147). Minneapolis: University of Minnesota Press.

EDITORIAL COMMENTARY

The issues with studies in psychology that the authors have identified are all applicable to medical studies, as well. Far too few investigators remember to include the point of view of the study participant. Far too many investigators take the attitude, "This is MY study, not the 'subject's.'"

I have found another problem with many of the questionnaires that are used in medical studies: Total lack of training of the investigator. Many young faculty are under great pressure to "publish or perish." Often, when they are at a loss for a project, they decide to "send out a questionnaire." It is obvious from the quality of the ones that I receive (and currently there seems to be no shortage of questions to ask department chairs) that there is a perception that "anyone can make up a questionnaire." It is common in the ones that I receive for at least 25 percent of the questions to be so vague that they are impossible to answer. I wind up throwing many of them away out of frustration. And most of the time, I see the results printed somewhere!

For more than 30 years I have been involved with questionnaire research. I have great experience in the science of writing questions, choosing possible responses, and avoiding vagary. Nonetheless, I would never think of using a questionnaire without pretesting it first. Obviously, based on the quality of the material I receive in the mail, that is a concept that is foreign to many.

—Kenneth L. Noller

Chapter 18

DIVERSITY IN UNITY: STANDARD QUESTIONS AND NONSTANDARD INTERPRETATIONS

Jaan Valsiner, Rainer Diriwächter, and Christine Sauck

Human communication seems very simple: what can be easier than asking people for information about themselves? This happens everywhere—doctors ask patients about their pains, psychologists ask people about their worries, sociologists conduct opinion polls, and so on. Our social lives are filled with myriads of questions we are constantly being asked—some very general, some very specific. We do answer those, some of the time, but how?

OBVIOUSNESS OF QUESTIONS AND INDETERMINACY OF ANSWERS

In line with issues in this volume, consider the questions asked within a legal or medical domain, where answers to specific questions could have a profound impact on an individual's future well-being. The perceived consequences of answers themselves contribute to how the person answers questions solicited from a legal or medical team. Thus, a seemingly simple question

"Do you take any drugs?"

when asked in a medical setting gets a lead different from that when asked in a legal context. Furthermore, what a "drug" means—among many substances the person takes into his or her biological body—differs both across persons and changes within one (Joerchel & Valsiner, 2003). It depends upon who is asking—a researcher, a lawyer, a friend, a rival, a doctor, a parent—and for what goal orientation the question is asked. Given the respondent's perception of the implied goal orientation of the question, the answer can be generated in a multitude of ways (Rommetveit, 1992). These ways reflect the different meaning construction processes that are involved (Josephs, Valsiner, & Surgan, 1999). Yet the study of mental processes has been rare in psychology. It is only in those areas of cognitive science that grow out from the work of the "Würzburg School" that thinking processes have been analyzed through a focus on them as process (Frijda & DeGroot, 1982; Simon, 1999). The focus on mental processes has been most effectively developed within German holistic tradition (Diriwächter, 2003).

Field-Theoretic Look at Responding to Questions

How can one analyze the whole? Everything that belongs to the totality of interest for analysis is never unrelated, and the relatedness is always dynamic. This creates a substantial hurdle for analytic schemes in any science, most of which are framed in terms of categories of entities and their relations. For holistic analytic schemes, a different direction is needed: a field-theoretic terminological system.

How can such perspective be built? In fact, it is already in existence in the area of *sematology* introduced by Karl Bühler (1934/1965, 1990). Bühler's sematology—general theory of signs—entails the copresence of three levels of "representational fields" in the communicative act. The *primary representational field* is the field that a communicative message immediately evokes when it is actualized. The sign—given its form— evokes a particular field of relations of meanings by the interpreter. If in a questionnaire a question is asked about "experiences," that sign leads to the activation of the whole field of personal phenomena that the respondent would consider as fitting into that field. Thus, "imagining monsters" may belong to it, but "being an elephant" might not.

The *secondary representational field* entails the field of personal memories and productive fantasies that the question evokes in the respondent. Here, episodes of personal past and anticipated future are merged into one whole, guided by the meanings network of the primary field (Bühler, 1990, pp. 65–66).

Finally, the *tertiary representational field* entails the interpretation of the intentionality of the communicator: why is this question asked? The respondent to a question "have you had strange experiences?" would interpret the asker's motives for asking this question and take that into account in responding. Bühler's account leads to the key of any research process: the centrality of the communicative act between the researcher and the subject and between the doctor and the patient.

RESEARCH WITH HUMAN PARTICIPANTS AS A COMMUNICATIVE ACT

In each act of research with human subjects, the researcher is involved in an act of bi-directional communication (Valsiner, 2000, chap. 4). Both the researcher and the researched are active constructors of meanings through their common encounter. The research encounter involving inventories or questionnaires is as much an episode of communication as an interview or focus group is. The difference here is in the fixity of the communicative messages by the researcher.

The items in questionnaires or standard personality inventories artificially fix the message from the researcher's side while leaving wide open the different constructions for the subjects. The latter are not involved in one-sided responding to questions but interpreting these questions as part of a wider whole of what the researcher is assumed to try to understand.

MEANINGS OF ITEMS IN STANDARD PERSONALITY INVENTORIES

Psychology of personality is an area where the discrepancy between studies of the universal and the particular have gone astray. While striving to make sense of the general picture of individual's systemic functioning, researchers often use the inter-individual comparison frame ("individual differences") in their empirical studies. The latter are often based on standardized measurement instruments. This perspective is unabashedly atheoretical and prides itself in its psychometric prudence, yet it entails a set of assumptions about the nature of the research procedure that remain hidden in the measurement practices. All kinds of personality research methods that ask persons to answer questions about themselves and to record the answers are capitalizing upon the outcomes of persons' psychological processes. They are based on a number of general assumptions:

Assumption 1: Local Independence of Test Items

Standard questionnaires, like other psychological tests, are built on the assumption that the respondent's answers to different items in a test are statistically independent—answering an item X in a certain way does not have an impact on any of the items from X to final item N of the questionnaire. This assumption may be difficult to satisfy in the case of personality questionnaire items that pull for a person's self-narrative disclosure that has continuity over time (and sequence of questions).

Assumption 2: Minimization of Response Process Is a Goal

This assumption is built into any standard method where subjects are instructed to respond as quickly as possible, or on the basis of their first impression. In case of a person's confronting with any psychological test, especially personality questionnaires, the fictional and real meanings of the terms brought into the situation by the researcher's formulating a single item become related with the read-out from the person's present interpretation of the situation and of one's past life story. A personality test item touches upon the depth of private experience (see Singer & Bonnano, 1990)—yet in ways that are minimized by the constructors of the test.

Minimization is given by the constraining of the response format: any step away from "free reply" (unbounded narrative)—such as sentence completion, rating scale, and "true/false" (or "yes/no") forced choice—entails some version of minimization of the contact of the researcher's message and that of the respondent. Such minimization is not an oversight (or "error"); it is a purposeful filter that allows the researcher to focus one's attention upon selected aspects of the issues under study. Yet each step in this method construction process—deciding upon the phrasing of a questionnaire item and deciding upon the answer format—necessarily limit the access to the phenomena.

Assumption 3: The (Maximal) Reality behind Minimized Responding

It is assumed that quick and immediate responding to an item can reflect the respondent's "true state" more adequately than a lengthy process of meaning construction. Considering a decision to use the minimalistic "forced choice" response format ("true/false," "yes/no") eliminates any access to the respondent's uncertainty in the responding process. That uncertainty cannot be reconstructed from data analyses later on; any uncertainty data surfacing from the aggregated responses (for the same person) cannot represent the uncertainty that was there in the responding process.

A DIALOGICAL ALTERNATIVE: RESPONDING AS A DISAMBIGUATION PROCESS

The assumptions of the traditional testing practices are not tenable if we look at the questionnaires as arenas for communication. Elsewhere, we have shown that uncertainty about what is to be responded to, and how the responding proceeds, can be generated in many ways (Wagoner & Valsiner, 2003). Here is the importance of the item format. By suggesting that some item *can and should be* answered considering the TRUE ↔ FALSE opposition, two kinds of responding processes can be triggered: that using the assumption of exclusion of opposites {TRUE < exclusive *or* > FALSE} and the other using inclusion of opposites {TRUE < inclusive *or* > FALSE}. The latter responding process leads to a dialogical opposition: where the meanings of TRUE and FALSE become unified in a whole where they operate as poles of tension. The object of rating is "pulled" from both poles, and if the strength of forces of such "pull" remains equal, the rating outcome is necessarily that of some mark in the middle region. By limiting the response format to a multiple choice—and demanding quick making on marks on the scale— the researcher has irreversibly closed one's door of access to the phenomena of dialogical interpretation processes. This decision to eliminate the access to responding process may follow from the theoretical framework of the researcher (and thus be consistent within the "methodology cycle"; Branco & Valsiner, 1997). However, it is a serious methodological problem if such consistency is not the case.

MEANING CONSTRUCTION WHILE RESPONDING TO THE MMPI

We are interested in demonstrating how unique individual human beings, when put into a comparable yet always new setting of filling out personality questionnaires, create meaning around selected items from a regular, standardized personality inventory. The Minnesota Multiphasic Personality Inventory (MMPI) is a classic theory-free personality task, available both in a card-sorting and paper-and-pencil formats, originally for psychiatric application. Over the last 60 years, its uses have spread far beyond clinical contexts. It contains classic forced choice tasks that require "true" versus "false" responses for each of the 550 personality-descriptive statements. For example:

- I brood a great deal
- I frequently have to fight against showing that I am bashful
- I have had very peculiar and strange experiences
- It makes me feel like a failure when I hear of the success of someone I know well

The originators of the MMPI, Starke Hathaway and J. C. McKinley, opted for an empirical keying method to construct the MMPI clinical scales. This approach, innovative in the 1940s, entailed (1) collecting hundreds of personality statements that were independent of one another, (2) selecting appropriate criterion for "normal" versus clinical subjects, (3) administering the 550 item test to both groups, and (4) conducting an analysis to determine which items were most endorsed by individuals belonging to either group (Graham, 1987). It was a quintessentially American, Midwest, cultural invention—an example of extreme belief in empirical data. The MMPI was constructed without any conceptual basis, relying strictly on the empirical analysis of survey results to design a personality assessment instrument.

In the clinical setting for taking the test, the clinician may provide a brief explanation of why it is being given. Once the client has been judged capable of completing the test by the clinician—who sees the client as sufficiently literate and willing—or at least not resisting—to perform the test-taking task, the test booklet and answer sheet are given to the client. The MMPI-2, a more current version of the MMPI test booklet, includes following instructions:

> Read each statement and decide whether it is *true as applied to you or false as applied to you* . . . If a statement is *true* or *mostly true*, as applied to you, blacken the circle marked *T*. If a statement is *false* or *not usually true,* as applied to you, blacken the circle marked *F*. If a statement does not apply to you or if it is something that you don't know about, make no mark on the answer sheet. But try to give a response to every statement. Remember to give *your own* opinion of yourself. (Hathaway & McKinley, 1989, p. 2, emphases added)

It is important to emphasize that this MMPI-2 instruction forces the respondent to polarization of possible answers—by insisting upon a 4-point rating scale that becomes finalized in 2-valent ("true" versus "false") forced choice. This simplification of the responding framework

that is encoded already in the instruction is a perfect example of minimization of the responding process. Furthermore, the instruction calls
forth the culture-specific folk model of persons "*having*" their "*own opinion.*" Thus, it becomes obvious that the traditions of MMPI are set out
to create personally constructed, context-freed, dichotomous "own opin-
ions." However, this procedure is not foreign to the participants. Ninety
percent of individuals taking the test do not need further clarification
from the clinician and complete the test in 60 to 90 minutes (Greene,
2000).

In our study, respondents were asked to take an abridged and slightly
modified version of the original MMPI. In the interest of brevity, only
72 questions were used from the original 550. We selected items from
the introversion/extroversion, or social isolation subscale of the MMPI
(i.e., "I don't mind meeting strangers" or "I easily become impatient
with people"). Another modification was made in the answer format. In
addition to the polarized "true" and "false" choices, we included opportunities for the participants to elaborate on their responses. In doing so,
we included varying degrees of "true" and "false" ratings as well as a
space in which the participants could make additional comments to justify or supplement their ratings, as in Figure 18.1.

As is clear from Figure 18.1, the "traditional" MMPI response format
(minimized TRUE versus FALSE dichotomy) is maintained at the first
step of responding but is then immediately followed up by differentiation

Figure 18.1
**Modified MMPI response format with true/false dichotomy and differentiated min-
imized response to "I wish I were not so shy."**

I wish I were not so shy

         TRUE   FALSE

                        Please rate your response

       |----------|----------| |----------|----------|
    LITTLE   MEDIUM   VERY   LITTLE   MEDIUM   VERY

Describe your thoughts & feelings while giving this answer: _____

---

of the minimized response and the provision of a qualitative externalized report of the meaning of the answer.

In line with our difference with standard personality investigations, our instructions were also modified to adapt to the new answer format of our questionnaire. They read as follows:

> For each of the following statements, please circle the response that seems to describe you the closest. First, decide whether it is TRUE or FALSE (circle one of the two) in respect to you, and then evaluate how false or true it is (circle either (LITTLE/MEDIUM/VERY). For example, if you feel that a statement describes you fairly closely, then circle first TRUE and then MEDIUM (always circle both). If you feel that a statement does not describe you at all, then circle first FALSE and then VERY. In addition to circling the responses that most closely describe you, **please also give us a short statement** (for each item!) **that explains your response to us.**

The present investigation included undergraduate students enrolled in an introductory personality course at a Massachusetts university. Three men and eight women between the ages of 20 and 25 years participated in this study. Our version of the questionnaire was administered to the participants during class at two separate time periods. The students completed the questionnaire once at the beginning of the semester (September) and then once again four months later (December). Identical versions of the questionnaire were administered at both time periods.

In addition, one set of questionnaires (in September) was administered to 13 undergraduate students enrolled in a cultural psychology seminar in Massachusetts. Three men and 10 women between the ages of 20 and 22 years filled out the same version of questionnaire as mentioned above, however, without filling it out again at time 2 (December).

Bashfulness and How One Deals with It

Consider the following item:

"I frequently have to fight against showing that I am bashful."

This seemingly simple everyday language statement has high psychological complexity, as the schematic structure of the statement entails (Figure 18.2). The use of this scheme can be illustrated by a list of different possible inventory statements:

Figure 18.2
High psychological complexity of the statement "I frequently have to fight against showing that I am bashful."

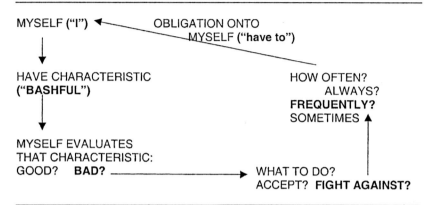

I am bashful.

I am glad I am bashful.

I feel bad because I am bashful.

I feel bad because I am bashful but this is the way I am.

I feel bad because I am bashful and I (sometimes/frequently/always) fight
   it.

I am glad I am bashful but I have to fight against that.

It is clear that this generative scheme leads to a field of phenomena (Bühler's first-level representational field), each of which would give the respondent a different suggestive starting point. Yet it is the coordination of these starting points with secondary representational fields (subjective episodes of life experiences) and the tertiary field ("why is this suggestion made and what it does for me to answer it one way or another?").

The data from individual subjects provide rich evidence of how this psychological structure of the item is handled by the same persons over time (Figure 18.3 and Table 18.1). The data include examples of seemingly opposite shifts (from "false" to "true"), which are clearly results of different highlighting of the parts of the item scheme (above). Consider Subject P2 (whose rating moved from "little TRUE" to "very FALSE" between test-taking times). This is linked with the person's bringing into the responding context two other personality features that are not present in the item itself ("shy" at Time 1, "boisterous" at Time

2) and using them as semiotic catalysts to generate the final answers. The action scheme takes different directions—in Time 1 it moves away from the MYSELF FIGHTING AGAINST X into SINCE I AM Y, MYSELF MAKES EFFORT FOR X (with "side effect" rating of the item as "little true." In Time 2 the MYSELF FIGHTING AGAINST X is taken but is channeled by the meaning "boisterous" being brought into the response-generating scheme. Again, the outcome rating—response to the manifest item—is almost a "side effect" (set up by the OPPOSITE of "bashful").

Elaborating the Idea Complex of "Strange Experiences"

Another example from the formation of complex-like meanings in the course of being confronted by an MMPI item is the way in which different subjects deal with something vague that is communicated to them in an affirmative statement:

"I have had very peculiar and strange experiences."

Here, the analysis of the structure of the item might take the following form (Figure 18.4).

To ask anybody to agree (or disagree) with generic statements pertaining to one's past creates a special task for the personal self-analysis system. Not only is one expected to scrutinize the whole set of "*experiences*" (assuming these are discrete events that stand out from the general ongoing flow of *experiencing* the world as one lives one's life), but the minimal (null) case of such experiences could be the taking of the MMPI and being queried by the present experience (of answering question about "*strange* experiences"). Triggering the recollection process of one's life course then proceeds as a sieve: what is "experience," and what is "strange" (or "peculiar") in relation to or comparison with whom or what. The data (from total of 24 participants, tested once) appear in Table 18.2.

As can be seen from Table 18.2, the answers indicate the distribution of the thinking processes into two basic classes—remembering oneself (reporting particulars or not) versus comparisons with others. The first crucial point in the data is the explication of the *disclosure boundary* in relation to the self report. The person discloses in writing that one avoids disclosing something in the same writing.

Table 18.1
Thoughts of Subjects while Giving Their Answers (Ratings in Parentheses)

Participant	Time 1	Time 2
1	I don't understand the question (No Answer)	I don't think I am bashful (5).
2	(1) <u>I'm a shy person</u> **I have to,** make an **effort** to introduce myself and speak to people.	(6) I **have to fight** against being **too boisterous**, I'm <u>not bashful</u> at all just the opposite
3	(5) No real thought	(3) I can be a shy person
4	(3) I try to work on being more outgoing + confident.	(2) I am shy which I don't like because it's a hindrance so I try to become more outgoing, but it is hard.
5	(5) <u>I don't fight it</u> because I <u>know I'm bashful</u>	(2) Usually, when I'm embarrassed my cheeks become bright red
6	(3) <u>I'm shy</u> in certain circumstances and <u>I try not to be</u>	(1) I <u>can be very shy</u> in certain situations
7	(4) I am not bashful <u>most of the time</u>	(6) I don't think I am bashful
8	(5) I'm <u>not very</u> bashful at all	(6) I am not bashful
9	(6) Bashfulness is <u>not</u> an emotion I <u>would be afraid of letting show</u>	(2) I <u>try to</u> overcome it
10	No Idea what it means (No Answer)	(4) I am not sure what bashful is
11	(5) I am not bashful in most situations	(4) I'm not usually shy

Figure 18.3
Individual subjects' data on two testing occasions of Item 16 of the SI scale ("I frequently have to fight against showing that I am bashful").

RATING TASK FORMAT

TRUE

|-----------|-----------|

LITTLE(3) MEDIUM(2) VERY(1)

FALSE

|-----------|-----------|

LITTLE (4) MEDIUM(5) VERY(6)

Figure 18.4
Analysis of the response structure of the statement "I have had very peculiar and strange experiences."

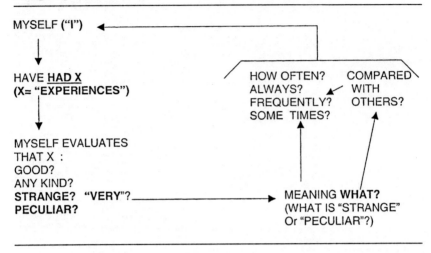

Myself and the Others: Coping with Their Failures

Jealousy and envy are basic human feelings that require interpersonal comparisons. Consider the following item:

> "It makes me feel like a failure when I hear of the success of someone I know well."

The meaning structure of this item could be written as shown in Figure 18.5.

The complex of feelings/meanings that this item unleashes is interesting in itself because it can be seen how the personal–cultural background that the subject brings into this scheme can take few, clearly specifiable states in this system. These states are

1. Other's Success → My Failure (suggested by the item)
2. Other's Success → My Success (contrary to the social suggestion) [*feeling good for* the other; *being proud of* the other]
3. Other's Success → Inconsequential for Me

Obviously, in the case of a person who is in exaggerated competition with others, state 1 applies. But since human beings—even in a supposedly hypercompetitive society such as the U.S.—vary in their relations with others, we can see the dominance of state 2 or state 3 (see Table 18.3).

Table 18.2
Subjects' Reflections upon Answering the Question about Experiences

Compare to others
(2) Has anything weird happened to me? *What will people think of me if I disclose that.*
(2) I think everybody has strange experiences Not a real advocate of normal
(4) everyone has peculiar + strange experiences (therefore I have) but I have not had <u>very</u> peculiar + strange experiences
(2) I have had strange experiences, but not as strange as people I have met.
(3) I believe I have had experiences in my life that deviate from the "normal college student."
(2) Some things I have gone through seem either unique to myself or things many others haven't faced.
(3) I think everyone has had at least some.
(2) I feel that everyone has such unique and original experiences and stories and I consider myself equally blessed with lots of opportunity to have peculiar + strange experiences
(3) I feel that I have had experiences that are different from others.
(3) There have been experiences which I sometimes think are different than the norm.
(3) Very strange things have happened to me but in relation to other people/world regions, they don't seem as peculiar.
(4) How weird have my experiences really been when compared with other individuals I know.
(3) Very arbitrary question. I couldn't imagine anyone answering False or True and the Very.
(2) I'm sure that everyone has experiences which they would deem "strange", but I'm considering encounters that make me feel awkward / uncomfortable also.

Self / Remembering
(3) I was thinking of a few peculiar experiences I've had
(1) I thought back to past experience where strange things occurred.
(1) some of the experiences that I have gone through / mostly the ones that marked a great change in my life
(3) I feel like I've had some odd experiences in my life, funny things that have happened.
(3) I tried to think about strange things and at first thought none, but realized *some were strange to me.*
(5) I seem to think that my life has not been "very" strange.

Other
(5) I can't think of it right now, so what would suggest that I hadn't.
(2) My thoughts were: peculiar and strange compared to who or what?
(4) I don't know what the definition of peculiar or strange is
(6) I can't think of any strange experiences in my life.

(Item: "I have had very peculiar and strange experiences"; Time 1 data, with ratings in parentheses before the descriptions)

GENERAL DISCUSSION

We emphasize that our intention in this investigation was not to discredit personality inventories such as the MMPI nor was it to devalue the efforts of the creators of such assessment tools. Instead, our aim was to shed light on the various mechanisms involved in the answering process of an individual completing such questionnaires. Furthermore, we do not intend to discourage the use of assessment tools in clinical settings or for research purposes. Instead, we caution the users of such standard-

Figure 18.5
Meaning structure of the statement "It makes me feel like a failure when I hear of the success of someone I know well."

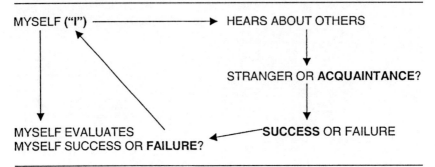

Table 18.3
Describing One's Responding to Others

True	False
(3) I wish it were me, even though I know I should just be proud.	(4) It makes me feel proud that I know of some one w/ success.
(2) I feel like I am not succeeding fast enough and that I should be better	(5) I don't judge myself in this way.
(4) I know I am successful too (P7)	(6) I would feel happy for them.
(3) Only a little but, mostly I feel very good for them and happy	(6) people are different
(2) I guess I get a little jealous and feel this way	(5) It makes me work harder
(3) Maybe envious, but depends on who it is & what they've accomplished	(6) I am usually proud to know them
(2) I often wish I could be as successful as others and it makes me feel inferior.	(4) I am glad they made it would like to do better myself as well
(3) honestly it can but I am getting better at dealing with that.	(6) I feel I am successful, no mater what anyone else does.
	(4) It makes me happy for them
	(5) I congratulate others for their successes
	(6) b/c I am proud of them
	(6) I am more proud of them then thinking of me
	(5) It makes me happy (unless I don't like that person) wow... that sounds really mean
	(4) I'm happy for them
	(5) It makes me happy for them
	(5) definitely compare to myself, but I don't feel like a failure.

(Item: "It makes me feel like a failure when I hear of the success of someone I know well"; Time 1 data, with ratings in parentheses before the descriptions)

ized methods to make their goals—in research and in practice—clear and consistent with the ways in which the methods are usable. Because clinicians making assessments are asked to both answer specific questions about the client and to help in making relevant decisions about him or her, assessment tools such as personality inventories become quite useful because they produce *working* descriptions of peoples' series of traits or abilities. These working descriptions may be sufficient for some practical clinical purposes, but not for a scientific study of the human psyche. Such tests are merely one method of collecting data on individuals within groups.

Psychological assessment, therefore, places questionnaire-derived information within a larger perspective: problem solving and decision making about the client (Groth-Marnat, 1997). It is important to note that within psychological assessments, contextual (i.e.. why the assessment is being conducted: school, forensic purposes, etc.) and historical information gathered from the client via an interview are gathered in addition to questionnaire results, which are used to provide supplementary information about the individual. In psychological studies, however, we encourage researchers to provide similar opportunities for participants to reveal such information (contextual and historical dimensions) that may temper test scores (i.e., providing space for an open-ended explanation of rating). In addition, we also highlight the perils of drafting complex statements that are difficult to process or open to different interpretations (i.e., "I believe that the 'new morality' of permissiveness is no morality at all"). As we have shown, even the simplest verbal statements that can be given to a subject can become highly complex communicative messages that are open to a multitude of interpretations.

The item-by-item analysis paints a world that is anything dichotomous ("true" versus "false"). Behind the forced choice answers, such as true/false, or any human experience, for that matter, lie complex psychological processes of complex qualities (Diriwächter, 2003). Humans are not static entities whose development occurs in jumps (from a to b), rather we undergo a moment-by-moment transformation that occurs simultaneously on several levels. The notion of sameness is a theoretical as well as practical impossibility since the axiom of development implies constant change (i.e., we are not the same at Time B as we are at Time A). This fact has been highlighted through our discussion of the item "*I frequently have to fight against showing that I am bashful*," where in certain cases a seemingly opposite shift in responses (from "false" to "true") occurred. A careful examination of the context indicates that seemingly opposite answers may actually be manifestations of the same underlying processes of personal meaning construction.

Our intention for highlighting this item was not so much to show changes in the responding process but to demonstrate a shift in what is attended to by the participant. If we reject the notion of a black-and-white world and replace it with a world that consists of obscurity and lack of differentiation from which we must abstract a certain component (i.e., to differentiate) from the whole in order to process it in a meaningful way, then we come to understand the relevance of semiotic catalysts that are incorporated into the context (i.e., responding to questionnaire items) in order to generate final answers. We always proceed from the whole (which is unclear at first) to the elements by abstracting certain components that are meaningful to us and thus contribute to a concrete experience. Bühler's three-level representational field is the interpretive system that mediates the generation of answers.

All human beings are historically and contextually driven. That is, we draw upon past experience in order to create meaning in the present context. The present context is further driven by institutional forces. For example, when filling out a questionnaire, participants are placed in a framework set up by researchers or clinicians that allows for a limited set of responses. If the contextual setting is too diffuse (i.e., the general nature of the question is not understood) or if the present cannot be contrasted with the past, we either withdraw from the process (i.e., by answering with "hard-to-say" or leaving the answer blank) or we engage in a forced answer in order to follow through with the framework that expects each question to have an answer. After all, we have a certain notion of what the process of filling out questionnaires entails.

We are faced with finite reality (something any method of inquiry faces) as to what participants choose to disclose (provided that participants respond truthfully), that is, the participant sets a disclosure boundary in relation to self-reports. As was shown in Table 18.2, this disclosure boundary can be contingent upon what other people may think of the participant, how other people, particularly clinical assessors, will judge his or her experience, or how the experience compares to other peoples experiences (e.g., strange compared to the norm). However, the disclosure boundary can also revolve around self, without regard to other people's judgments or norms, thus drawing a circle around the individual that excludes others. This boundary can only be understood through qualitative analysis.

The relationship between participant and imagined scenario also reveals a form of positioning of self vis-à-vis others or self. Similar to what Diriwächter and Hughes (2000) have reported, storytelling involves a myriad of positions the self can take. For example, in Table 18.2 we can see how participants position their imagined selves vis-à-vis imagined others (e.g., "What will *people* think of *me* if I disclose that") or vis-à-vis themselves (e.g., "*I* was thinking of a few peculiar experiences *I've* had"). Furthermore, what may go unnoticed is that there is also a level of positioning of self toward the questionnaire, or better put, toward the researcher. This form of positioning is implicit in all responses made by the participant. However, unlike the social constructionist approach as advocated by Holstein and Gubrium (2000), we see the self *transformed* and not as being constructed. Construction implies a *bricolage*— using anything at hand as building blocks to construct self from any experience encountered. However, how does one proceed from the elements when we are already dealing with a whole? No analysis makes sense (void of meaning) until the whole has been revealed. In that sense, construction is at best reconstruction—based on the secondary representational field (of episodes of personal experiences) and interpretation of the goals implied by the question, meanings of responses may vary widely behind the same mark a person has made on paper. Psychology needs to see the forest of meaning making behind the specific trees of responses.

REFERENCES

Branco, A. U., & Valsiner, J. (1997). Changing methodologies: A co-constructivist study of goal orientations in social interactions. *Psychology and Developing Societies, 9*(1), 35–64.

Bühler, K. (1934/1965). *Sprachtheorie* [Theory of language]. Jena-Stuttgart: Gustav Fischer.

Bühler, K. (1990). *Theory of language: The representational function of language.* Amsterdam: John Benjamins.

Diriwächter, R. (2003). *What really matters: Keeping the whole.* Paper presented at the 10th Biennial Conference of the International Society for Theoretical Psychology (ISTP), Istanbul, Turkey, June 24, 2003.

Diriwächter, R., & Hughes, M. (2000, February). *I am not who you think I am: Identity construction in narrative interviews.* Paper presented at the Clark University Conference for Cross-Discipline Research Exchange, Worcester, MA.

Frijda, N. H., & DeGroot, A. D. (Eds). (1982). *Otto Selz: His contribution to psychology.* The Hague: Mouton.

Graham, J. R. (1987). *The MMPI: A practical guide* (2nd ed.). New York: Oxford University Press.

Greene, R. L. (2000). *The MMPI-2: An interpretive manual* (2nd ed.). Boston, MA: Allyn and Bacon.

Groth-Marnat, G. (1997). *Handbook of psychological assessment* (3rd ed.). Oxford, England: John Wiley & Sons

Hathaway, S. R., & McKinley, J. C. (1989). *Minnesota Multiphasic Personality Inventory-2.* Minneapolis, MN: The University of Minnesota Press.

Holstein, J. A., & Gubrium, J. F. (2000). *The self we live by: Narrative identity in a postmodern world.* New York: Oxford University Press.

Joerchel, A. C., & Valsiner, J. (2003). Making decisions about taking medicines: A social coordination process [79 paragraphs]. *Forum Qualitative Sozialforschung/Forum: Qualitative Social Research* [On-line journal], *5*(1). Available at http://www.qualitative-research.net/fqs-texte/1-04/1-04joerchelvalsiner-e.htm

Josephs, I. E., Valsiner, J., & Surgan, S. E. (1999). The process of meaning construction. In J. Brandtstätdter & R. M. Lerner (Eds.), *Action & self development* (pp. 257–282). Thousand Oaks, CA: Sage.

Rommetveit, R. (1992). Outlines of a dialogically based social-cognitive approach to human cognition and communication. In A. H. Wold (Ed.), *The dialogical alternative: Towards a theory of language and mind* (pp. 19–44). Oslo: Scandinavian University Press.

Simon, H. (1999). *Karl Duncker and cognitive science. From past to future. 1*(2), 1–11.

Singer, J. L., & Bonanno, G. A. (1990). Personality and private experience: Individual variations in consciousness and in attention to subjective phenomena. In L. Pervin (Ed.), *Handbook of personality* (pp. 419–444). New York: Guilford Press.

Valsiner, J. (2000). *Culture and human development.* London, U.K.: Sage Publications.

Wagoner, B., & Valsiner, J. (2003). *Rating tasks in psychology: from construction of static ontology to dialogical synthesis of meaning.* Poster presented at 10th Biennial Conference of the International Society for Theoretical Psychology (ISTP), Istanbul, Turkey, June, 24, 2003.

EDITORIAL COMMENTARY

I had two thoughts after reading this nice chapter. The first is that I have always been impressed that one never knows whether the person taking a test is telling the truth. Most clinicians (certainly including myself) are not well trained in the diagnosis of psychiatric diseases. Many of us rely on one of the well-known multiple choice instruments to help us determine who might need further evaluation. Yet a smart patient could certainly manipulate the outcome. When I was a resident, the facility where I trained made great use of the MMPI. There were stacks of the booklets all over the hospitals and clinics. On several occasions when we were somewhat bored, waiting for something to happen on the Obstetrics ward in the middle of the night, we would grab a box of the booklets and fill them out with an alias, with the intent of trying to manipulate the interpretation of the answers in a given direction. One night we might try to score a "major depressive illness" outcome, while on another we might try to hit the "schizophrenia" jackpot. We never could wind up with a "sociopath" profile, and often the computer would tell the "clinician" that there was some reason to believe that the answers were not truthful. While I'm certain that we wasted some dollars, the fact that the results could be manipulated made an important and lasting impression on me.

My other thought concerns the great difference between an "odd" and "even" number of choices when opinion questions are asked. The classic is the MMPI type of question that only allows a "true" or a "false" or a "yes" or "no" response. However, I believe that it is much easier to choose between those TWO answers than to have FOUR choices, and, of course, FIVE choices is the easiest. For example, if the statement is "Politicians are corrupt" it is relatively easy to choose from among these five options: "strongly agree—somewhat agree—neither agree nor disagree—somewhat disagree—strongly disagree." It is much harder if the choices are limited to an even number: "strongly agree—somewhat agree—somewhat disagree—strongly disagree." Even the "agree—disagree" two-choice option is easier than four options. I found it interesting that the authors changed the MMPI "true" statements into three subcategories and treated the "false" statements similarly.

—Kenneth L. Noller

INDEX

ABOUT THE EDITORS AND CONTRIBUTORS

ROGER BIBACE is a Professor of Psychology at Clark University, Chief of the Division of Behavioral Science, Adjunct Professor of the Department of Obstetrics and Gynecology at Tufts University Medical School, and Adjunct Professor of Family and Community Health at University of Massachusetts Medical School. He has developed the Partnership Model for understanding doctor–patient and researcher–subject relationships.

JAMES D. LAIRD is a psychology professor at Clark University. His research explores feelings: how they arise, affect behavior, and may be controlled and organized. Other ongoing research explores personality factors that predict medical outcomes and adherence to medical advice.

KENNETH L. NOLLER is Professor and Chair of Obstetrics and Gynecology at Tufts University School of Medicine and Gynecologist-in-Chief at the Tufts–New England Medical Center. He is the leader in the field of colposcopy and has been the principal investigator of a longitudinal study of reproductive risks at the Mayo Clinic over three decades.

JAAN VALSINER is the founding editor of the Sage Publications journal, *Culture & Psychology*. His research interests are in semiotic mediation of human psychological processes and in the general methodology of science—how generalizations from individual cases are possible.

MARY ALSTON KERLLENEVICH is finishing her Ph.D. in clinical psychology at Clark University. She has been Editorial Associate of the journal *Culture & Psychology*. Her research interests concentrate on emotion regulation in children and adults and in doctor–patient relationships.

KATIA S. AMORIM is a child psychiatrist and psychologist in research and practice, leading a research group of CINDEDI at the Faculty of Letters of the University of São Paulo at Ribeirão Preto, Brazil. She is interested in the intricate relations between health issues of children and their embeddedness in everyday life contexts.

SOFIE BÄÄRNHIELM is a Medical Doctor at the Transcultural Consultation Centre in Stockholm, Sweden. She studies psychosocial factors to promote, or counteract, the successful integration of immigrants and refugees into the host society.

DAVID CHELMOW is the Program Director of Obstetrics and Gynecology Residency Program and Associate Professor at the Division of General Obstetrics and Gynecology at Tufts–New England Medical Center in Massachusetts. He is a member of a number of medical societies, including the American College of Obstetricians and Gynecologists and the American Medical Association.

RAINER DIRIWÄCHTER is finishing his Ph.D. in social psychology at Clark University. He is interested in restoring contemporary psychological science's focus on *Ganzheitspsychologie,* and works on the role of music in the regulation of social conduct.

GERD GIGERENZER is the Director of the Center for Adaptive Behavior and Cognition at the Max Planck Institute for Human Development in Berlin, Germany. He is the originator of the concept of Fast and Frugal Heuristics in contemporary cognitive psychology.

JEREMY GOLDING, M.D., is a family physician teaching and practicing at the University of Massachusetts Medical School. He is Associate Professor of Family Medicine, Inpatient Director, and Associate Residency Director for the Worcester Family Medicine Residency. He is married, and the father of three remarkable daughters who remind him constantly that "listening is not hearing."

BOB HEYMAN is the Associate Dean for research at St. Bartholomew School of Nursing and Midwifery in West Smithfield, London. His research interests include analyzing professional and service user perspectives about health and health care.

ULRICH HOFFRAGE of the Max Planck Institute for Human Development in Berlin, Germany, is a research scientist with a Ph.D. in Habilitation in Psychology. His research interests include risk communication and analytic study of simple heuristics. Project focuses include bounded rationality and ecological rationality.

STEPHANIE KURZENHÄUSER is a research scientist for Adaptive Behavior and Cognition at the Max Planck Institute for Human Development in Berlin, Germany. Her research interests include risk management and the legal and political implications of bounded rationality. Her project focus is on ecological rationality.

TALIA LaPUSHIN was an undergraduate honors student in the Psychology Department at Clark University at the time of the work done on the chapter in this book. Her interests are in health psychology and health administration.

ROBERT LEEMAN is finishing his Ph.D. at the University of Pennsylvania, after having been a Gurel–Bell Prize-winning undergraduate psychology major at Clark University. His research interests include concepts of health and undergraduates' alcohol use. He is also interested in other addictions, such as smoking cessation, and in moral judgment, particularly regarding health.

MARIA CLOTILDE ROSSETTI-FERREIRA is Professor of Developmental Psychology and Head of the Department of Psychology and Education at the Faculty of Philosophy, Sciences, at the University of São Paulo at Ribeirão Preto, Brazil. Her research interests include social interaction in early childhood, the process of construction and the role of the physical and social contexts, and mother–infant attachment and the child's and the family's adaptation to the day-care center.

PETER SALOVEY is a Yale University Professor of psychology and also a lead researcher at the Center for Disciplinary Research on AIDS (CIRA). Research focus is in the health promotion area concerning the effectiveness of interventions designed to promote prevention and early detection behaviors for cancer and HIV/AIDS.

CHRISTINE SAUCK is a doctoral student in clinical psychology at Clark University, with a research interest in the dynamics of family functioning in everyday life contexts.

MICHELINE SILVA is a post-doctoral fellow of pediatric psychology at Ohio State University. She has worked extensively on mother–infant interaction (together with Maria Lyra at Federal University of Pernambuco, Brazil) and is currently interested in the social environments of children with terminal illness.

DAVID STEVENS is a psychology professor at Clark University. He is currently involved in studies on adult's perception of baby cries and of resident physicians' perception of heart murmurs.

AARO TOOMELA is a Professor in Special Education at the University of Tartu in Estonia. He is a neuropsychologist, pediatrician, and cultural psychologist. His interests are in the theoretical heritage of Lev Vygotsky and the role of concept use in human reasoning.